To Bill Meyer

With Regard.

Joe Brady

PRINCIPLES, PRACTICES,
AND POSITIONS
IN NEUROPSYCHIATRIC RESEARCH

The papers in this volume are reprinted from the *Journal of Psychiatric Research* Volume 8, No's. 3 and 4.

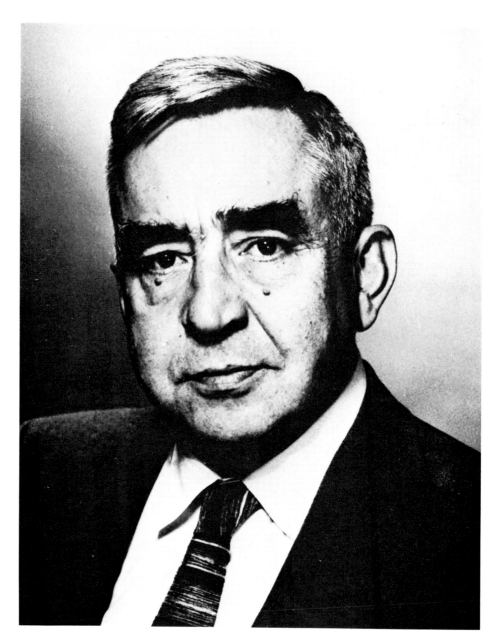

Dr. David McKenzie Rioch

PRINCIPLES, PRACTICES, AND POSITIONS IN NEUROPSYCHIATRIC RESEARCH

A Volume in Honor of Dr. David McKenzie Rioch

Edited by

JOSEPH V. BRADY
WALLE J. H. NAUTA

Proceedings of a Conference held in June 1970 at the Walter Reed Army Institute of Research, Washington, D.C., in tribute to Dr. David McKenzie Rioch upon his retirement as Director of the Neuropsychiatry Division of that Institute.

PERGAMON PRESS
OXFORD · NEW YORK · TORONTO
SYDNEY · BRAUNSCHWEIG

Pergamon Press Ltd., Headington Hill Hall, Oxford

Pergamon Press Inc., Maxwell House, Fairview Park, Elmsford,
New York 10523

Pergamon of Canada Ltd., 207 Queen's Quay West, Toronto 1

Pergamon Press (Aust.) Pty. Ltd., 19a Boundary Street,
Rushcutters Bay, N.S.W. 2011, Australia

Vieweg & Sohn GmbH, Burgplatz 1, Braunschweig

First edition 1972

Library of Congress Catalog Card No. 72–86256

Printed in Great Britain by A. Wheaton & Co., Exeter

08 017007 2

CONTENTS

Contents

PREFACE

DURING the summer of 1970, David McKenzie Rioch attained his seventieth birthday, and completed 20 years as Director of the Division of Neuropsychiatry at the Walter Reed Army Institute of Research. To mark the occasion, a group of the Walter Reed "alumni" and many other friends and colleagues gathered in Washington, D.C. to attend a two-day scientific conference arranged in his honor as an expression of gratitude for the leadership and support he provided his associates over the two lively decades of his pioneering research stewardship. Along with the twenty or more original contributions presented on that occasion, the present volume incorporates several invited papers which could not be programmed at the meeting because of the usual limitations imposed by such time-locked affairs. Taken together, the contributions to this volume may serve to reflect, in some measure at least, the remarkable range of bio-social research interest and competence represented in the unusually productive career of the man to whom they are dedicated.

Almost half a century ago, as a medical student at Johns Hopkins, David Rioch published his first scientific paper. The subject of this single-authored début in the *Anatomical Record* is rather remote from his later endeavors, but in hindsight it could seem almost prophetic that the words 'morphology' and 'behavior' appear in its title. Following several years of training in Medicine and Surgery in the middle 1920's at the Peter Bent Brigham Hospital in Boston, he accepted a National Research Council Medical Fellowship and took up residence at the University of Michigan for the fruitful years which produced the now classical anatomical *Studies on the Diencephalon of Carnivora*, published in the *Journal of Comparative Neurology* over the period from 1929 to 1931. A year or more in Sherrington's laboratory at Oxford, followed by an associateship in Physiology at Johns Hopkins, preceded the productive span of the 1930's at Harvard during which he made his fundamental contributions to our current knowledge of the relationship between forebrain mechanisms and behavior.

In 1938, David Rioch accepted the Chair in Neurology at Washington University School of Medicine in St. Louis, where he continued his anatomical and physiological analysis of central nervous function, and meanwhile became more directly concerned with the psychological and psychiatric implications of his endeavors. Significantly, his first formal publication in these latter fields appeared during this period in the August 1941 issue of *Psychiatry: a Journal of the Biology and Pathology of Interpersonal Relations*. And by 1951, following almost a decade of intensive clinical and research involvement with the Washington School of Psychiatry and Chestnut Lodge in the nation's capital, he documented his involvement in problems of interpersonal relationships with a treatise on psychotherapeutic theories, published in a volume entitled *Current Trends in Psychological Theory*.

A unique conceptual coalescence of these varied biological, psychiatric and social domains can be seen as David Rioch's crowning achievement, an accomplishment of which all who were associated with him at the Walter Reed Army Institute of Research became the fortunate beneficiaries. In the course of these two decades, he himself authored fifty scientific papers, but many times that number of publications that issued from his Division of Neuro-psychiatry bore the mark of his sophisticated, ever unobtrusive sponsorship. The range and quality of this inspired intellectual leadership is eloquently, if only too incompletely, expressed by the individual contributions to this volume.

Over the course of his distinguished career as a scientist, physician, teacher, author, and above all, as a humanist, David McKenzie Rioch has been the recipient of many honors. It is probably fair to say, however, that none can have pleased him more than the tribute to his enduring contributions that is offered him by the contents of this volume.

JOSEPH V. BRADY
WALLE J. H. NAUTA

DAVID McKENZIE RIOCH—A CHIEL O' MONY PAIRTS

Text of an address delivered by Dr. Donald M. Mackay, Professor of Communication, The University of Keele, Staffordshire, England, on the occasion of a banquet held in Dr. Rioch's honor in the course of the Conference.

I first made the acquaintance of David Rioch through our mutual friend, Warren McCulloch. This was in 1951, which must have been soon after David took up the post which he has held with such distinction for the past twenty years. We were both to be guests at the Macy meeting on Cybernetics. Warren McCulloch, who was chairman of the meeting, was describing the folk I would meet. "One of them is a real honey," he said; "he's a typical Scot, one of God's angry men: David McKenzie Rioch." As a fellow Scot, I don't think I am qualified to comment on Warren's description, but what I soon found was that David is one of God's great human beings; and it has been one of the great pleasures of my life to have got to know and respect him over these past two decades.

The significant thing about David is, that with all his remarkable encyclopedic knowledge he has combined, in the most natural way, the humility to want to put it at the disposal of all comers. Whenever I have felt discouraged or doubtful about something I have been trying to work out, a session with David would have two sorts of effects: on the one hand, a lot of the nonsense trimmed off, and on the other hand, tremendous encouragement to get on with the things that he felt to be worth while. Evidence of his encyclopedic range is, I think, sufficiently offered by the program of the present symposium. There can be few men of science today in whose honor it could have seemed more entirely appropriate to assemble this galaxy of scientific talent from so many different fields. It is perhaps even more significant that the pioneering experiment in interdisciplinary cooperation for which his Division at Walter Reed is so well known should have produced this remarkable array of talent. For him, the idea of narrow, parochial specialization simply did not exist. If data were good and relevant, it did not matter from what field they came; David was interested and wanted to get support for more of the same.

I have referred to the Macy meetings and to the famous or notorious term "Cybernetics," which grew up in all our vocabularies about the time these meetings began. Over the years, the term has taken on various prefixes, and I suppose one description of the program represented in this volume might be "neurocybernetics." Obviously, terms like this have their dangers. Most of us here would probably agree that it is a continuing battle in any interdisciplinary field to keep the scientific standards high. It is difficult to say just why this should be. I think there are a number of factors. For one thing, interdisciplinary activity is attractive for a number of nonscientific reasons. There is the delicious flavor of the other man's jargon rolling over your lips, and there is an almost prurient interest in discovering what these other people do behind their closed doors. I can still recollect, from my days as a "pure" physicist, the feeling that there was an element almost of professional indecency involved in collaborating with medical men, and things of that sort; perhaps the sort of

ix

feeling that one has when wandering into an establishment normally reserved for the opposite sex.

Then, there is the difficulty of cross-checking credentials. It's relatively easy in the company of people from another discipline to gain credit and have nobody call your hand, as it were, in the way it would be called when you are among your peers. And then there is the appeal, the very natural appeal to our hearts, of searching for the grand generalization, the key to all things. This is the obverse, I suppose, of the very proper search of scientists for unity in multiplicity, for general principles that might somehow unify disparate fields.

All these factors are potentially unhealthy, however much good there may be in them. And, of course, the question is what antidote can one have against the dangers that go with such interdisciplinary effort. It sems to me that perhaps the only antidote, certainly the best antidote, is a strong spirit of respect for hard data and an eager readiness to be corrected by fact. I think it is this kind of antiseptic toughmindedness that, as far as my observation goes, has been the secret of David Rioch's success in making the work in his Division of Walter Reed over the last twenty years so well known for its fruitfulness in the inter-disciplinary field. This kind of integrity, when properly understood, is not inhibitory of adventurous innovation; it is rather more like a pruning knife, a means of encouraging the stronger and more promising shoots of the imagination of those with whom it comes in contact.

Looking back over the twenty years, and looking at the way we talked so lightheartedly at the Macy meeting in 1951, I suppose many of us might ask ourselves what's become of the things we were then so keen about. At that time, the theory of information was thought by many to be the missing link that would unify all our disciplines. David Rioch, I think, was one of those who never fell into the trap of looking to the theory of information in its mathematical form as a short-cut to the development of imposing theoretical structures in fields other than those for which it was developed. I think that it is a very natural thing for those of us who become interested in a field where mathematics hasn't been used, to feel that physics, which uses mathematics as its main tool, is the archetype of a science, and that our own field won't really be respectable until it's got the sort of mathematical framework that has given physics the rock-bottom respectability that I suppose most of us would say it has. But, in most areas in which information theory was applied in that sense, I think it's fair to say that after a few years of happy flirtation with the communication engineers, the end-point came with a very large "so what?"

What David saw, and has continued to maintain, over these twenty years, is that there *is* a function for the thinking of the communication engineer in a wide range of fields outside engineering, and particularly in the field of brain research and psychiatry, both individual and social; but that it is in the application of the *qualitative* concepts of goal-directed in-formation systems, their ecology, and the principles on which they have to be organized for optimal efficiency. This theme, as I need not tell any of you here, occurs again and again in David's writing and thinking. In this respect, he was one of those who perceived the real unifying influence that the development of cybernetics at the hands of Wiener and Shannon and others did bring, and one may hope will continue to bring, to the initially disparate fields which are represented here tonight: the enduring value of the qualitative notions, their generality, and their focusing power. What they offer is essentially a conceptual tool of research, a framework on which to hang data as they accumulate in such a way that these data don't merely gratify one's desire to predict, but rather develop further one's curiosity, by raising new experimental questions which are better focused than they would be without such a framework.

Finally, I would like to refer to one further characteristic of David's thinking which I have particularly appreciated, and which I believe has meant a great deal to the spirit of the research program that he has directed. I refer to his clear and often-stated appreciation of the complementarity of the personal and the mechanistic categories which he, in his position, finds it necessary to use in the understanding of human beings. In many areas, and not least in the areas which are sometimes labeled cybernetic, the feeling is sometimes expressed that personal categories, the traditional categories of human values and our human conceptions of one another as persons, have a kind of interim character—tolerable only until the engineers can come up with a more rigorous and professionally well-disciplined equivalent, at which time these categories will fade away. David, I think, has been entirely clear in his mind that, instead of regarding these two sets of categories, the personal and the mechanical, as rivals, where the one fights for its existence only in the gaps of the development of the other, the two have to be regarded as complementing one another, two different but equally essential aspects of the mysterious unity that is a human being.

Attempts to make rivals of these two aspects always make me think of the old story of the earthworm who was burrowing through some particularly hard clay and heard the unmistakable sounds of another earthworm ahead. As he broke through into the tunnel, he growled furiously, "Get out of the way, I was here first," and received the reply, "Don't be silly, I'm your other end." It seems to me that this is a parable of the stupidity of regarding the mechanistic analysis of the machinery of our brains as, in any fundamental sense, antagonistic to the traditional values of our human and spiritual nature around which our culture has developed. I believe there is a great need in our day to divest our science in the public mind of this illusory aura of antagonism to the spiritual significance of human beings.

In the preservation of all his humane and broad understanding of what it is to be a man, as in much else, I believe that David's charming wife, Margaret, has had a great part to play. I am sure that no scientist could be more fortunate in having such a partner to help maintain his balance in the rough seas of the scientific analysis of human nature. It is with great warmth of feeling then that I would ask you to include her in the toast which I now propose, the toast of a man whom we delight to honor, a master of many crafts—or, as we put it in Scotland—a "chiel o' mony pairts"—David McKenzie Rioch.

LIST OF PUBLICATIONS BY DAVID McKENZIE RIOCH

1. The morphology and behavior of the migratory cells in tissue cultures of the chick's spleen. *Anat. Rec.* **25**: 41–57, 1923.
2. The refractometric determination of serum proteins (with B. S. Neuhausen). *J. Biol. Chem.* **55**: 353–6, 1923.
3. Experiments on water and salt diuresis. *Arch. Int. Med.* **40**: 743–56, 1927.
4. Studies on the diencephalon of carnivora. Part I. The nuclear configuration of the thalamus, epithalamus and hypothalamus of the dog and cat. *J. Comp. Neurol.* **49**: 1–119, 1929.
5. Studies on the diencephalon of carnivora. Part II. Certain nuclear configuration and fiber connections of the subthalamus and midbrain of the dog and cat. *J. Comp. Neurol.* **49**: 121–53, 1929.
6. Studies on the diencephalon of carnivora. Part III. Certain myelinated-fiber connections of the diencephalon of the dog (*Canis familiaris*), cat (*Felis domestica*) and arvisa (*Croesarchus obscurus*). *J. Comp. Neurol.* **53**: 319–88, 1931.
7. The influence of experimental lesions of the spinal cord upon the knee-jerk and crossed extensor reflexes (with F. J. Fulton and E. G. T. Liddell). *J. Physiol.* **69**: 12–17, 1930.
8. The influence of experimental lesions of the spinal cord upon the knee-jerk. I. Acute lesions (with J. F. Fulton and E. G. T. Liddell). *Brain* **53**: 311–26, 1930.
9. Water diuresis. *J. Physiol.* **70**: 45–52, 1930.
10. "Dial" as an anaesthetic for surgical operations on the nervous system (with J. F. Fulton and E. G. T. Liddell). *Proc. Physiol. Soc.*, 1930; *J. Physiol.* **70**.
11. "Dial" as a surgical anaesthetic for neurological operations; with observations on the nature of its action (with J. F. Fulton and E. G. T. Liddell). *J. Pharm. & Exp. Therapeutics.* **40**: 423–32, 1930.
12. The influence of unilateral destruction of the vestibular nuclei upon posture and the knee-jerk (with J. F. Fulton and E. G. T. Liddell). *Brain* **53**: 327–43, 1930.
13. A note on the centre median nucleus of luys. *J. Anat.* **65**: 324–7, 1931.
14. Zur Frage der sympathischen Beeinflüssung des cerebrospinalen Nerven-systems (with H. Altenburger). *Pflügers Archiv f. d. ges. Physiol.* **229**: 473–85, 1932.
15. Relation of the cerebrum to the cerebellum (with J. F. Fulton and E. G. T. Liddell). *Arch. Neurol. Psychiat.* **28**: 542–67, 1932.
16. Electrical excitation of multifibered nerves (with A. Rosenblueth). *Am. J. Physiol.* **104**: 519–29, 1933.
17. Temporal and spatial summation in autonomic systems (with A. Rosenblueth). *Am. J. Physiol.* **106**: 365–80, 1933.
18. The responses to changes in environmental temperature after removal of portions of the forebrain (with J. O. Pinkston and P. Bard). *Am. J. Physiol.* **109**: 515–31, 1934.
19. The nature of the responses of smooth muscle to adrenin and the augmentor action of cocaine for sympathetic stimuli (with A. Rosenblueth). *Am. J. Physiol.* **103**: 681, 685, 1933.
20. Inhibition from the cerebral cortex (with A. Rosenblueth). *Am. J. Physiol.* **113**: 663–76, 1935.
21. Paths of secretion from the hypophysis. *Res. Publ. Ass. nerv. ment. Dis.* **17**: 151–71, 1936.
22. A study of four cats deprived of neocortex and additional portions of the forebrain (with P. Bard). *Bull. of the Johns Hopkins Hosp.* **60**: 73–174, 1937.
23. A physiological and histological study of the frontal cortex of the seal (*Phoca vitulina*). *Biol. Bull.* **73**: 591–602, 1937.
24. The influence of the forebrain on an autonomic reflex (with R. S. Morison). *Am. J. Physiol.* **120**: 257–76, 1937.
25. Certain effects of prolonged stimulation of afferent nerves on the reflexes evoked (with C. Nelson and E. W. Dempsey). *J. Neurophysiol.* **1**: 533–42, 1938.
26. Experiments on the corpus striatum and rhinencephalon (with Ch. Brenner). *J. Comp. Neurol.* **68**: 491–507, 1938.
27. Certain effects of prolonged stimulation of afferent nerves on the reflexes evoked (with C. Nelson and E. W. Dempsey). *J. Neurophysiol.* **1**: 533–42, 1938.
28. The influence of the cerebral cortex on peripheral circulation (with J. O. Pinkston). *Am. J. Physiol.* **121**: 49–54, 1938.

29. Certain aspects of the behavior of decorticate cats. *Psychiatry: a J. of Biol. & Pathol. of Interpersonal Relations.* **1**: 339–45, 1938.
30. The localization in the brain stem of the oestrous responses of the female guinea pig (with E. W. Dempsey). *J. Neurophysiol.* **2**: 9–18, 1939.
31. Spinal pathways for nictitating membrane reflexes in the cat (with S. Howard Armstrong, Jr.). *J. Neurophysiol.* **2**: 526–32, 1939.
32. Neurophysiology of the corpus striatum and globus pallidus. *Psychiatry: a J. of Biol. & Pathol. of Interpersonal Relations* **3**: 119–39, 1940.
33. A précis of preoptic, hypothalamic and hypophysial terminology with atlas (with G. B. Wislocki and J. L. O'Leary). *Res. Publ. Ass. nerv. ment. Dis.* **20**: 3–30, 1940.
34. Functions of the brainstem in preparations with extensive lesions of the neocortex. *Res. Publ. Ass. nerv. ment. Dis.* **21**: 133–49, 1941.
35. Consideration of the registrant as a person (with C. F. Jacobsen, H. H. Fingert and S. R. Warson). *Psychiatry: a J. of Biol. & Pathol. of Interpersonal Relations.* **4**: 331–6, 1941.
36. Theories of psychotherapy: frames of reference in which psychotherapeutic events have been conceptualized. *Current Trends in Psychological Theory.* Pittsburgh, U. Pittsburgh Press, pp. 140–64, 1951.
37. Summary of papers on ascending systems and on those dealing with higher cerebral functions. *Res. Publ. Ass. nerv. ment. Dis.* **30**: 548–52, 1952.
38. Résumé: The EEG in relation to psychiatry. *EEG. Clin. Neurophysiol.* **4**: 457–62, 1952.
39. Disturbances in blood sugar regulation in animals subjected to transection of the brain stem (with E. Anderson and W. Haymaker). *Acta Neurovegetativa* **5**: 132–64, 1952.
40. Milieu therapy (with A. H. Stanton). *Psychiatry: a J. for the Study of Interpersonal Relations* **16**: 65–72, 1953; *Res. Publ. Ass. nerv. ment. Dis.* **31**: 94–105, 1953.
41. Disorders associated with disturbance of brain function (with E. A. Weinstein and E. C. Alvord, Jr.). *Ann. of Am. Acad. of Polit. Soc. Science,* 34–44, 1953.
42. Nervous system. *The Americana Annual.* New York, Americana Corp., pp. 501–2, 1954.
43. Psychopathological and neuropathological aspects of consciousness. In: *Brain Mechanisms and Consciousness.* Oxford, England, Blackwell Scientific Publ., pp. 470–3, 1954.
44. The brain and consciousness. In: H. E. Himwich (ed.): *Biological Foundations of Psychiatry.* Dedicatory Address at Thudichum Psychiatric Research Laboratories, Galesburg State Research Hospital, Galesburg, Ill., October 1953.
45. Certain aspects of "conscious" phenomena and their neural correlates. *Am. J. Psychiatry* **3**: 810–17, 1955.
46. The influence of the central nervous system on metabolism and endocrine activity as based on transection of the brain stem in dogs (with E. Anderson, K. Knowlton, Wm. T. Spence, S. M. McCann, G. Lacqueur and W. Haymaker). *Acta Neurovegetativa* Bd. XII, Heft 1–2, 53–94, 1955.
47. Alterations of adrenal cortical and ovarian activity following hypothalamic lesions (with G. Laqueur, S. M. McCann, L. Schreiner, E. Rosenberg and E. Anderson). *Endocrinology* **57**: 44–54, 1955.
48. Problems of preventive psychiatry in war. *Psychopathology of Childhood* (Vol. X of *Trans. of Am. Psychopathol. Ass.*), New York, Grune & Stratton, pp. 146–165, 1955.
49. Psychiatry as a biological science. *Psychiatry: a J. for the Study of Interpersonal Relations.* **18**: 313–21, 1955.
50. The application of the experimental method to psychiatric therapy. *J. of the Hillside Hospital* (Glen Oaks, N.Y.) **5**: 3–16, 1956.
51. Experimental aspects of anxiety. *Am. J. Psychiatry* **113**: 435–42, 1956.
52. Discussion of Chapters 13–16, *Experimental Psychopathology.* New York, Grune & Stratton, pp. 255–261, 1957.
53. The effects of midbrain and spinal cord transection on endocrine and metabolic functions with postulation of a midbrain hypothalamic-pituitary activating system (with E. Anderson, R. W. Bates, E. Hawthorne, W. Haymaker, K. Knowlton, W. T. Spence and H. Wilson). *Recent Progress in Hormone Research,* XIII: 21–66, 1957. New York, Academic Press, Inc.
54. Summary. *Brain Mechanisms and Drug Action* (W. S. Fields, ed.) Springfield, Ill., Charles C. Thomas, pp. 142–7, 1957.
55. Metabolic changes following transection of the spinal cord in dogs (with K. Knowlton, W. T. Spence, W. Haymaker, A. Laskey, L. Kedda, R. Bahn and E. Anderson). *Acta Neurovegetativa* **15**: 374–403, 1957.
56. Research in psychiatry: certain problems and developments in multi-disciplinary studies. New York, Thomas W. Salmon Lecture, 1957.

57. The biological roots of psychoanalysis. Part I. An interdisciplinary survey of psychoanalysis. *Science and Psychoanalysis*. New York, Grune & Stratton, 28 pp., 1958.
58. Some experimental observations on gastrointestinal lesions in behaviorally conditioned monkeys (with R. Porter, J. V. Brady, D. Conrad, J. W. Mason and R. Galambos). *Psychosomatic Med.* **XX**: 379–94, 1958.
59. Multidisciplinary methods in psychiatric research. *Am. J. Orthopsychiat.* **28**: 467–82, 1958.
60. Etiology of duodenal ulcer. II. Serum pepsinogen and peptic ulcer in inductees (with P. G. Yessler and M. F. Reiser). *J.A.M.A.* **169**: 451–6, 1959.
61. Résumé of Chapter 24: The effect of pharmacologic agents on the nervous system. *Res. Publ. Ass nerv. ment. Dis.* **37**: 412–16, 1959.
62. Problems of "Perception" and "Communication" in mental illness. *A.M.A. Arch. Gen. Psychiat.* **1**: 81–92, 1959.
63. The psychophysiology of death. Panel Discussion. *Proc. of Symposium on The Physiology of Emotions*. Springfield, Ill., Charles C. Thomas, 1961.
64. Dimensions of behavior. *Lectures on Experiment Psychiatry*. University of Pittsburgh Press, pp. 341–61, 1961.
65. Recent contributions of neuropsychiatric research to the theory and practice of psychotherapy. *Am. J. Psychoanalysis* **XX**, No. 2, 1960.
66. Foreword to *Delusional Systems and Cultural Factors* by E. A. Weinstein, 1961.
67. Discussion of: I. Page: Neurohumoral and endocrine aspects of shock. *Fed. Proceed.* **20**, No. 2, Part III, 1961.
68. Psychiatric problems of man in the Arctic. *Symposium on Man in the Arctic*. National Acad. of Sciences—National Research Council, Washington, D.C., 1961.
69. The sense and the noise. *Psychiatry* **24**, Suppl. to No. 2, May, 1961.
70. The future of psychiatry from the standpoint of physiology. *Proc. Am. Psychopathol. Ass.*, 1961. Reprinted in *The Future of Psychiatry*. New York, Grune & Stratton, 1962.
71. The future of psychiatry in view of recent developments. Lecture at William Alanson White Institute of Psychiatry, New York, 20 Jan. 1962.
72. The problem of consciousness in the clinic and the laboratory. Lecture at San Francisco Medical Center, San Francisco, 10 April 1962.
73. Behavioral approach to the problem of self-control. Presented at Interdisciplinary Conference on Individual Self-Control Under Stress. Bureau of Social Science Research, Inc., Washington, D.C. 9–10 Sept. 1962.
74. Communication in the laboratory and communication in the clinic. Fromm–Reichman Memorial Lecture. Washington School of Psychiatry. *Psychiatry* **26**: 209–21, 1963.
75. The role of violence in behavior (Introduction). Proc. Am. Ass. Adv. Sci., Philadelphia, 27–30 Dec. 1962. Reprinted in *Science and Psychoanalysis*. New York, Grune & Stratton, 1963.
76. Foreword to *An Introduction to the Science of Human Behavior*, edited by J. I. Nurnberger, C. B. Forster and J. P. Brady. New York, Appleton-Century-Croft, 1963.
77. Psychological considerations related to disaster. *Amer. Ass. of Indus. Nurses* **IX**, June 1963.
78. Modern concepts of the brain and behavior. Presented to Danish Society of Natural Sciences, Copenhagen, 12 June 1963.
79. Introduction to disorders of communication. *Res. Publ. Ass. nerv. ment. Dis.* **42**, 1964.
80. Social interaction among primates. Proceedings, International Conference and Symposium on *Communication and Social Interactions in Primates*, Montreal, Canada, December 1964.
81. Leadership and motivation: an operational formulation applicable to unconventional situations. *Forsvarsmedicin (Military Medicine)* **3**: 71–84, 1967.
82. Introduction to: C. W. Sem-Jacobsen, *Brain Stimulation and Behavior in Man* (in press).
83. Military psychiatry—a prototype of social and preventive psychiatry in the United States (with W. Hausman). *Arch. Gen. Psychiat.* **16**: 727–39, 1967.
84. Prevention: the major task of military psychiatry. *Proc. 7th International Congress of Psychotherapy*, Wiesbaden, 1967.
85. Categories of sexual phenomena with particular reference to symbolic behavior. *Science and Psychoanalysis* (in press).
86. Mental health research in military psychiatry. *Am. J. of Orthopsychiatry* (in press).

J. psychiat. Res., 1971, Vol. 8, pp. 167–187. Pergamon Press. Printed in Great Britain.

THE PROBLEM OF THE FRONTAL LOBE: A REINTERPRETATION

WALLE J. H. NAUTA

Department of Psychology, Massachusetts Institute of Technology, Cambridge, Mass.

INTRODUCTION

THE FRONTAL lobe, despite decades of intensive research by physiologists, anatomists and clinicians, has remained the most mystifying of the major subdivisions of the cerebral cortex. Unlike any other of the great cerebral promontories, the frontal lobe appears not to contain a single sub-field that could be identified with any particular sensory modality, and its entire expanse must accordingly be considered association cortex. It should, perhaps, not be surprising in view of this circumstance alone that loss of frontal cortex, in primate forms in particular, leads to a complex functional deficit, the fundamental nature of which continues to elude laboratory investigators and clinicians alike. The purpose of this paper is, to review some aspects of this deficit in animals and man, and to inquire to what extent the consequences of frontal-lobe lesion can be evaluated in neurological terms.

It is unfortunate that the search for neural substrata of the frontal lobe syndrome is hampered by a nearly complete absence of data obtained by modern neurophysiological methods. As a consequence, no entirely satisfactory hypothesis concerning the neural mechanisms of the frontal lobe would seem attainable at present. On the other hand, largely as a result of several excellent anatomical studies reported within the past 5 years, the neural associations of the frontal lobe, in particular those with other regions of the cerebral cortex, have come into sharper focus, and it is on the basis of these anatomical findings that an attempt could be made to formulate a general and preliminary notion of the major neural mechanisms in which the frontal lobe is involved. Needless to say, no concept so exclusively based upon neuroanatomical data can be stated in any but very general terms, for the value of anatomical studies lies largely in the identification of specific questions that can be explored by physiological methods.

FUNCTIONAL CONSIDERATIONS

1. *Observations in animals*

Monkeys subjected to extensive bilateral ablation of granular frontal cortex have long been noted to exhibit hypermotility and hyperreactivity to external stimuli. Little further information concerning their functional impairment was obtained until in 1935 JACOBSEN[1] reported his now classical observation that primates deprived of their prefrontal cortex

A

perform little better than at the level of chance in the so-called *delayed-response test*. In this simple task, that is quickly mastered by intact chimpanzees, monkeys, cats and dogs, the animal is shown under which one of two or more identical covers food is placed, but it is forced to postpone retrieval of the food for a short period (usually $\frac{1}{2}$–2 min) during which the scene of the choice is hidden from its view by an opaque screen. The initial impression that the 'frontal animal' suffers from a memory loss, and while waiting for the screen to go up 'forgets' where he saw the food being hidden, has been effectively refuted, and it now seems certain that frontal-lobe ablation affects a response-guidance other than memory in the customary sense. In this test, as also in the somewhat related delayed-alternation (alternative baiting of the left and right one of an identical pair of containers) and multiple-choice tests (all covers marked by a differently-shaped object, one of which serves as the clue for bait in one block of trials, another one in a contiguous trial-block, and so on), 'frontal' animals exhibit a characteristic tendency to perseverate a particular choice, despite the obviously poor reward average. It has been suggested that this 'rigidity of central sets' actually constitutes the fundamental deficit[2] but KONORSKI and LAWICKA,[3] on the basis of a remarkable series of experiments in dogs and cats, arrived at a somewhat different interpretation according to which the *conditioning signal* (e.g. the being shown which box contains bait) undergoes an abnormally rapid decay during the delay, and is thus overcome by the essentially unguided *release response* triggered by the actual presentation of the choice. Perseveration, according to Konorski and Lawicka, is a relatively unspecific phenomenon that is encountered in a variety of functional impairments (often, for example, in aphasia). As an alternative hypothesis, Konorski and Lawicka suggest an abnormally strong release-response overriding a normal signal trace, a suggestion which would appear compatible with another observation made in 'frontal' monkeys[4,5] in the so-called *go–no go* tests. In this testing procedure the animal must learn not only to respond to a particular signal (either auditory or visual) but also, to withhold response to another signal that randomly alternates with the first. Under such conditions, monkeys deprived of their frontal cortex score more errors of commission than do normal monkeys. It must be remarked, however, that it still appears uncertain to what extent this deficiency is due to an actual perceptual impairment rather than to the nature of the go–no go test proper.

Last to be mentioned here is the observation that, in object-discrimination tests, 'frontal' monkeys show an increased tendency to prefer any novel object over a tried, familiar one, even if the experiment is so arranged that the choice of a novel object is never rewarded. Although this novelty-preference would at first glance seem incompatible with the choice-reiteration noted above, both could conceivably result from one and the same guidance failure in a response that in normal subjects is more stably determined by the previously experienced consequence of the choice.

2. *The frontal-lobe syndrome in man*

Complex and difficult of analysis as are the consequences of frontal lobe ablation in animals, the frontal lobe syndrome in man is even more bewildering. As a result of its complexity, current concepts concerning the function of man's frontal lobes range between two widely separate extremes: on the one hand the notion that this part of the brain is crucially involved in man's highest mental faculties;[6,7] on the other extreme the conclusion that the only defects objectively demonstrable in frontal-lobe patients are of a perceptual nature, all other impairments being too variable and vague to serve as reliable characteristics of frontal-lobe dysfunction.[8]

The wide divergence between these two views may be attributable in part at least to the common difficulty of determining clinically the precise extent and location of the cerebral tissue damage in human patients. As emphasized by TEUBER,[9] tumors of the frontal lobe are likely to have reached considerable size by the time the patient is seen by a neurologist, and in such cases it is difficult to determine whether the symptomatology may not have become complicated by a more general impairment of brain function. Penetrating traumatic lesions of the frontal lobes are only rarely explored surgically, and their result in tissue loss thus as a rule remains undetermined. In fact, the only category of patients in whom the extent of the tissue defect is usually known with reasonable accuracy are those who have been subjected to surgical ablations performed in order to alleviate epileptic disorders.

Most controversial among the symptoms of frontal-lobe disorder in man are the psychiatric signs, in particular mood changes (euphoria, irritability or its opposite: emotional indifference), and character changes (boastfulness, impetuousness, lack of initiative and other behavioral disorders). Significant and practically important though such general personality changes may be, they show much individual variation and for the present must therefore remain somewhat at the periphery of the search for common denominators in the frontal-lobe syndrome. This search is still directed largely toward an evaluation of the patient's perceptual and motor capacities, and his strategies in performing certain relatively simple tasks. Some results of such analyses will be reviewed in the following account.

In the course of detailed studies of patients with gunshot wounds of the frontal lobe, TEUBER and his associates[8,9] have identified certain perceptual impairments, notably such affecting the maintenance of the perceived vertical during passive tilt of the body, the interpretation of line drawings with ambiguous perspective, and the capacity of reversing standpoint in dealing with mirror images of the body. Their tests, in addition, disclosed in frontal-lobe patients a significant impairment in the speed and efficiency with which a visual array is scanned for detail (see also LURIA[10]). In discussing these functional deficits, TEUBER[9] arrives at the important suggestion that all are attributable to the loss of a mechanism of 'corollary discharge', i.e. a flow of impulses from the central effector organization to central sensory structures, ". . . presetting the latter for those predictable changes of input that will be the consequences of the particular motor output."*

Among the results obtained with more complex testing procedures, the observations reported by MILNER[11] and LURIA[10,12] are particularly noteworthy. Milner's findings have demonstrated a profound and characteristic inability of frontal-lobe patients to achieve normal scores in the Wisconsin modification of the Weigl card-sorting test, a test in which the patient is asked to sort 128 cards on the basis of any one of three arbitrary criteria

---

* Some mechanism of this nature must be postulated to explain the well-known phenomenon that actively executed eye movements do *not* cause the illusion that the visual scene is moving, whereas by contrast, passive displacements of the eyeball, e.g. by finger push, do cause such an impression. In the 'active' case there must have been some form of forewarning to the effect that the perceived shift of images over the retina should be attributed to the impending eye movement.

(color, shape or number of the figures shown on the cards). The patient is given no verbal instruction as to which criterion is valid, and is required to determine the criterion pragmatically, on the basis of being told at each placement whether his choice is right or wrong. It is remarkable that frontal-lobe patients in this testing situation show no noteworthy difficulty in deducing the required strategy from the signals given by the observer. Their characteristic deficit appears when, at some point in the procedure, the observer arbitrarily changes the criterion (e.g. from color to number), thus requiring the patient to identify and follow a new ordering system. Under such conditions, frontal-lobe patients tend to perseverate the original strategy, even in the face of an ever-mounting score of errors. In the words of MILNER[11]: " . . . it does not seem accurate to attribute this poor test performance to a loss of abstract thought, since such patients often state spontaneously that 'it has to be the color, the form or the number,' although they seem unable to recognize the possibility of a change once a particular pattern of response has become established. They thus show a curious dissociation between the ability to verbalize the requirements of the test and the ability to use this verbalization (and other verbal cues) as a guide to action." Superfluous to say that the perseveration shown by frontal-lobe patients in the card-sorting test strongly recalls the high score of reiterative errors recorded for 'frontal' monkeys in various testing procedures.

LURIA and his colleagues[10,12] have identified a similar perseverative tendency in frontal-lobe patients. When asked to draw a sequence of simple figures, for example, "a cross, two circles and a triangle," the frontal-lobe patient may simply draw four crosses. This 'inertia' may declare itself dramatically when the patient is asked to perform a task requiring an orderly sequence of separate steps. In such cases, he may perseverate an early phase of the action, but it is important to note that he may, instead, be side-tracked in a direction that could have been appropriate in the context of another task. LURIA and HOMSKAYA[12] note that such patients evince no dismay at their failure to achieve the required goal, and suggest ". . . a deficit in matching of action carried out with the original intention . . ." as a central characteristic of the frontal-lobe syndrome. Particularly interesting among Luria and Homskaya's findings is their observation that this derailment of programmed behavior is remarkably refractory to the normally quite compelling effect of repeated verbalization of the required steps by the observer, or even by the patient himself, throughout the process. Such dissociation of the verbal signal from the subject's action appears closely related to MILNER'S[11] observations in frontal-lobe patients in the card-sorting test. As an electrophysiological corollary of this behavioral disconnection, LURIA[10] cites the following important observation by his co-workers Homskaya and Simernitskaya: frontal-lobe patients—but not patients with more posterior cerebral lesions—fail to show an effect that in normal subjects characteristically follows a verbal instruction to await a visual or tactile signal, namely, an enhancement of the electrical potentials evoked in the corresponding sensory area by the signal. LURIA[10] concludes from this observation ". . . that the frontal lobes play a significant part in the regulation of the active states started by a verbal instruction."

Of considerable significance among the test results reported for frontal-lobe patients appear to be MILNER'S[11] findings in the so-called stylus-maze test. According to Milner, the poor performance of frontal-lobe patients in this tracing task is attributable not to any form of spatial disorientation but, instead, to an apparent inability to comply reliably with the 'rules of the game'. Such patients often seem unable to curb a propensity for taking illegal shortcuts (such as moving the stylus diagonally across the board); as in the card-sorting test, they appear aware of their mistakes (in the sense that they can verbalize these) but unable to modify their strategy accordingly.

3. *Comment*

It is clear even from the foregoing highly fragmentary review that the frontal-lobe disorder is characterized foremost by a derangement of behavioral programming. One of the essential functional deficits of the frontal-lobe patient appears to lie in an inability to maintain in his behavior a normal stability-in-time: his action programs, once started, are likely to fade out, to stagnate in reiteration or to become deflected away from the intended goal. The fact that even his self-admitted awareness of a mis-match between the purpose and the result of his actions fails to affect his strategy suggests an inadequate 'internalization' of all those error—or error-approach signals, including even self-directed verbal commands, that normally modulate the evolvement of behavioral programs. The same failure to register (i.e. to furnish a stable constraint) could be thought to be involved in his tendency to break game-rules. If this indeed be the case, it would seem probable that 'feed-back' of opposite sign likewise would fail to become incorporated in the mechanisms of behavioral guidance. It could be asked, for example, if the reiterative phenomena illustrated so forcefully by Luria and his co-workers could not be due in part at least to a 'getting lost' of a message reporting successful accomplishment of initial or intermediate stages of the program.

A state of affairs as here suggested would amount to one in which action programs can be aimed at their intended goal, but must evolve under conditions of severely impaired functioning of some guidance mechanism associated (but not necessarily identical) with that determining the subject's affective responses to the apparent success or failure of his approach. Depending on circumstances, the effect of such inadequate guidance could be either an abnormal inflexibility of the program or an excessive vulnerability to interfering events.

NEURAL ASSOCIATIONS OF THE FRONTAL LOBE

In view of the complex and evasive character of the frontal-lobe syndrome it is appropriate to ask what the nature might be of the neural information normally received and processed by the frontal cortex, and what efferent channels might account for its unique role in behavioral programming.

Obviously, nothing short of a comprehensive analysis of the response determinants of single cortical units can be expected to answer the question as to the informational content of neural impulses converging upon the frontal cortex. Studies of this sort (exemplified by Hubel's contribution to this volume) recently have provided extremely valuable insights into the feature-extracting mechanisms of the visual, somatosensory and auditory fields of the cerebral cortex. However, the problems encountered in exploring these modality-specific cortical fields are likely to be multiplied many times over in regions such as the frontal cortex which are certain to be associated with more than one sensory modality.

Especially the problem of identifying the natural stimuli consistently capable of eliciting responses by a sufficiently large number of cortical units in such regions might prove quite elusive. However that may be, explorations of this sort have not yet provided the data which alone could identify the nature of the information received, and the manner in which it is processed by the frontal cortex. Consequently, little more than anatomical data are currently available from which to draw inferences related to this question. This anatomical information, as the following account is intended to show, is by no means negligible.

1. *Anatomical definition*

The term, frontal lobe or 'prefrontal cortex', has come to denote the cortical field that extends forward of the 'premotor' area 6 and is projected upon by the mediodorsal nucleus of the thalamus. In primates and carnivores, this large cortical expanse covers the frontal pole of the hemisphere, but in the rat, and probably in other rodent species as well, the corresponding and relatively smaller region is composed of two widely separate sub-fields: one confined to the medial surface of the hemisphere, the other occupying the dorsal bank of the rhinal sulcus, and neither extending forward far enough to cover the frontal pole[13]. Apart from such differences of relative size and topography, there is another reason to believe that the prefrontal cortex reaches vastly different stages of development in different mammalian lineages: Only in primates does the larger rostral part of the field exhibit the cytoarchitectural features of a granular cortex. In the cat, dog, sheep, and rat, apparently the only non-primate species in which the prefrontal cortex has been delimited by experimental methods, the field is throughout of an agranular structure; in the rat its laminar pattern is so poorly differentiated that it is nearly indistinguishable from the anterior cingulate cortex with which its medial sub-field is caudally continuous. In fact, on cytoarchitectural grounds alone the existence of a non-primate homologue of the primate prefrontal cortex could be questioned, and it is largely the constancy of its afferent relationship with the mediodorsal nucleus of the thalamus that has allowed a prefrontal cortex to be identified in non-primate forms.

Since the anatomical account to follow is based very largely upon observations in the rhesus monkey, a brief description of the main anatomical features of the prefrontal cortex of this species would seem relevant. As shown in Fig. 1, the caudal border of the prefrontal cortex is marked by the deep *arcuate sulcus* which delimits it from the agranular 'motor cortex' of the precentral gyrus (areas 4 and 6 of Brodmann). The only other macroscopic features of importance are: (1) the general shape of the frontal lobe which allows a fairly flat medial surface to be distinguished from a concave ventral (or orbital) aspect and a lateral convexity, and (2) the deep *principal sulcus* which divides the lateral convexity into a dorsal and a ventral field.

The cortex forming the most caudal part of the prefrontal region, i.e. the rostral bank of the arcuate sulcus, is structurally speaking something of a transition zone between the agranular 'motor cortex' behind it and the distinctly granular cortex that occupies the large rostral remainder of the frontal lobe. This crescent-shaped 'dysgranular' zone of the prefrontal cortex, labelled area 8 by Brodmann, is customarily referred to as the 'frontal eye field'. The justification for this label lies in the fact that electrical stimulation of the region elicits conjugate contraversive eye movements, whereas its ablation is followed by a *transitory* inability of the monkey to turn its eyes to the contralateral side, and a concomitant failure to pay attention to stimuli delivered in the contralateral half of the visual field ('contralateral visual neglect'). Tempting as it would seem to assume that area 8 is the oculomotor area of the 'motor cortex', recent findings concerning the temporal relationship between eye movements and the activity patterns of single neurons of area 8 flatly contradict such a notion and appear to suggest that the area is involved in the *monitoring* rather than the effectuation of eye movements.[14,15] It is here included in the 'prefrontal' rather than the 'motor' cortex for the reason that its thalamo-cortical afferents come from the mediodorsal thalamic nucleus.[16]

The large remainder of the prefrontal region is distinctly granular in type. A varying number of cytoarchitectural subdivisions have been recognized in this large granular territory, but the structural differences have been too subtle to permit anything resembling agreement among individual observers (see AKERT[16]). Whether or not manifested by cytoarchitectural contrasts, however, a functional parcellation of the region appears virtually certain from the observation that different sub-fields of the granular frontal cortex have markedly different afferent and efferent relationships (see below).

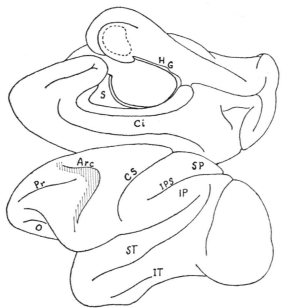

FIG. 1.   Line drawing representing the lateral (lower half of figure) and medial aspect of the cerebral hemisphere of a rhesus monkey. The lateral view shows the arcuate sulcus (Arc) which marks the caudal boundary of the region here called 'the frontal lobe', and the principal sulcus (Pr) which divides the frontal convexity in a dorsal and ventral half. The shaded region forming the rostral bank of the arcuate sulcus represents the dysgranular area often referred to as 'frontal eye field.' A small rostral part of the orbital surface of the frontal lobe (O) is visible in the lateral view. The broken line in the upper half of the figure indicates the approximate position of the amygdala, a structure largely hidden from view by the overlying olfactory cortex. Other structures labelled are: Ci: cingulate gyrus; CS: central sulcus; HG: hippocampal gyrus; IP: inferior parietal lobule; IPS: intraparietal sulcus; IT: inferior temporal region; S: septum; SP: superior parietal lobule.

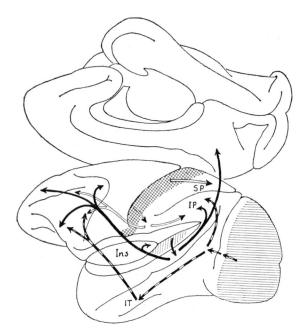

FIG. 2. Schematic representation of some of the major association pathways extending away from the great primary sensory fields of the cortex. The visual area 17 is indicated by horizontal shading, the auditory area by vertical shading, and the somatic sensory cortex by cross-hatching. Afferents to the frontal lobe presumably conveying auditory information are indicated by solid-black arrows, those conveying visual information, by black and white arrows, and presumably somatosensory afferents by open arrows. Note that pathways representing all of these three modalities also converge upon the inferior parietal lobule (IP). The substantial projections from this parietal region to the frontal cortex are indicated separately in Fig. 3.

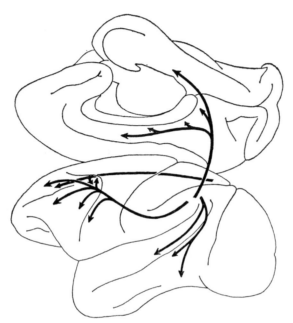

FIG. 3.   Schematic representation of parieto-frontal connections originating from the inferior and superior parietal lobules. Those from the inferior lobule can be thought to convey visual, auditory and somatosensory information. Note that the inferior parietal lobule also has substantial efferent connections with the cingulate and hippocampal gyri, and with all of the temporal gyri (see also Petras' contribution to this volume).

2. *Afferent connections of the frontal lobe*

Recent experimental findings with respect to the afferent connections of the frontal lobe have combined to suggest that the frontal cortex is a common end-point for generally long neuronal chains that extend away from the primary sensory regions of the cerebral cortex. Some such conduction routes are composed entirely of cortico-cortical links, and could therefore be classified as associative connections throughout. Others, by contrast, involve the mediodorsal nucleus of the thalamus and thus have their last link in the thalamo-frontal projection system.

2 (a) *Afferents from the visual, auditory and somatic sensory areas.* Associative chains linking the primary cortical fields of the visual, auditory and somatic sensory systems with the frontal cortex have been outlined in a series of recent experimental studies by KUYPERS *et al.*,[17] PANDYA and KUYPERS[18] and PANDYA *et al.*[19] in the rhesus monkey. As shown in extremely schematic form by Figs. 2–3, in each of these three sensory systems the connection in question initially involves one or more cortical zones adjoining the primary sensory field ('belt zones', for example areas 18 and 19 of the visual cortex), and spreads from there to either or both the inferior parietal lobule and the rostral half of the temporal neocortex. The latter two fields are major sources of direct cortico-cortical afferents to the frontal cortex (for a more detailed accounting of parieto- and temporo-frontal connections the reader is referred to Petras' contribution to this volume).

An interesting detail reported by the aforementioned authors is that, whereas virtually no fibers to the frontal cortex appear to originate in the primary sensory fields, some can be traced from the immediately adjoining field (such as area 18 of the visual cortex) and a considerably larger number from the field 'next in line' (e.g. area 19 of the visual cortex). It thus appears that the association of each of these three sensory systems, although largely organized so as to involve a lineal sequence of intermediate cortical processing stations, includes some additional conduction lines originating in parallel from such intercalated way-stations.

It is remarkable that the direct associative connection of the anterior temporal cortex to the frontal lobe by way of the uncinate bundle is paralleled by a pathway from lower temporal regions (middle and inferior temporal gyri) via the so-called inferior thalamic peduncle to the particular (medial, magnocellular) subdivision of the mediodorsal thalamic nucleus[20] that is known[16,21] to project to the cortex covering the orbital surface of the frontal lobe (Fig. 4). The field of origin of this transthalamic temporo-frontal conduction route overlaps that of the uncinate bundle to some extent at least, but whereas the latter, direct connection appears to involve a very large part of the frontal cortex,[18] the temporo-thalamo-frontal pathway must be limited in its distribution to the orbital surface. The functional significance of the mediodorsal nucleus as an intermediary in the path to the frontal lobe must for the present remain a matter of conjecture, but it is interesting that the lower temporal gyri share this efferent way-station with the olfactory cortex (see below).

It must be emphasized that the various cortical and thalamic intermediaries in these sensory-frontal conduction routes cannot be viewed as mere 'relay stations' along the path to the frontal lobe. There can be little doubt that fundamental input-transformations take place at each step along the transcortical way, and there is thus reason to suspect that the information content of the impulse flow arriving at the frontal cortex can be little more than a remote derivative of the neural events taking place in the primary sensory areas. Nonetheless, the systematic progression of associative conduction routes toward the frontal lobe suggests that all of the three major sensoria represented by modality-specific areas in the neocortex find some form of re-representation in the frontal cortex, however abstracted or compounded that form may be.

2 (b) *Afferents from the olfactory system.* It is of interest to note here that the frontal lobe is not the only neocortical region in which association systems related to the visual, somesthetic and auditory systems converge. For example, at earlier stages of cortico-cortical processing a similar confluence, or at least a partial spatial overlapping of these three modalities* appears to take place in the inferior parietal lobule. However, nowhere but in the frontal lobe does this convergence appear to be augmented by an afferent connection from the *olfactory system.* The unexpected evidence of a close relationship of the frontal lobe with the olfactory sensorium came from studies in the rat by SANDERS–WOUDSTRA[22] and POWELL et al.[23] that convincingly demonstrated a substantial projection from the prepirifrom (olfactory) cortex via the inferior thalamic peduncle to the medial, magnocellular subdivision of the mediodorsal nucleus of the thalamus. This olfacto-thalamic connection, schematically illustrated in Fig. 4, implies the theoretical possibility that the posterior orbitofrontal cortex is not more than a few synapses removed from the olfactory receptor neurons. No less interesting is the fact that the projection to the mediodorsal nucleus appears to be only one subdivision of a wider projection from the olfactory cortex that includes substantial connections to the lateral hypothalamic region.

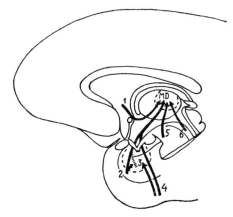

FIG. 4. Schematic drawing indicating some of the subcortical afferents of the mediodorsal nucleus of the thalamus (MD). Arrow 1 represents afferents from the septum, arrow 2: such from the olfactory cortex; arrow 3 (shaded because of uncertainty mentioned in the text): fibers from the amygdala; arrow 4: fibers from the inferior temporal region; arrow 5: fibers from the ventromedial area of the midbrain tegmentum, and arrow 6: fibers ascending through the dorsal region of the tegmentum. The connections 2, 3 and 4 are components of the inferior thalamic peduncle.

---

* The term, *overlap,* is here used without prejudice as to the question whether two or more afferent systems converging upon a given cortical region establish synaptic contacts with the same, or different, neuronal constituents of the region.

One could wonder whether perhaps, by these short routes to the frontal lobe and hypo-thalamus, the olfactory system—no less than other sensoria involved in learning and memory—may be giving us a basic anatomical 'flow-diagram' of telencephalic signal-processing, a model which other sensory modalities complicate by the interposition of a series of neocortical processing stations beyond the primary cortical receiving area.

2 (c) *Other afferent connections of the frontal lobe.* All of the evidence summarily reviewed above suggests the frontal lobe as a neocortical region representing the external environ-ment as reported by all exteroceptive sensoria. But even this encompassing statement may not adequately describe its afferent relationships, for it does not take into account a remarkable diversity of further fiber systems connected to the frontal cortex by way of the mediodorsal nucleus.

Such additional afferents include connections to the medial subdivision of the medio-dorsal thalamic nucleus from the septal region and from a ventral-paramedian zone of the mesencephalic tegmentum.[24] It is likely, but not certain, that the same medial component of the mediodorsal nucleus also receives afferents from the amygdala.*

Only sparse data are available with respect to the afferent connections of the con-siderably larger *lateral* subdivision of the mediodorsal thalamic nucleus, a cell territory known to project to the *convexity* of the frontal lobe.[16,21] The observation that it receives fibers originating in the intralaminar thalamic nuclei[26] holds little clue-value, for such fibers appear to be distributed widely among specific thalamic nuclei. Neither is much informa-tion to be derived from the fact that the nucleus receives numerous thalamic fibers from the frontal convexity: reciprocity appears to be a common, if not indeed universal, property of thalamo-cortical relationships. In a recent experimental study in the rat, however, CHI[27] has demonstrated a discrete fiber system that ascends beneath the ventrolateral border of the central grey substance of the midbrain, and terminates with dense arborizations in a circumscript region of the more lateral zone of the mediodorsal nucleus. The cells of origin of this well-defined, lemniscus-like fiber system have not been identified, but the position of the bundle in the midbrain suggests that it may be a transsynaptic continuation of a projection system ascending from the nucleus of the solitary tract, a projection which follows a comparable mesencephalic trajectory[28] but appears not to extend into the thalamus directly.

It is difficult to evaluate the functional nature of these various afferents of the medio-dorsal nucleus on the basis of anatomical evidence alone. At present, only the projection from the olfactory cortex can be identified in terms of sensory modality. There is none-theless ample reason to suspect that several at least of the remaining afferent fiber systems mentioned above convey information concerning the organism's internal milieu. Such a relationship would seem likely in particular for the fiber systems originating in the septum

---

* The lingering uncertainty concerning this point is due to the efferents from the overlying olfactory cortex that traverse the amygdaloid complex in passage to the hypothalamus and mediodorsal nucleus, and thus are unavoidably involved in lesions of the amygdala. Although, as a consequence, direct proof of an amygdalo-thalamic projection is lacking, the existence of this connection appears nonetheless likely in the context of current knowledge concerning temporal-lobe efferents contained in the ansa peduncularis and its thalamic extension, the inferior thalamic peduncle. As summarized in Fig. 4, such connections include efferents from both the inferior temporal region[20] and the olfactory cortex[23,25] to both the amygdaloid complex and mediodorsal thalamic nucleus.

and in paramedian zones of the midbrain tegmentum, brainstem regions prominently involved in the circuitry of the telencephalic limbic structures and hypothalamus. It would not seem far-fetched to interpret such conduction systems as conveyors of neural codes related to motivational states and their visceral concomitants.

3. *Efferent connections of the frontal lobe*

Much like most other subdivisions of the cerebral mantle, the frontal cortex has been found to be connected by a great variety of efferent pathways to other cortical regions as well as to subcortical structures. In both categories of connections, indications are found that the frontal lobe is closely associated with the limbic system, but there are other efferent relationships that cannot be so classified.

3 (a) *Efferent cortical associations of the frontal lobe.* Major cortico-cortical efferents connect the frontal lobe with the anterior temporal cortex, with the inferior parietal lobule, and with the cingulate and parahippocampal gyri (Fig. 5). The two former of these efferent connections to some extent at least appear to reciprocate the prominent afferent association

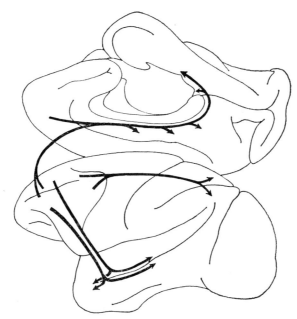

FIG. 5. Schematic representation of afferent connections of the frontal lobe with both parietal lobules, upper and middle temporal gyri, and cingulate and hippocampal gyri. This figure is based in parts on reports by PANDYA and KUYPERS[18], in part also on personal communications from Dr. D. N. Pandya.

of the frontal lobe with the anterior temporal and inferior parietal regions. The findings of PANDYA and KUYPERS[18] suggest that the connection to the inferior parietal lobule originates most massively in the caudal frontal region approximately corresponding to the 'frontal eye field', whereas fronto-temporal fibers appear to arise more evenly throughout the frontal convexity and are organized topographically in such fashion that the dorsal half of the convexity (i.e. the field dorsal to the principal sulcus) projects to the superior temporal gyrus, the ventral half to the dorsal bank of the middle temporal gyrus. It is important to note that a substantial projection to the amygdaloid complex arises from the inferior temporal region[20] (Fig. 4). The fronto-temporal connection could therefore be thought to permit the frontal cortex to modulate not only the activity patterns of the temporal cortex but also those of the amygdala.

The frontal efferents to the limbic cortex (cingulate and parahippocampal gyri) originate largely from dorsal convexity cortex, and there is evidence (Pandya, personal communication) that the field of origin has its center in the dorsal bank lining the middle one-third of the principal sulcus. The fronto-limbic association is established by a fairly compact fiber bundle that follows the white matter of the cingulate gyrus caudalward, issuing fibers to the overlying cortex throughout its extent. The longest fibers curve around the splenium of the corpus callosum into the hippocampal gyrus, and are distributed in this region as far as the presubiculum hippocampi. By virtue of this fronto-limbic connection the frontal cortex stands in very close relationship with the hippocampal formation, but it must be emphasized that the frontal lobe is not unique in this regard, for PANDYA and KUYPERS'[18] study has demonstrated that substantial direct projections to the cingulate and parahippocampal gyri originate also from rostral temporal regions and from the inferior parietal lobule. The remarkable conclusion can be drawn from these observations that neocortical projections to the limbic (cingulate and juxtahippocampal) cortex originate largely at least from three interconnected cortical regions among which the frontal cortex appears to occupy a central position.

3 (b) *Subcortical projections of the frontal cortex.* Nowhere more remarkably than in its subcortical connections does the frontal lobe declare its close association with the limbic system. This relationship is most explicitly expressed by the substantial projections that have been traced from the frontal cortex[29,31] to the preoptic region and hypothalamus and, beyond these diencephalic structures, to a paramedian zone of the mesencephalic tegmentum that includes the ventral half of the central grey substance, the ventral tegmental area, and the nucleus centralis tegmenti superior of Bechterew. Together with the septal region, these subcortical structures and their interconnections compose a highly differentiated meso-diencephalic continuum that also is a major distribution zone for projections arising in various components of the limbic telencephalon, the hippocampus and amygdala in particular.[32,33]

By entertaining subcortical projections in such extensive overlap with those of the limbic forebrain, the frontal lobe distinguishes itself sharply from all other regions of the neocortical mantle. It must be noted, however, that this unique neocortical projection apparently does not arise from all subdivisions of the frontal lobe equally. A frontal projection to the lateral preopticohypothalamic region, for example, has been traced from caudal regions of the orbital surface,[30] whereas a second projection, apparently originating dorsal to the principal sulcus, distributes itself not only to lateral regions of the hypothalamus, but also to the so-called dorsal hypothalamic area and to the posterior hypothalamic nucleus, central grey substance, ventral tegmental area, and Bechterew's nucleus (personal, unpublished observations). In a recent article JOHNSON et al.[34] have described an additional projection passing from the dorsal bank of the principal sulcus to the septum. Few if any comparable projections appear to arise from convexity cortex ventral to the principal sulcus. It must be noted, however, that the fronto-hypothalamic and fronto-mesencephalic projections have not yet been analyzed in adequate detail with respect to either origin or distribution.

Besides these projections to the hypothalamus and associated brainstem structures, the frontal lobe has been found to emit fibers to the striatum, to the subthalamic region, and to the mesencephalic region lateral and dorsal to the red nucleus. The fronto-striatal projection involves a rostroventral part of the caput nuclei caudati as well as certain regions of the fundus striati (i.e. the zone of confluence of the caudate nucleus and putamen).

Any functional significance of the fronto-striatal connections must lie hidden in its topographic characteristics, for all or nearly all cortical regions project to particular zones of either the caudate nucleus or putamen, or both. No functional mosaic of the striatum appears to be known at present, but it may eventually prove significant that, in the cat, extensive lesions of the general region of the caudate nucleus receiving the frontal lobe projection have been found to cause a peculiar hyperkinetic dyskinesia[35] that has been compared tentatively to athetosis. The functional implications of the fronto-subthalamic and fronto-tegmental projections are obscure, except for the obvious likelihood that the frontocortical mechanism, by virtue of these connections, can affect general activity levels.

DISCUSSION

In hindsight it is possible to argue that, even in the absence of any but elementary physiological knowledge, the general functional associations of many cortical regions could have been inferred from anatomical relationships. Such a statement would be not at all presumptuous in reference to the sensory areas or the sensorimotor cortex, and perhaps not even much so if it were made with respect to certain associative areas such as the parietal cortex. Whether it can be applied to cortical regions functionally as complex as the frontal cortex remains to be considered. In any event, in attempting to elucidate a unique functional attribute of a given cortical region, it would seem appropriate, in a first approach, to look for unusual features in the anatomical relationships of that region.

The unique feature of the neural circuitry outlined in the foregoing account is, that it places the frontal cortex in a reciprocal relationship with two great functional realms, namely: (1) *parietal and temporal regions of the cerebral cortex involved in the processing of visual, auditory and somatic sensory information, and* (2) *the telencephalic limbic system and its subcortical correspondents, in particular the hypothalamus and meso- and diencephalic structures associated with the hypothalamus.* The reciprocal nature of both of these two relationships deserves particular emphasis, for it entails a need to view the frontal lobe at once as a 'sensory' and as an 'effector' mechanism. In the following part of this discussion an attempt will be made to interpret part at least of the frontal-lobe syndrome as the consequence of loss of a senso-effector organization involved in mechanisms of both perceptual processing and behavioral programming.

The frontal lobe is characterized so distinctly by its multiple associations with the limbic system, and in particular by its direct connections with the hypothalamus, that it would seem justified to view the frontal cortex as the major—although not the only—neocortical representative of the limbic system. The reciprocity in the anatomical relationship suggests that the frontal cortex both monitors and modulates limbic mechanisms.

All of the experimental and clinical evidence leads to the conclusion that the telencephalic limbic structures and their subcortical correspondents are centrally involved in functions related to the organism's internal milieu. Not only do they receive neural and chemical signals emanating from that environment, they also modulate it by the medium of complex endocrine and neural effector systems. Moreover, it now appears certain that their functional states manifest themselves subjectively in the form of affects and motivations. In view of the fact that the frontal lobe is closely associated with the limbic system and hypothalamus, extensive lesions of the frontal cortex could be expected to have a marked effect upon the range and differentiation of the subject's viscero-endocrine, affective and motivational responses to his environment. This suggestion from anatomical data is compatible with Homskaya's observation (reported by LURIA[10]) of diagnostically significant anomalies in the conditioning of the galvanic skin reaction of frontal-lobe patients.

The physiological nature of the fronto-limbic relationship cannot be postulated *a priori* and would have to be identified by animal experimentation. It would seem of interest, for example, to determine whether perhaps the limbico-hypothalamic axis, no longer afferented by the frontal cortex, functions at a permanently changed level, a change that might reveal itself, among others, in anomalous viscero-endocrine responses even to vital-stress factors such as cold. Such a condition would be comparable to the enduring changes observed in certain kinesthetic and cutaneous reflexes following lesions of the sensorimotor cortex, a comparison that comes to mind readily because of the existence of a direct fronto-hypothalamic connection. However, whether or not loss of the frontal lobes so gravely affects the intrinsic mechanisms of the limbic system and hypothalamus, it is certain to eliminate important pathways by which the neocortex could be thought to modulate the organism's affective and motivational states. It may be of particular importance that such pathways include the fronto-hypothalamic connection, the only known direct route from the neocortex to the hypothalamus. The failure of the affective and motivational responses of the frontal-lobe patient to match environmental situations that he nonetheless can describe accurately could thus be tentatively interpreted as the consequence of a loss of a modulatory influence normally exerted by the neocortex upon the limbic mechanisms via the frontal lobe.

However, the reciprocity in the fronto-limbic association urges consideration of an opposite, perception-oriented (i.e., corticipetal) interpretation of the frontal-lobe syndrome. Viewed along that line, part at least of the behavioral effects of frontal-lobe destruction could be seen as the consequence of an 'interoceptive agnosia', i.e., an impairment of the subject's ability to integrate certain informations from his internal milieu with the environmental reports provided by his neocortical processing mechanisms. It may be recalled that the available anatomical evidence indicates the frontal cortex as one, and perhaps the only realm of the neocortex where neural pathways representing the internal milieu converge with conduction systems re-representing the external environment as reported by *all* exteroceptive modalities. The two opposite points of view are by no means mutually exclusive; in fact, both conditions are likely to exist together in the frontal-lobe patient.

It should be stressed at this point that even complete ablations of the frontal lobes are unlikely to block all impulse traffic between the neocortex and the limbico-hypothalamic complex. Under such conditions, interoceptive information would still be likely, by way of the anterior thalamic nucleus, to reach the cingulate and parahippocampal gyri, where it could conceivably be integrated with information reaching the same gyri (Fig. 5) from the temporal and inferior parietal regions. Although, therefore, complete ablations of the frontal lobes alone do not dissociate the neocortex from the limbic system and hypothalamus, such lesions may nevertheless severely impair the normal interplay between these two forebrain levels.

It is tempting to speculate that the reciprocal fronto-limbic relationship could be centrally involved in the phenomenon of *behavioral anticipation,* and elucidate the 'loss of foresight' that has so long been recognized as one of the most disabling consequences of massive frontal-lobe lesions. The normal individual decides upon a particular course of action by a thought-process in which a larger or smaller number of strategic alternatives are compared. It could be suggested—admittedly on purely introspective grounds—that the comparison in the final analysis is one between the affective responses evoked by each of the various alternatives.* The strategy ultimately elected would thus be one that has already passed censure by an interoceptive sensorium. It is entirely conceivable that this anticipatory selection process is severely impaired in the absence of the frontal cortex.

A somewhat similar, or at least related, frontal mechanism could be postulated to explain the phenomenon of *temporal stability* in behavioral programs. In an earlier section of this paper it was mentioned that TEUBER[9] has found reasons to attribute the visual and proprioceptive defects associated with frontal-lobe lesions to the loss of a mechanism of *corollary discharge* that pre-sets sensory processing mechanisms for such input changes as would predictably result from the impending motor output. Teuber's notion essentially postulates an effector function of the frontal lobe, even though that function would have its primary impact on perception rather than movement. The substantial efferent connections of the frontal lobe with the temporal cortex and the inferior parietal lobule could well form part of the anatomical substratum of such a function. It could be asked, however, if not perhaps a wider aspect of the frontal-lobe syndrome could be interpreted in terms of a corollary discharge. More specifically, it would seem possible to envisage a pre-setting not only of exteroceptive processing mechanisms, but also of those mechanisms dealing with interoceptive information. Such a pre-setting could be thought to establish a temporal sequence of affective reference points serving as 'navigational markers' and providing, by their sequential order, at once the general course and the temporal stability of complex goal-directed forms of behavior.

---

* The incorporation of an interoceptive intuitive element in decision-making, earlier suggested by Henri Bergson (for example, Chapter 2 of *L'Evolution Créatrice*), is emphasized by Charles DeGaulle in *Le Fil de l'Epée*. Collective awareness of this ultimate sensorium undoubtedly far antedates these explicit formulations, and is expressed in a variety of idioms (" . . . the mere thought of doing such a thing makes me ill").

It could be suspected—so far on no more than introspective grounds—that the itineraries of anticipated behavior require being registered and 'kept on hand' not only in somatic sensorimotor mechanisms but also in structures subserving the organism's affective responsiveness, and thus, that a plan for action cannot be kept in abeyance intact for any length of time unless it is represented in matching somatic and affective registries. If this were indeed the case, it would be readily understandable that loss of the frontal cortex as a major mediator of information exchange between the cerebral cortex and the limbic system is followed not only by an impairment of strategic choice-making, but also by a tendency of projected or current action programs to 'fade out' or become over-ridden by interfering influences. This notion would seem to be somewhat in line with KONORSKI and LAWICKA'S[3] suggestion that the poor performance of 'frontal' animals in the delayed-response task may be caused by an abnormally rapid decay of signal traces. In this context it could even be suggested that the 'frontal' animal has suffered a memory impairment after all, even though this loss affects the storage of its action plans rather than that of its external-perceptual images.

It cannot be correct to interpret the frontal lobe exclusively as a structure modulating sensory, viscero-endocrine, and affective mechanisms, for the frontal cortex also projects to structures that may be involved primarily in somatic effector functions. For example, as mentioned earlier in this paper, it has efferent connections with the caudoputamen, and PANDYA and KUYPERS'[18] findings suggest that it is also connected—even though perhaps not massively—to the premotor cortex. It would therefore seem likely that, as already suggested above, the role of the frontal lobe also manifests itself in the realm of somatic motor function. LURIA and HOMSKAYA[12] have observed patients with tumors causing massive frontal-lobe destruction who were often unable to initiate a movement required by the examiner, even though audibly repeating to themselves the examiner's instruction. It remains to be determined whether such akinetic and hypokinetic consequences of massive frontal-lobe tumors reflect a motivational loss or an effector deficit in the more restricted sense, and if the latter should be the case, whether they may not be due to a direct involvement of the caudoputamen or premotor cortex in the pathological process.

Up to this point in the discussion, the frontal lobe has been dealt with as if it were a homogeneous structure. There is, however, ample evidence that the input–output relationships of the monkey's frontal cortex vary considerably from one subregion of the field to the next, and some of these variations have been noted in the anatomical account. To recapitulate, it seems certain that those afferent associations likely to convey visual, auditory and somesthetic information primarily affect the caudal half of the monkey's frontal convexity, and particularly the region of the frontal eye-field. Olfactory information, by contrast, would seem to be distributed via the mediodorsal nucleus entirely to the caudal half of the orbital aspect of the lobe, and the same is probably true of the transthalamic afflux of impulses here interpreted as representing the internal milieu, except for that part conveyed through the mesencephalon by way of the lateral division of the mediodorsal nucleus to a yet undisclosed region of the frontal convexity. Further 'interoceptive' afferents to the frontal cortex are likely to come from the cingulate cortex, but their distribution remains to be determined. As to the efferent connections of the frontal lobe, the great conduction route to the hippocampal gyrus appears to originate largely from the dorsal bank of the sulcus principalis, whereas associations with the amygdala by way of the temporal cortex are more likely to arise from ventral convexity areas. The fronto-hypothalamic connection apparently originates from two widely separated fields: the caudal orbitofrontal region and some region dorsal to the sulcus principalis, whereas the 'feedback' association with the multimodal processing areas of the parietal lobe arises largely in and near the frontal eye-field. This anatomical mosaic suggests a great functional differentiation of the frontal region, a suggestion that has begun to be borne out by the results of some recent behavioral studies in the monkey. In one of these, the monkey's ability to perform at normal levels in the spatial delayed-alternation test was found to depend on the integrity of the cortex lining the principal sulcus, whereas his capacity to integrate auditory, visual and kinesthetic information was found impaired by lesions in the 'peri-arcuate' region, i.e. the general area of the frontal eye field.[37] In another study, the region crucially involved in the mechanisms required for the delayed-alternation task could be further localized to the cortex lining the middle one-third of the principal sulcus.[38] Further studies of this nature may disclose yet other instances of differential functional localization in the frontal lobe. One must hope that such and other laboratory experiments may eventually be extended so as to provide records not only of the overt behavior of animals with variously located frontal-lobe lesions but also of its visceral and endocrine concomitants, and of contemporaneous activity states in such structures as the hippo-campus, the amygdala, the caudate nucleus, and parietal and temporal regions of the cortex. Several tantalizing, but as yet anecdotal, findings pertinent to this general question have already been reported from both animal[36] and clinical[10] studies. From such inquiries a clearer picture of the physiological nature of frontal-lobe function may be expected eventually to emerge.

Acknowledgements—The author expresses his sincere appreciation to Drs. H.-L. TEUBER and STEPHEN M. SHEA for valuable guiding comments, to Dr. D. N. PANDYA for providing several important data prior to publication, and to Miss ELIZABETH B. JONES for her efficient technical assistance in the pre-paration of this article. His greatest debt, however, accumulated over two decades, is to Dr. DAVID McKENZIE RIOCH for providing not onlymaterial support but, above all, an unexcelledi ntellectual milieu for inquiries into problems of brain and mind.

REFERENCES

1. JACOBSEN, C. F. Functions of the frontal association area in primates. *Archs Neurol. Psychiat.* **33**, 558, 1935.
2. MISHKIN, M. Perseveration of central sets after frontal lesions in monkeys. In: *The Frontal Granular Cortex and Behavior*, WARREN, J. M. and AKERT, K. (Eds.), p. 219. McGraw-Hill, New York, 1964.
3. KONORSKI, J. and LAWICKA, W. Analysis of errors by prefrontal animals on the delayed-response test. In: *The Frontal Granular Cortex and Behavior*, WARREN, J. M. and AKERT, K. (Eds.), p. 271. McGraw-Hill, New York, 1964.
4. WEISKRANTZ, L. and MISHKIN, M. Effects of temporal and frontal cortical lesions on auditory discrimination in monkeys. *Brain* **81**, 406, 1958.
5. BÄTTIG, K., ROSVOLD, H. E. and MISHKIN, M. Comparison of the effects of frontal and caudate lesions on delayed response and alternation in monkeys. *J. comp. physiol. Psychol.* **53**, 400, 1960.
6. RYLANDER, G. *Personality Changes after Operations on the Frontal Lobes.* Oxford University Press, London, 1939.
7. HALSTEAD, W. C. *Brain and Intelligence: a Quantitative Study of the Frontal Lobes.* The University of Chicago Press, Chicago, 1947.

8. TEUBER, H.-L. Some alterations in behavior after cerebral lesions in man. In: *Evolution of Nervous Control from Primitive Organisms to Man*, BASS, A. D. (Ed.), p. 157. Am. Ass. Adv. Sci., Washington, D.C., 1959.

9. TEUBER, H.-L. The riddle of frontal lobe function in man. In: *The Frontal Granular Cortex and Behavior*, WARREN, J. M. and AKERT, K. (Eds.), p. 410. McGraw-Hill, New York, 1964.

10. LURIA, A. R. *The Origin and Cerebral Organization of Man's Conscious Action*, Evening lecture to the XIX Int. Congress Psychol., London 1969. Moscow Univ. Press, Moscow, 1969.

11. MILNER, B. Some effects of frontal lobectomy in man. In: *The Frontal Granular Cortex and Behavior*, WARREN, J. M. and AKERT, K. (Eds.), p. 311. McGraw-Hill, New York, 1964.

12. LURIA, A. R. and HOMSKAYA, E. D. Disturbance in the regulative role of speech with frontal lobe lesions. In: *The Frontal Granular Cortex and Behavior*, WARREN, J. M. and AKERT, K. (Eds.), p. 352. McGraw-Hill, New York, 1964.

13. LEONARD, C. M. The prefrontal cortex of the rat. I. Cortical projection of the mediodorsal nucleus. II. Efferent connections. *Brain Res.* 12, 321, 1969.

14. BIZZI, E. Discharge of frontal eye field neurons during saccadic and following eye movements in unanesthetized monkeys. *Expl Brain Res.* 6, 69, 1968.

15. BIZZI, E. and SCHILLER, P. H. Single unit activity in the frontal eye fields of unanesthetized monkeys during eye and head movements. *Expl Brain Res.* 10, 151, 1970.

16. AKERT, K. Comparative anatomy of frontal cortex and thalamofrontal connections. In: *The Frontal Granular Cortex and Behavior*, WARREN, J. M. and AKERT, K. (Eds.), p. 372. McGraw-Hill, New York, 1964.

17. KUYPERS, H. G. J. M., SZWARCBART, M. K. and MISHKIN, M. Occipitotemporal cortico-cortical connections in the rhesus monkey. *Expl Neurol.* 11, 245, 1965.

18. PANDYA, D. N. and KUYPERS, H. G. J. M. Cortico-cortical connections in the rhesus monkey. *Brain Res.* 13, 13, 1969.

19. PANDYA, D. N., HALLETT, M. and MUKHERJEE, S. K. Intra- and interhemispheric connections of the neocortical auditory system in the rhesus monkey. *Brain Res.* 13, 49, 1969.

20. WHITLOCK, D. G. and NAUTA, W. J. H. Subcortical projections from the temporal neocortex in Macaca mulatta. *J. comp. Neurol.* 106, 183, 1956.

21. FREEMAN, W. and WATTS, J. W. Retrograde degeneration of the thalamus following prefrontal lobotomy. *J. comp. Neurol.* 86, 65, 1947.

22. SANDERS-WOUDSTRA, J. A. R. Experimenteel anatomisch onderzoek over de verbindingen van enkele telencefale hersengebieden bij de albino rat. Doctoral Dissertation, Groningen, 1961.

23. POWELL, T. P. S., COWAN, W. M. and RAISMAN, G. The central olfactory connexions. *J. Anat. (Lond.)* 99, 791, 1965.

24. GUILLERY, R. W. Afferent fibers to the dorsomedial thalamic nucleus in the cat. *J. Anat.* 93, 403, 1959.

25. VALVERDE, F. *Studies on the Piriform Lobe*. Harvard University Press, Cambridge, Mass., 1965.

26. NAUTA, W. J. H. and WHITLOCK, D. G. An anatomical analysis of the non-specific thalamic projection system. In: *Brain Mechanisms and Consciousness*, DELAFRESNAVE, J. F. (Ed.), p. 81. Blackwell, Oxford, 1954.

27. CHI, C. C. An experimental silver study of the ascending projections of the central grey substance and adjacent tegmentum in the rat, with observations in the cat. *J. comp. Neurol.* 139, 259, 1970.

28. MOREST, D. K. Experimental study of the projections of the nucleus of the tractus solitarius and the area postrema in the cat. *J. comp. Neurol.* 130, 277, 1967.

29. DE VITO, J. L. and SMITH, O. E. Subcortical projections of the prefrontal lobe of the monkey. *J. comp. Neurol.* 123, 413, 1964.

30. NAUTA, W. J. H. Neural associations of the amygdaloid complex in the monkey. *Brain* 85, 505, 1962.

31. NAUTA, W. J. H. Some efferent connections of the prefrontal cortex in the monkey. In: *The Frontal Granular Cortex and Behavior*, WARREN, J. M. and AKERT, K. (Eds.), p. 397. McGraw-Hill, New York, 1964.

32. NAUTA, W. J. H. Hippocampal projections and related neural pathways to the midbrain in the cat. *Brain* 81, 319, 1958.

33. NAUTA, W. J. H. Fibre degeneration following lesions of the amygdaloid complex in the monkey, *J. Anat.* 95, 515, 1961.

34. JOHNSON, T. N., ROSVOLD, H. E. and MISHKIN, M. Projections from behaviorally-defined sectors of the prefrontal cortex to the basal ganglia, septum, and diencephalon of the monkey. *Expl Neurol.* 21, 20, 1968.

35. LILES, S. L. and DAVIS, G. D. Permanent athetoid and choreiform movements after small caudate lesions in the cat. In: *Psychotropic Drugs and Dysfunctions of the Basal Ganglia*, CRANE, G. E. and GARDNER, R. (Eds.), p. 98. U.S. Public Health Service Publication No. 1938, 1969.

36. HOCKMAN, C., TALESNIK, J. and LIVINGSTON, K. E. Central nervous system modulation of cardiovascular reflexes. *Proc. Int. Un. physiol. Sci.* 7, 196, 1968.

37. GOLDMAN, P. and ROSVOLD, H. E. Localization of function within the dorsolateral prefrontal cortex of the rhesus monkey. *Expl Neurol.* 21, 20, 1968.

38. BUTTERS, N. and PANDYA, D. N. Retention of delayed-alternation: effect of selective lesions of sulcus principalis. *Science* 165, 1271, 1969.

J. psychiat. Res. ,1971, Vol. 8, pp. 189–201. Pergamon Press. Printed in Great Britain.

CONNECTIONS OF THE PARIETAL LOBE

J. M. PETRAS

Department of Neurophysiology, Division of Neuropsychiatry, Walter Reed Army Institute of
Research, Washington, D.C. 20012

INTRODUCTION

THE PARIETAL lobes of the brains of primates exhibit an increase in fissuration and gyral complexity when comparing prosimians with New World and Old World monkeys, and some species of ceboids and cercopithecids with the apes and man. [1-4] Increases in fissuration and gyration can be seen among the New World species themselves. [4] Ample attention has been given to the great increase in size of the frontal lobes among primates, but a similar importance clearly should be attached to the parietal lobes of primates, and most probably to the temporal lobes as well. Our findings with respect to the anatomy of the parietal lobe suggest that the posterior part of the parietal lobe, i.e. the expanse of parietal cortex adjoining the somatic sensory region on the caudal side, undergoes an equally rapid development in several primate lines, such as ceboids and anthropoids, and that this development may indeed proceed somewhat in concert with the growth of the frontal lobes. The present account will serve to report and discuss evidence that the parietal lobe is connected with (i) the granular frontal cortex, directly as well as via a transcortical and transthalamic circuit with the temporal cortex, and (ii) the limbic system, more especially the cingulate gyrus, by direct associations and also more indirectly by way of a transthalamic pathway involving the nucleus lateralis dorsalis thalami.

Severe agnosias, apraxias and aphasias may beset man following infarction of the parietal lobes. [2,5,6] Cerebrovascular accidents and cerebral tumors commonly cause tissue destruction extensive enough to involve both parietal lobules as well as adjoining regions of the occipital or temporal isocortex. Clinico-pathological studies have led to the identification of polyesthesias, hallucinations, graphesthesia, ahylognosia, amorphognosia and constructional apraxia as symptoms attributable to parietal lobe involvement. Dyscalculia, dysgraphia, finger-agnosia, right and left-sided disorientation (Gerstmann's syndrome) have been found symptomatic of lesions involving the supramarginal and angular gyri of the inferior parietal lobule together with adjacent occipital gyri, with or without additional involvement of the adjoining superior temporal convolution. In such cases, visual agnosias and disorientation are also commonly present. Disorders of body-image such as lack of awareness or complete denial of one-half of the body may be caused by lesions of the posterior parietal cortex and adjacent cortical territories. In experimental studies in the rhesus monkey and chimpanzee [7,8] tactile agnosias such as barognosis, amorphogenesis and ahylognosia have been found to follow ablations of the posterior parietal cortex. It thus appears that in such anthropoids as well as in man, the integrity of the parietal association cortex is required if tactile and proprioceptive signals are to gain emotional color and qualitative value.

Disconnection of the parietal lobes severely impairs the association of the somatic sensorium with visual, auditory, or olfactory informations obtained from the environment. The anatomical basis of such cortical syndromes requires elaborate study, a time-consuming and tedious process because of the enormous amount of labor involved in the tracing of widely distributed fiber connections by the use of fiber degeneration techniques. The present report represents but a brief beginning of this task.

MATERIALS AND METHODS

This report is based on findings made in ten rhesus monkeys (*Macaca mulatta*) in which various parts of the superior (areas 5 and 7 of Brodmann) and inferior (area 7 of Brodmann) parietal lobules had been removed by aspiration of cortical gray matter. All operations were performed under aseptic conditions in animals deeply anesthetized with Nembutal, and every precaution was taken to minimize damage to the subjacent white matter. The superior lobules were lesioned unilaterally in three monkeys, and bilaterally in one animal. Five monkeys sustained lesions of the inferior lobule; in one monkey the inferior lobule was lesioned on both sides. Area 5 of the left hemisphere and area 7 of the right hemisphere were lesioned in one other monkey.

The animals were allowed to survive from 12 to 18 days, except for one animal which received bilateral lesions of the inferior parietal lobule (area 7) on separate days and was subsequently sacrificed to provide survival times of 13 and 4 days after surgery. All animals were killed in deep anesthesia by exsanguination and transcardial perfusion with physiological saline followed by 10 per cent formalin for fixation. The brains and spinal cords were removed immediately after the perfusion, and further fixed in 10 per cent formalin.* Serial transverse sections of the brain were cut on the freezing microtome at 26μ and 52μ, and collected in 10 per cent formalin. Serial sections were stained for degenerated fibers using the Nauta uranyl nitrate modification of the NAUTA-GYGAX[9-11] techniques, and the FINK–HEIMER[12] methods. In some instances the ALBRECHT–FERNSTROM[13] phosphotungstic acid modification of the NAUTA–GYGAX[11] method was used. Alternate sets of adjacent serial sections were stained for cell bodies with cresylechtviolett, and for myelinated fibers with the Weil method. These supplementary series provided an important aid in determining the cytoarchitectonic and myeloarchitectonic identity of the structures shown by the silver methods to contain degenerating nerve fibers. Additional material available for the study of the normal anatomy of the cortex and subcortical nuclei included brains cut frozen at 200μ thickness or after celloidin embedding cut at 36μ thickness.

The distribution of degenerated fibers of passage and the location of terminal degeneration in the cortex and subcortical nuclei were determined microscopically and recorded in projection drawings of the actual sections.

---

* This study was performed in strict adherence to the Guide for Laboratory Animal Facilities and Care, published by the Institute of Laboratory Animal Resources, National Academy of Sciences-National Research Council.

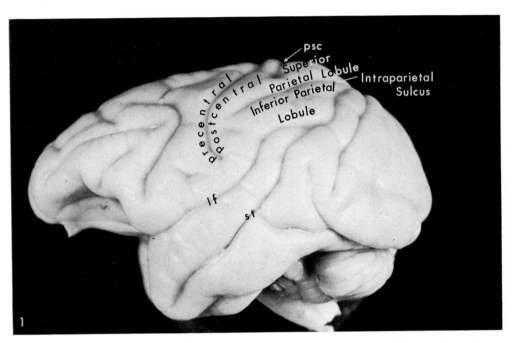

FIG. 1.   Photograph of the left cerebral hemisphere of the rhesus monkey. The superior post-central dimple (or sulcus; psc), seen near the dorsal margin of the hemisphere, approximately corresponds to the caudal border of the postcentral gyrus and thus demarcates the somatic sensory cortex from the superior parietal lobule. The long, almost horizontally disposed, intraparietal sulcus separates the superior parietal lobule from the inferior parietal lobule. The lateral fissure (lf) marks the ventral border of the inferior lobule and separates the parietal lobe from the temporal isocortex. The caudal border of the inferior lobule is bounded by the superior temporal (st) sulcus.

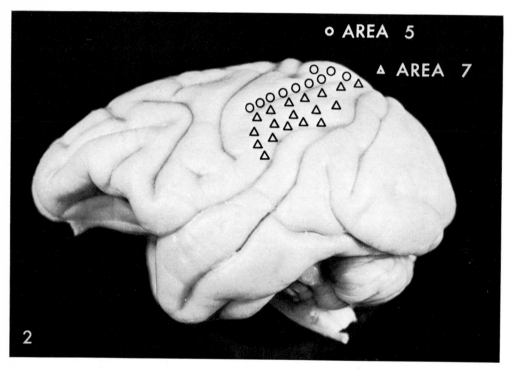

FIG. 2.

FIGS. 2 and 3. Lateral (Fig. 2) and dorsal (Fig. 3) views of the left hemispheres showing the approximate cytoarchitectonic limits of areas 5 and area 7 of Brodmann. These figures were prepared on the basis of Brodmann's architectonic map of the hemisphere of an Old-World monkey of the genus *Cercopithecus*. VON BONIN and BAILEY[20] have labelled the superior parietal lobule PE and subdivided it into a rostral PEm and a caudal PE region. The same authors divide the inferior parietal lobule into a rostral PF and a caudal PG region. In *Cercopithecus*, and perhaps also in *Macaca mulatta*, that portion of the superior temporal sulcus bounding the inferior parietal lobule contains on the very edge of its rostral bank the rostral limit of area 19 of Brodmann (not shown in this figure).

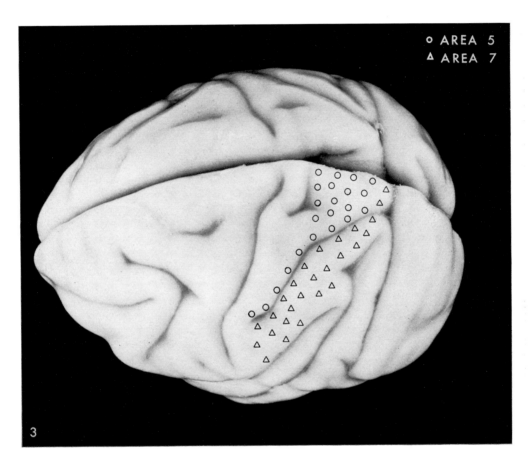

Fig. 3.

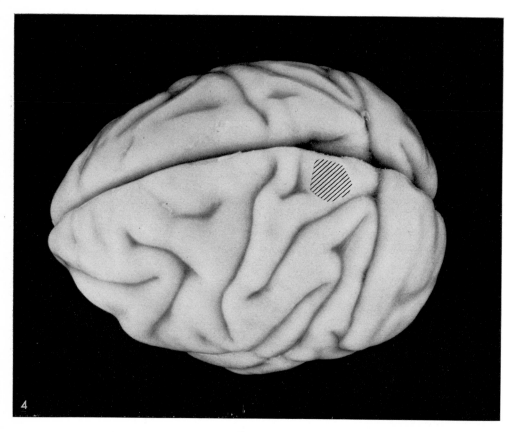

FIG. 4.

FIGS. 4 and 5. These photographs illustrate two of our cases, each representing the extent of cortical ablations made within the confines of areas 5 and 7, respectively.

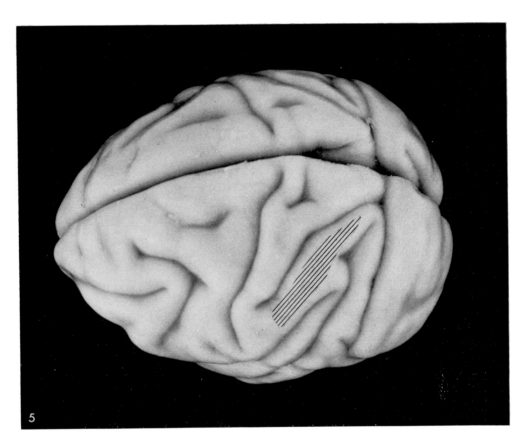

Fig. 5.

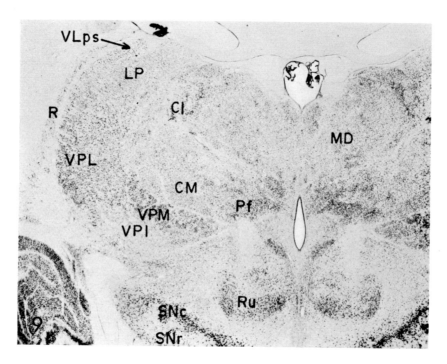

Fig. 9.   This Nissl-stained section of the monkey's thalamus passes through the level of the
nucleus lateralis posterior (LP). The cells of the nucleus at this level begin to merge with those
of the nucleus lateralis dorsalis and are easily distinguished from the dorsally located nucleus
ventralis lateralis pars postrema (VLps) and the ventrally situated nucleus ventralis posterior
lateralis (VPL). Abbreviations: Cl, n. centralis lateralis; CM, n. centrum medianum; LP, n.
lateralis posterior; MD, n. medialis dorsalis; Pf, n. parafascicularis; R, n. reticularis thalami;
Ru, n. ruber; SNc and SNr, n. substantia nigra pars compacta et pars reticularis; VLps, n.
ventralis lateralis pars postrema; VPI n. ventralis posterior inferior; VPL, n. ventralis posterior
lateralis; VPM, n. ventralis posterior medialis.

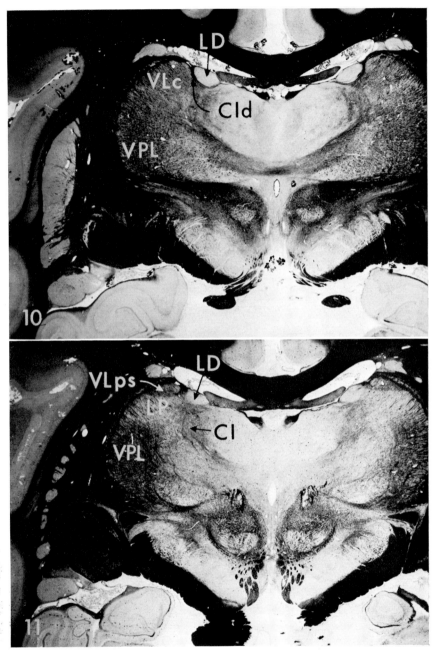

FIGS. 10 and 11. Myelin-stained sections of the rhesus monkey thalamus. In the upper photograph the capsule (Cld) of the n. lateralis dorsalis (LD) can be seen clearly. At more caudal levels of the thalamus, cells of the nucleus lateralis posterior (LP) and n. lateralis dorsalis are no longer separated by a dense myelinated fiber bundle. A comparison of figs. 9 and 11 clearly shows the close correspondence between cytoarchitectonic and myeloarchitectonic characteristics of the thalamic territories VLps, LP and VPL.

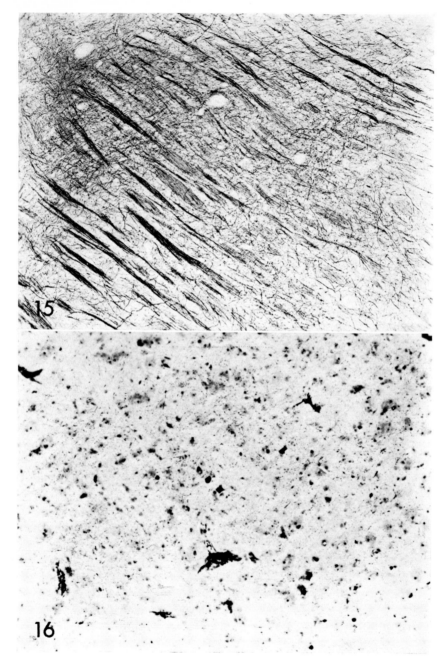

FIGS. 15 and 16. Low and medium-power photomicrographs of fiber degeneration in the nucleus lateralis posterior following ablations of area 5. Figure 15 is a photograph of the nucleus stained according to the uranyl nitrate modification of Nauta, while fig. 16 shows the corresponding area stained according to procedure I of Fink and Heimer.

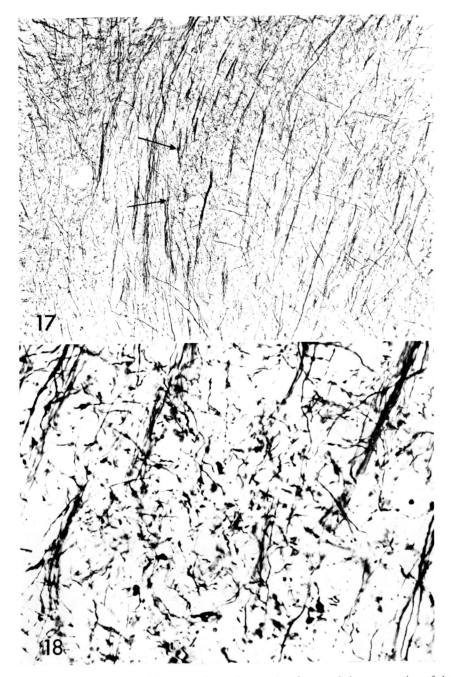

FIGS. 17 and 18.   Low and high-power photomicrographs of one and the same region of the pretectal area. Both figures show fiber degeneration in this region following ablation of area 5 bilaterally. The sections were stained according to the uranyl nitrate modification of the Nauta method.

RESULTS AND DISCUSSION

This report can be considered a somewhat preliminary documentation of current studies concerning the efferent connections of the parietal lobules of the rhesus monkey. The material available is still being analyzed, and only the clearest evidence of parietal lobe connections with other cortical regions and with the basal ganlia, the thalamus and the midbrain will here be reported and discussed.

The superior parietal lobule

A large bundle of degenerated fibers leaves the superior parietal lobule and traverses the centrum semiovale before entering the internal capsule. Some of these fibers leave the superior lobule in a nearly vertical direction to enter the extreme and external capsules which they follow as routes to their distribution fields in the claustrum and putamen. Additional degenerating fibers coursing through the extreme capsule enter the dorsal portion of the insular cortex which contains numerous degenerating axon ramifications, especially abundant in the infragranular layers. A field of very dense terminal degeneration occupies the dorsal two-thirds, and tapers to a narrow lateral zone in a more ventral part of the putamen. Terminal degeneration is also present in the body of the caudate nucleus, but no degenerating fibers can be identified in the globus pallidus.

Dense terminal degeneration is present in the nucleus lateralis posterior (LP) of the thalamus (Fig. 6) and extends among the adjacent cells of the nucleus reticularis thalami (R). The degenerated fibers enter the nucleus lateralis posterior from the internal capsule as components of the lateral thalamic peduncle by recurving in a medial and dorsal direction. The fibers are interspersed with medium-sized lightly stained neurons which are easily distinguished from the larger cells of the nucleus ventralis lateralis pars postrema (VLps), a cell group receiving cerebellothalamic fibers[4] and fibers originating in the precentral (motor) gyrus.[14-16] Ventral to the nucleus lateralis posterior is the nucleus ventralis posterior lateralis (VPL), composed of a mixed population of neurons, some of which are large and deeply chromatophilic, while others are smaller and of lighter color. The mixing of the dark cells with medium-sized lighter cells distinguishes VPL conspicuously from the nucleus lateralis posterior which has a somewhat denser population of more evenly spaced medium-sized round cells lacking an admixture of large cells (Fig. 9). The cytoarchitectonic differences between VLps, LP and VPL coincide well with the myeloarchitectonic structure of the same nuclei (compare Figs. 9–11). In myelin-stained sections LP is characterized by being extremely lightly stained (Fig. 11); in contrast with VLps and VPL it contains only sporadic bundles of heavily myelinated fibers. The fiber plexus of VLps appears much darker in myelin stains. The nucleus ventralis posterior lateralis (VPL) is richly populated with myelinated bundles oriented in nearly horizontal planes, but the nucleus is also penetrated by numerous dorsoventrally oriented myelinated fibers entering through its ventral border. Some of these fibers are components of the medial lemniscus, while others are cerebellofugal fibers destined for VLps and VLc (Fig. 14). The correspondence between the cytoarchitectonic and myeloarchitectonic appearance of these cell groups and the pattern of fiber degeneration in LP following superior parietal lobule lesions is remarkable.

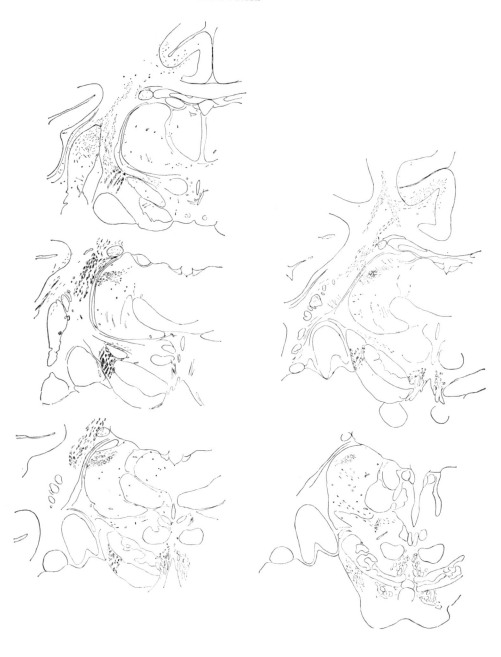

FIG. 6. Fiber degeneration following ablation of the superior parietal lobule (area 5) in the rhesus monkey as described in the text. Degenerating fibers are indicated as thin, broken lines.

Numerous degenerating axons descend from the lesion in the superior parietal lobule through the internal capsule into the cerebral peduncle. At rostral levels of the subthalamic region such fibers can be seen to terminate in moderate numbers in the zona incerta and field H_2 of Forel, but no degenerated terminal fibers can be identified in the subthalamic nucleus.

A more massive termination of this brainstem projection is evident in the pretectal area, superior colliculus, and pontine nuclei, but no degenerated terminal fibers can be identified in the substantia nigra. Terminal degeneration is dense in the pretectal region just medial or medioventral to the nucleus limitans of OLSZEWSKI,[17] and also surrounds the regio pretectalis anterior of OLSZEWSKI[17] (nucleus olivarius of KUHLENBECK and MILLER[18]). Dense terminal degeneration occupies an approximately vertical field at the transition between the superior colliculus and pretectal area. In the absence of an adequate cytoarchitectonic study, it is not clear to what extent the cellular organization of the simian pretectal region corresponds to the description of the region in the rat. In the latter species, BUCHER and NAUTA[21] outlined three major cell groups, viz., a nucleus pretectalis, nucleus pretectalis medialis and nucleus pretectalis profundus. In the present cases of lesion of the superior parietal lobule (area 5), a very dense terminal degeneration appeared in the ventrolateral part of the pretectal area bounded by the nucleus limitans and the nucleus suprageniculatus laterally, the mesencephalic reticular formation ventrally, and the superior colliculus and nucleus of the posterior commissure medially. It seems possible that this area corresponds to the nucleus pretectalis profundus of the rat.

The corticocortical connections of the superior lobule have not been fully mapped. It can nevertheless be demonstrated that lesions of the superior parietal lobule elicit degeneration of fibers extending to the contralateral superior and inferior parietal lobules, the ipsilateral premotor cortex, precentral and postcentral gyri, arcuate cortex, granular frontal cortex along the dorsal and ventral banks of the principal sulcus, cingulate gyrus (areas 23 and 24), inferior parietal lobule, insular cortex and superior temporal gyrus. The parieto-cingulate projection (to area 23 of BRODMANN;[19] LC of VON BONIN and BAILEY[20]) is substantial. PANDYA and KUYPERS[21] traced ipsilateral fibers of the superior lobule to the same areas: arcuate cortex, granular frontal cortex along the dorsal and ventral banks of the principal sulcus, premotor and motor cortex, postcentral gyrus, inferior parietal lobule, superior temporal gyrus, cingulate gyrus, and additional fibers to the preoccipital gyrus.

The inferior parietal lobule

Fiber degeneration can be traced from lesions of the inferior parietal lobule through the centrum semiovale of the cerebral hemisphere and into the internal capsule and cerebral peduncle. At the base of the lobule, degenerating fibers enter the dorsal parts of the insular cortex, forming a dense terminal plexus in the deep cortical cell layers IV–VI. The claustrum is invaded by degenerating fibers from its lateral and medial sides, the putamen by way of both the external and internal capsule. The dorsal two-thirds of the putamen contains a dense terminal degeneration. The body of the caudate nucleus is infiltrated by degenerated fibers which appear to terminate in greatest number in its lateral parts. No evidence of direct parietal projections to the globus pallidus was found in any of the cases studied.

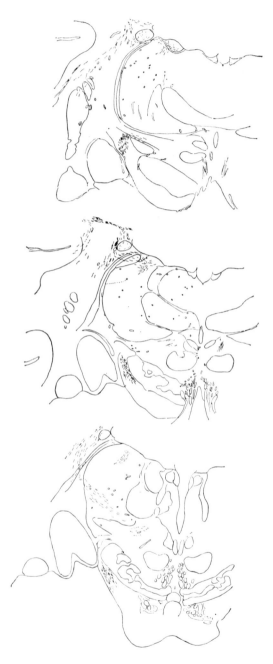

Fig. 7. Axon degeneration following ablation of the inferior parietal lobule (area 7) of the rhesus monkey, as described in the text. Note dense terminal degeneration in the nucleus lateralis posterior of the thalamus immediately ventral to the nucleus lateralis dorsalis. Abundant terminal degeneration is also present in the nucleus lateralis dorsalis.

The parietothalamic fibers from the inferior lobule enter the thalamus from the internal capsule by curving under the caudate nucleus, and subsequently sweep over the nuclei VLps and VLc before entering the capsule of the nucleus lateralis dorsalis (LD) and terminating in that cell group. Other degenerated fibers pass directly through VLps and subsequently curve ventralward by bending inward from the capsule of the nucleus lateralis dorsalis prior to entering the nucleus lateralis posterior. The terminal distribution of fibers from the inferior parietal lobule appears to be confined to the dorsomedial cells of the nucleus lateralis posterior (Fig. 7). The corresponding projection from the superior lobule, by contrast, appears to affect preferentially the ventrolateral part of the nucleus.[22]

In the ventral thalamus moderate fiber degeneration is seen in the zona incerta and field H_2 of Forel, but no evidence was found for the presence of terminal fibers in the subthalamic nucleus.

The corticocortical efferents of the inferior lobule have not been fully analyzed in these experiments, but connections with the contralateral superior and inferior lobules are evident, as are fibers to the ipsilateral premotor cortex, precentral and postcentral gyri, and a substantial connection with the adjacent cingulate gyrus (area 23). Another prominent bundle was traced via the external capsule toward the ventral surface of the temporal lobe. This fiber system distributes axons to the superior, middle and inferior temporal gyri, and to the fusiform gyrus. A portion of the projection reaching into the cranial part of the inferior temporal gyrus extends beyond this gyrus, following a medial direction and passing the shallow rhinal sulcus to terminate in the parahippocampal gyrus. Fiber degeneration in this gyrus is restricted to a sector of isocortex situated immediately lateral to the hippocampal formation and identified as TH by von Bonin and Bailey.[20] Our preliminary data on intra- and interhemispheric connections, as also the fuller documentations of Pandya and Kuypers,[21] and Pandya and Vignolo,[23] suggest significant differences in the cortical associations of each of the parietal lobules. The projections from the inferior lobule involves particular regions of each of the gyri of the temporal lobe: superior, middle, and inferior temporal gyri, fusiform gyrus, and area TH of the parahippocampal gyrus. The superior parietal lobule, by contrast, entertains more limited connections with the temporal lobe that involve part of the ipsilateral superior temporal gyrus, and a small sector about midway rostrocaudally in the ventral bank of the contralateral superior temporal gyrus.[23]

The inferior parietal lobule gives rise to still another prominent ipsilateral corticocortical fiber bundle. This substantial fiber group runs cranially in the hemisphere and distributes itself in a zone of the granular frontal cortex along the ventral bank of the principal sulcus.

Pandya and Kuypers[21] reported evidence of similar ipsilateral corticocortical connections originating in the inferior lobule. They describe fibers to the superior parietal lobule, to a small cortical area in the caudal part of the superior temporal sulcus, the middle temporal gyrus, the postcentral and precentral gyri, the premotor and arcuate cortices, and to the granular frontal cortex ventral to the principal sulcus. Efferent connections to the contralateral insular cortex, cingulate gyrus, retrosplenial area, cortex along the occipitotemporal sulcus, and parahippocampal gyrus are also reported by Pandy and Vignolo.[23]

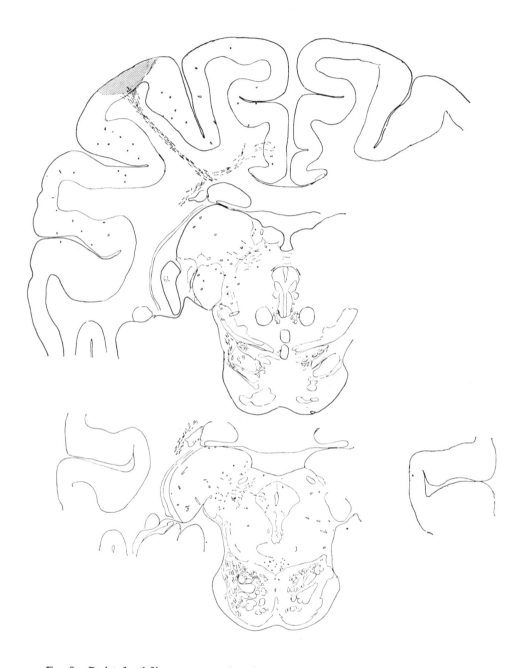

Fig. 8.   Parietofugal fibers were traced to the pretectal area and superior colliculus following
superior and inferior parietal lobule lesions. These chartings illustrate some of the projections
of the inferior lobule (area 7) to the pretectal area, to the central gray substance of
the mesencephalon, and to the nuclei pontis Varolii.

The possibility of *functional associations of the inferior parietal lobule with the limbic system* can be clearly appreciated from the present experiments. The lobule has efferent connections not only with the cingulate gyrus but also with the nucleus lateralis dorsalis and with the temporal isocortex. In the monkey, VALENSTEIN and NAUTA[24] have identified fibers to the nucleus lateralis dorsalis that appear to originate in either the septal region or hippocampus, or both. Projections of the inferior temporal gyrus have been traced by WHITLOCK and NAUTA[25] to the periamygdaloid part of the pyriform cortex, entorhinal area, amygdaloid complex (central, lateral, basal, and accessory basal nuclei), substantia innominata and, via the inferior thalamic peduncle, to the magnocellular part of the nucleus medialis dorsalis (MDmc of OLSZEWSKI[17]). The parieto-temporal connection thus appears to be associated with the granular frontal cortex by way of two pathways from the temporal lobe to the mediodorsal nucleus. One of these temporo-thalamic connections is direct, while the other one involves the amygdaloid complex as an intermediary way-station. A third, direct association of the temporal cortex with granular frontal fields is established by the prominent uncinate fasciculus. This direct temporofrontal association is reciprocated by fibers that originate in the cortex of the frontal convexity and follow the uncinate fasciculus to the superior and middle temporal gyri and to a lesser extent to the inferior temporal cortex.[26] The orbitofrontal cortex is reciprocally connected with the nucleus medialis dorsalis[26,27] by a fiber system of rather precise topographic organization, and some degree of connective reciprocity also appears to exist between the amygdaloid complex and the nucleus medialis dorsalis of the thalamus.[28] Numerous conduction routes are available, therefore, for the spread of somatic sensory information to the frontal granular cortex. Two of these routes are direct pathways and include fibers from the superior parietal lobule as well as a more massive projection from the inferior parietal lobule. Several further potential parieto-frontal conduction pathways involve the temporal lobe cortex, the temporo-thalamic and temporo-amygdalo-thalamic pathways, and the uncinate fasciculus.

Projections from the inferior parietal lobule to the mesencephalon are distributed to the pretectal area, the deeper layers of the superior colliculus, certain districts of the gray matter of the pons Varolii (Fig. 8), and the lateral densocellular central gray substance; but no evidence of a parieto-nigral projection was found in the present study. Parieto-pretectal and parieto-collicular fibers originating in both parietal lobules appear to involve to some extent at least the same general territories that are also projected upon by the retina, the cortical eye fields of the frontal lobe[29] and the middle temporal gyrus.[25] KUYPERS and LAWRENCE[30] found evidence of corticomesencephalic fibers to the superior colliculus originating in the premotor (area 6), arcuate (area 8), occipital and temporal cortices of the rhesus monkey. Such parietomesencephalic fibers could be thought to permit a direct dissemination of tactile and proprioceptive information to mesencephalic components of the visual system capable of integrating this information into mechanisms of visually guided behavior.

The multitude of cortical associations of the parietal lobules and their numerous sub-cortical connections makes it difficult to identify any one of them as the obvious explanation for parietal lobe syndromes. Some attention should be given, nevertheless, to the possible significance of parietal lobe connections with the cingulate gyrus, frontal granular

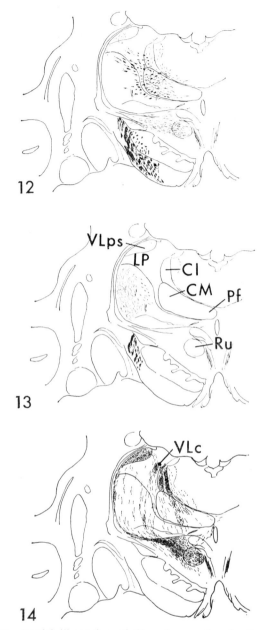

FIGS. 12, 13 and 14. Partial illustration of fiber degeneration in the thalamus following lesions of, respectively, the precentral gyrus[16] (Fig. 12), the postcentral gyrus[16] (Fig. 13) and the deep cerebellar nuclei[4] (Fig. 14). Compare with present findings concerning parieto-thalamic projections shown in figs. 6 and 7, and note the striking correspondence between intrathalamic degeneration patterns on the one hand, and cyto- and myeloarchitectural delineations on the other. The VLps is a recipient of numerous fibers from the motor cortex and cerebellum, while LP receives fibers from the parietal lobules, but fails to receive afferent connections from the precentral and postcentral gyri or the cerebellum. The VPL receives afferent connections from the postcentral gyrus but appears not to be a recipient of fibers from the motor cortex or the cerebellum. A massive cerebellothalamic connection is established with the nucleus centralis lateralis and the ventromedial part of VLc (Fig. 14). Cerebellothalamic fiber connections are summarized and discussed further by MEHLER[31] et. al., MEHLER[32] and MEHLER.[33]

cortex, and temporal isocortex. The efferent connections of the postcentral gyrus are more limited than those of the parietal lobules. The former projects to the posterior parietal lobules, precentral gyrus, premotor, arcuate, insular and cingulate cortices,[21,23] but appears not to establish connections with the occipital or temporal lobes. The parietal lobules, in contrast, project to a rostral sector of the occipital lobe, and to wide areas of the frontal and temporal lobes, thus disseminating their neural codes to all other lobes of the cerebral cortex. The direct parietofrontal connections appear to be augmented by additional, and more indirect parietofrontal pathways which utilize the temporal isocortex and thalamus to reach lateral and orbital areas of the frontal granular cortex.

The results of RUCH et al.[7,8,34,35] show that somatic sensory deficits may or may not follow parietal lobe lesions, depending upon the size of the lesion, the species involved, and the specific modality under consideration. Current evidence from animal experiments—chiefly in rhesus and mangabey monkeys—is inadequate to permit any definitive conclusion with respect to this comparative-neurological problem. Unfortunately, data from the human clinic are likewise often incomplete, for the histological analysis of lesions in the human brain is only rarely detailed enough to permit the identification or exclusion of deep infarctions of white matter involving connections of cortical areas other than the parietal lobules. Moreover, systematic and detailed functional testing of parietal-lobe patients is by no means a routine practice. Despite these handicaps, a clinical picture of severely debilitating agnosias, aphasias and apraxias appears well identified with parietal-lobe lesions.[2,5,6] The widespread efferent connections of the parietal lobules considered here, in particular the evidence of a variety of neural pathways reciprocally connecting the parietal lobules with the frontal[21], temporal[21,37] and occipital[21] cortices, emphatically suggests a multimodal nature of the parietal-lobe mechanisms. These anatomical data suggest that the parietal lobules may serve not only to augment the potential routes of spread of somatic sensory signals from the postcentral gyrus, but also, to extend vastly the range of connections subserving communication and interaction between all sensory modalities and their motor expression.

SUMMARY

The efferent connections of the posterior parietal cortex were studied in rhesus monkeys subjected to selective lesions of the superior and inferior parietal lobules, which correspond approximately to Brodmann's areas 5 and 7, respectively.

Following ablations of either the superior or inferior parietal lobule, axon degeneration, stained with the Nauta and Fink–Heimer methods, was traced into the extreme, external, and internal capsules, and into the cerebral peduncle. This degeneration extended into the ipsilateral insular cortex, cingulate gyrus, prefrontal and premotor cortices, and the precentral and postcentral gyri. In addition to these connections, the superior lobule sends fibers to the ipsilateral inferior parietal lobule and superior temporal gyrus, and via the corpus callosum to the contralateral superior and inferior parietal lobules, whereas the inferior parietal lobule sends fibers to the ipsilateral superior parietal lobule and to the contralateral superior and inferior parietal lobules. A prominent fiber system to the

c

ipsilateral temporal lobe degenerates following lesions in the inferior parietal lobule (area 7); in such cases fiber degeneration appears in the superior, middle and inferior temporal convolutions, and in the fusiform and parahippocampal gyri.

Both lobules evidently project to the claustrum and body of the caudate nucleus. Both, moreover, have massive efferent connections with the dorsal two-thirds of the putamen. By contrast, no evidence of projections from the parietal cortex to the globus pallidus was found in any of the cases studied.

A further subcortical projection from the posterior parietal cortex involves the nucleus reticularis thalami and the nucleus lateralis posterior thalami. The inferior lobule projects directly to the nucleus lateralis dorsalis and to the mediodorsal region of the nucleus lateralis posterior that closely adjoins two thalamic cell groups: the n. lateralis dorsalis and the intralaminar nucleus centralis lateralis. The superior parietal lobule, by contrast, projects massively to a ventrolateral district of the nucleus lateralis posterior.

Parietosubthalamic connections could be traced from areas 5 and 7 to the zona incerta and fields H_2 and H of Forel, but evidence for terminal connections with the n. subthalamicus (Luys) could not be found.

Both areas 5 and 7 project massively to the pretectal area and the deeper layers of the superior colliculus. This parieto-mesencephalic connection is amplified by a fiber connection from the inferior parietal lobule (area 7) to the lateral, densocellular region of the circumaqueductal gray matter. No evidence of parietal corticonigral fibers connections was found. Finally, both parietal lobules were found to project to the pontine nuclei.

Speculations regarding the associative functions of the parietal lobules at the cortical and subcortical levels are presented, with particular emphasis upon the possible significance of the projections from the inferior parietal lobule to insular, cingulate and temporal regions of the cortex.

Acknowledgements—The author gratefully acknowledges the unfailing technical assistance of Mrs. Michie A. Vane and Mr. Curtis King.

REFERENCES

1. Connolly, C. J. *External Morphology of the Primate Brain.* Charles C. Thomas, Springfield, Illinois, 1950.
2. Critchley, M. *The Parietal Lobes.* Edward Arnold, London, 1953.
3. Ingalls, N. W. The parietal region in the primate brain. *J. comp. Neurol.* 24, 291, 1914.
4. Petras, J. M. Unpublished observations.
5. Geschwind, N. Disconnexion syndromes in animals and man. *Brain* 88, 237, 1968.
6. Geschwind, N. Disconnexion syndromes in animals and man. *Brain.* 88, 585, 1968.
7. Ruch, T. C. Cortical localization of somatic sensibility. The effect of precentral, postcentral, and posterior parietal lesions upon the performance of monkeys trained to discriminate weights. *Res. Publs Ass. Res. nerv. ment. Dis.* 15, 289, 1935.
8. Ruch, T. C., Fulton, J. F. and German, W. J. Sensory discrimination in the monkey, chimpanzee, and man after lesions of the parietal lobe. *Archs Neurol. Psychiat., Chicago* 39, 919, 1938.
9. Nauta, W. J. H. and Ryan, L. F. Selective silver impregnation of degenerating axons in the central nervous system. *Stain Tech.* 27, 175, 1952.
10. Nauta, W. J. H. and Gygax, P. A. Silver impregnation of degenerating axon terminals in the central nervous system: (1) Technic, (2) Chemical notes. *Stain Tech.* 26, 5, 1951.
11. Nauta, W. J. H. and Gygax, P. A. Silver impregnation of degenerating axons in the central nervous system: a modified technique. *Stain Tech.* 29, 91, 1954.

12. FINK, R. P. and HEIMER, L. Two methods for selective silver impregnation of degenerating axons and their synaptic endings in the central nervous system. *Brain Res.* **4**, 369, 1967.
13. ALBRECHT, M. H. and FERNSTROM, R. C. A modified Nauta–Gygax method for human brain and spinal cord. *Stain. Tech* **34**, 91, 1959.
14. PETRAS, J. M. Some fiber connections of the precentral and postcentral cortex with the basal ganglia, thalamus and subthalamus. *Trans. Am. neurol. Ass.* **90**, 274, 1965.
15. PETRAS, J. M. Fiber degeneration in the basal ganglia and diencephalon following lesions in the precentral and postcentral cortex of the monkey (*Macaca nulatta*); with additional observations in the chimpanzee, p. 95. Eighth Int. Anat. Congr., Wiesbaden, Germany, 1965.
16. PETRAS, J. M. Some efferent connections of the motor and somato-sensory cortex of simian primates and felid, canid and procyonid carnivores. *Ann. N.Y. Acad. Sci.* **167**, 469, 1969.
17. OLSZEWSKI, J. *The Thalamus of Macaca mulatta.* S. Karger, Basel, 1952.
18. KUHLENBECK, H. and MILLER, R. N. The pretectal region of the human brain. *J. comp. Neurol.* **91**, 369, 1949.
19. BRODMANN, K. *Vergleichende Lokalisationslehre der Grosshirnrinde*, 2. Auflage. J. A. Barth, Leipzig, 1925.
20. VON BONIN, G. and BAILEY, P. *The Neocortex of Macaca mulatta.* The University of Illinois Press, Urbana, Illinois, 1947.
21. PANDYA, D. N. and KUYPERS, H. G. J. M. Cortico-cortical connections in the rhesus monkey. *Brain Res.* **13**, 13, 1969.
22. PETRAS, J. M. Some efferent connections of the superior and inferior pareital lobules with the basal ganglia, diencephalon and midbrain in the rhesus monkey. *Anat. Rec.* **163**, 243, 1969.
23. PANDYA, D. N. and VIGNOLO, L. A. Interhemispheric projections of the parietal lobe in the rhesus monkey. *Brain Res.* **15**, 49, 1969.
24. VALENSTEIN, E. S. and NAUTA, W. J. H. A comparison of the distribution of the fornix system in the rat, guinea pig, cat, and monkey. *J. comp. Neurol.* **113**, 337, 1959.
25. WHITLOCK, D. C. and NAUTA, W. J. H. Subcortical projections from the temporal neocortex in *Macaca mulatta. J. comp. Neurol.* **106**, 183, 1956.
26. NAUTA, W. J. H. Some efferent connections of the prefrontal cortex in the monkey. In: *The Frontal Granular Cortex and Behavior*, WARREN, J. M. and AKERT, K. (Eds.), p. 397. McGraw Hill, New York, 1964.
27. AKERT, K. Comparative anatomy of frontal cortex and thalamofrontal connections. In: *The Frontal Granular Cortex and Behavior*, WARREN, J. M. and AKERT, K., (Eds.), p. 372. McGraw Hill, New York, 1964.
28. NAUTA, W. J. H. Fibre degeneration following lesions of the amygdaloid complex in the monkey. *J. Anat.* **95**, 515, 1961.
29. ASTRUC, J. Corticofugal fiber degeneration following lesions of area 8 (frontal eye field) in *Macaca mulatta. Anat. Rec.* **148**, 256, 1964.
30. KUYPERS, H. G. J. M. and LAWRENCE, D. G. Cortical projections to the red nucleus and the brain stem in the rhesus monkey. *Brain Res.* **4**, 151, 1967.
31. MEHLER, W. R. Further notes on the centre median nucleus of Luys. In: *The Thalamus*, PURPURA, D. P. and YAHR, M. D. (Eds.), p. 109. Columbia University Press, New York, 1966.
32. MEHLER, W. R., VERNIER, V. G. and NAUTA, W. J. H. Efferent projections from the dentate and interpositus nuclei in primates. *Anat. Rec.* **130**, 430, 1958.
33. MEHLER, W. R. Idea of a new anatomy of the thalamus. *J. Psychiat. Res.* **8**, 203, 1971.
34. RUCH, T. C., FULTON, J. F. and KASDON, S. Further experiments on the somato-sensory functions of the cerebral cortex in the monkey and chimpanzee. *Am. J. Physiol.* **119**, 394, 1937.
35. RUCH, T. C., FULTON, J. F. and KASDON, S. Late recovery of sensory discriminative ability after parietal lesions in the chimpanzee. *Am. J. Physiol.* **129**, 453, 1940.
36. BUTTERS, N. and BARTON, M. Effect of parietal lobe damage on the performance of reversible operations in space. *Neuropsychologia* **8**, 205, 1970.
37. PANDYA, D. N., HALLETT, M. and MUKHERJEE, S. K. Intra- and interhemispheric connections of the neocortical auditory system in the rhesus monkey. *Brain Res.* **14**, 49, 1969.

J. psychiat. Res., 1971, Vol. 8, pp. 203–217. Pergamon Press. Printed in Great Britain.

IDEA OF A NEW ANATOMY OF THE THALAMUS

William R. Mehler

NASA, Ames Research Center, Moffett Field, California

"I have found some of my friends so mistaken in their conception of the object of the demonstrations which I have delivered in my lectures, that I wish to vindicate myself at all hazards. They would have it that I am in search of the seat of the soul; but I wish only to investigate the structure of the brain, as we examine the structure of the eye and the ear.

It is not more presumptuous to follow the tracts of nervous matter in the brain, and to attempt to discover the course of sensation, than it is to trace the rays of light through the humours of the eye, and to say, that the retina is the seat of vision. Why are we to close the investigation with the discovery of the external organ?"

Charles Bell[1]

Idea of a New Anatomy of the Brain

INTRODUCTION

At the turn of the 19th century one could have compared the available knowledge of the mammalian thalamus to man's knowledge of Africa about the time of Stanley's search for Livingstone. The coastal geography of the Dark Continent was well charted, but little was known about its interior or the origins and ramifications of its great rivers. To the explorers of the mid-Victorian era, discovery of the sources of the Nile were what the poles of the earth became at the turn of the century, and the moon at mid-century—a supreme goal. As geographic explorations of the Nile and Congo rivers threw new light on the Dark Continent, much of our knowledge of the organization of the thalamus stems from studies of the major afferent pathways of the brain that terminate in the thalamus.

For example, around the turn of the century neurological explorers such as Mott, Probst and Wallenberg, employing the then recently introduced Marchi method, traced the course of the secondary spinal and trigeminal afferent systems, the medial lemniscus and the branchium conjuctivum to the thalamus. These earliest experimental studies of the intrathalamic distribution of major thalamic afferent systems, coupled with normal cyto- and myeloarchitectural 'cartography', led to a beginning of understanding of the parcellation of the ventral tier of the 'lateral thalamic nuclei'. In the ensuing first half of the 20th century, studies of the patterns of retrograde degeneration in the thalamus elicited by selective cortical ablations provided additional insights into the organization of these ventral nuclei and suggested various functional relationships of other thalamic cell groups. However, since most of these reports were based upon studies in subprimate species, many questions of homology among mammalian species arose, some of which are still unanswered.

CLARK's[2] and WALKER's[3] studies and critical appraisals of the literature in the 1930's lent new impetus to experimental studies of the primate brain, but the absence of more sensitive experimental-anatomical methods retarded progress toward a more definitive analysis of the finer-fibered systems of the thalamus, especially those that interconnect the thalamus with various forebrain structures. Nevertheless, the introduction of improved neurophysiological methods during the 1940's and 50's progressively advanced our knowledge of other aspects of thalamic organization, and introduced new concepts of thalamic function that renewed interest in the thalamus (see AJMONE MARSAN[4]). Concurrently, the adaptation of the Horsley–Clarke stereotaxic instrument for neuro-surgical interventions in the human thalamus by SPIEGEL and WYCIS[5] created at once another important need for, and a potential new source of, knowledge of thalamic organization and function.

Concomitant with these developments, more sensitive silver-impregnation methods for the demonstration and tracing of degenerated axons were developed by GLEES[6] and NAUTA,[7,8] and it was this technological advance that ushered in a new epoch of neuro-anatomical analysis. The increasing application of these new experimental techniques during the past 15 years, together with a marked resurgence of activity in the use of the Golgi methods, and the more recently introduced experimental electron-microscopic techniques, has provided more detailed anatomical pictures of afferent and efferent thalamic relation-ships than were obtainable before. As a consequence, concepts of thalamic organization have changed considerably. In particular, cytoarchitectural differentiations heretofore of little more than descriptive interest have gradually begun to be clarified in terms of their functional significance.

NOMENCLATURE

In the following account, we will adhere largely to the topographical terminology of OLSZEWSKI.[9] The Olszewski terminology is an extended form of the nomenclature generally referred to as the WALKER[3] terminology. WALKER[10] recently reiterated that this nomencla-ture was based originally on that introduced by investigators at the University of Michigan who initiated the first systematic comparative anatomical studies of the thalamus in the United States. Notable among these studies were RIOCH's[11-13] three reports on the diencephalon of carnivora.

The present paper will be considerably more limited in scope than were Rioch's studies. We intend to discuss mainly the organization of certain ventral cell territories of the *dorsal thalamus*, a term denoting that subdivision of the diencephalon which is generally referred to as 'the thalamus'. Little mention will be made of such major diencephalic subdivisions as the hypothalamus or the ventral thalamus (subthalamus). With respect to the now generally accepted term, *subthalamus*, as a synonym for ventral thalamus, it is of interest

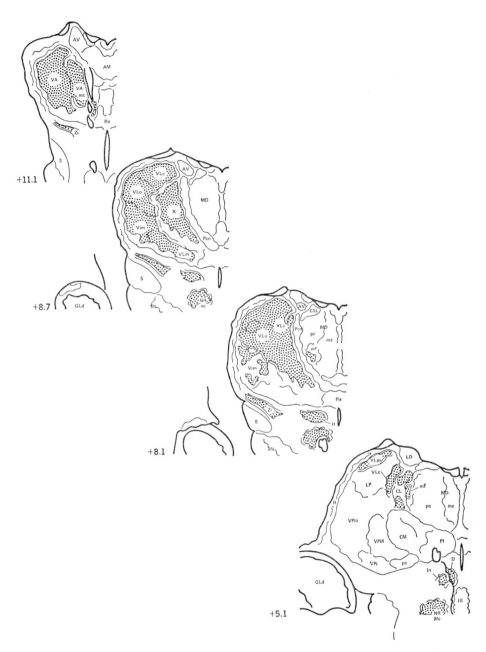

FIG. 1. Overall terminal distribution of cerebello-thalamic connections in the monkey.

to recall that RIOCH[14] was the first to call attention to the fact that this name is a Latin–Greek hybrid. KUHLENBECK[15] acknowledged this criticism, and pointed out that the term 'subthalamus' was introduced by no less a pioneer of neurology than FOREL[16], who also first described and named the zona incerta and the 'Haubenfelder' (H-fields), and later coined the term 'neuropsychiatry'.

There are many other nomenclature problems, some of which still continue to cause misunderstandings. Almost everyone who has devoted himself to studies of the thalamus has been confounded at one time or another by terminological discrepancies. Such leading contributors to our knowledge of thalamic organization as LE GROS CLARK[2,17] and WALKER[3,10] repeatedly commented on this problem and voiced the need for some kind of organized reform. We[18,20] also, have called attention to the cacophony of thalamic terms and its unfortunate sequel which we have characterized as 'atlas semantics'. Many of these difficulties stem from the lack of clear cytoarchitectonic boundaries between various nuclei, and the absence of objective means of establishing such borders.

It is remarkable that, from a cytoarchitectural point of view, the nuclear differentiation of the dorsal thalamus is, in a sense, inversely related to hypothalamic differentiation. In other words, in the brains of such non-primate species as the laboratory rat, the individuality of the hypothalamic nuclei is much more conspicuous than that of the dorsal thalamic nuclei. In the diencephala of advanced primate forms, this cytoarchitectural contrast appears in reversed form.[21,22] In spite of these morphological distinctions, by 1940 a number of different hypothalamic and thalamic terminologies had evolved from comparative anatomical studies, as well as from different studies in one and the same species, with the consequence that numerous semantical problems arose. To correct part of the terminological confusion, and thereby facilitate functional analyses of the hypothalamus, RIOCH et al.[14] in 1940 presented a precis of uniform nomenclature. Time has shown that this reformation served its intended purpose well.

CEREBELLO-THALAMIC CONNECTIONS

Figure 1 shows the overall terminal distribution of cerebello-thalamic connections in the monkey in accordance with the OLSZEWSKI[9] stereotaxic levels shown. The findings summarized in this figure were obtained in studies by the Nauta method initiated by the author and co-workers[23] at the Walter Reed Army Institute of Research. These studies have been supplemented and extended to include other species of mammals[24,25] in a long-range experimental comparative-anatomical investigation of cerebellofugal fiber projections that is still in progress.

Our observations have led us to conclude that cerebellar efferents connect with all of the subdivisions of the nucleus ventralis lateralis (VL) and 'area X' of Olszewski, with both the medial, magnocellular part of the nucleus ventralis anterior (VAmc) and the latter's smaller-celled lateral part (VA), and with the para- and intralamellar cell groups best identified as the nucleus centralis lateralis (Cl). Many of the latter's intralaminar clusters occupy the region often labelled pars multiformis of the nucleus medialis dorsalis (MDmf) (see MEHLER et al.[18]). The total distribution pattern of cerebello-thalamic fibers depicted in Fig. 1 emerges in cases of contralateral hemicerebellectomy. Partial lesions of the deep cerebellular nuclei or the brachium conjunctivum, by contrast, often elicit only part of this pattern of intrathalamic fiber degeneration, and in such cases the density of the degeneration in individual nuclear subdivisions varies somewhat with the localization of the lesion.

For example, lesions partially damaging deep cerebellar nuclei nearly always cause dense terminal degeneration in the medial aspects of the pars caudalis (VLc) and oralis (VLo) of the ventral lateral nucleus, in the VAmc and in the Cl, but VA, which appears to receive fibers of fine caliber, sometimes exhibits little or no terminal degeneration in such cases. Such observations might partially explain reports in the literature that deny cerebellar projections to the VA. The consensus based upon earlier studies of cerebellofugal projections in the monkey by the Marchi method regarded the VL, situated between the VA and the nucleus ventralis posterior (the somesthetic nuclear complex), as the main terminus of cerebello-thalamic fibers.[26,3,27] Such a restricted cerebello-thalamic fiber distribution was reported also in man by HASSLER[28] on the basis of observations in Marchi material. As HASSLER[29] and others have pointed out, precise data on the distributions of these afferent systems are needed to define functional subdivisions of the human thalamus more clearly.

Fourteen years ago, however, THOMAS et al.[30] in a study by the Nauta method, charted a wider distribution of the cerebello-thalamic projection in the cat, a distribution that extended over all region of VL and VA. MEHLER et al.[23] subsequently demonstrated the existence of an equally extensive cerebello-thalamic projection, involving corresponding thalamic nuclei, in the monkey. The projections in the monkey are schematically summarized in Fig. 1.

Observations in earlier studies of fiber-degeneration patterns (Nauta method) in humans having survived basal thalamotomies or lesions in the region of the pre-rubral field H of Forel for short time periods suggested to us that the distribution of cerebello-thalamic fibers in man are comparable to those we had observed in sub-human primates. Current Nauta studies (MEHLER et al. in preparation) of cerebellofugal fiber projections in man appear to confirm this impression. In a case of extensive therapeutic destruction of the dentate nucleus[31] massive cerebello-thalamic fiber degeneration could be traced in the VL- and VA-like territories which HASSLER[29] had labelled pars ventro-intermedius, pars ventro-oralis and pars latero-polaris of the lateral nuclear region. According to our observations, the nucleus ventro-oralis, pars internus (V.o.i.) for example, situated at the level of entrance of the mammillo-thalamic tract into the dorsal thalamus and described by HASSLER[29] as containing " . . . large very plump nerve cells," is a major locus of cerebello-thalamic fiber distribution. This experimental finding, considered together with the cytoarchitectural evidence, strongly suggest that the V.o.i. is anatomically homologous with VAmc in the monkey. Additional evidence suggesting that VAmc receives projections from the substantia nigra, but is avoided by pallido-thalamic fibers, will be discussed later. The thalamocortical projection arising from VAmc is still a controversial matter. HASSLER[28,32] found evidence in Marchi studies that indicated the ventral half of the posterior part of the nucleus ventro-oralis (V.o.p.) as the principal thalamic terminus of the brachium conjunctivum. On the basis of these observations, HASSLER[29,32] later concluded that V.o.p. alone was the homologue of the simian VL complex. The ventro-intermediate (V.im.) nucleus, situated between the ventro-oral and ventrocaudal complexes of HASSLER's[29] definitions, appears to be analogous with the oral part of VPL, a transitional area which blends imperceptibly with caudal VL regions receiving cerebellar connections. HASSLER[28,29] believes that vestibular relay projections terminate in V.im., but TARLOV[33] in more recent studies by the Nauta method was unable to confirm Hassler's earlier findings. Instead, Tarlov's observations in the macaque, baboon and chimpanzee, confirmed by findings in our own macaque material, suggest that the region corresponding to the human V.im. receives mainly cerebellar projections. It should be noted that Tarlov in all of these higher primate forms confirmed our earlier finding that cerebello-thalamic connections extend into the VA region at the rostral pole of the thalamus.

PALLIDO-THALAMIC CONNECTIONS

Figure 2 schematically depicts the distribution of pallido-thalamic fibers, all of which originate from the internal or medial segment of the globus pallidus. In its distribution to VA, VLo and VLm, this pallido-thalamic projection overlaps to some extent the cerebellar projection to the thalamus. We indicated the incomplete nature of this overlap in Table 1 of our re-evaluation study of the projections of the lentiform nucleus in the monkey.[34] At first, we attributed the apparent lack of complete coextensiveness of the two projections to the fact that none of our lesions involved the entire medial segment of the globus pallidus. However, it soon became evident that the pallidal projection selectively involves the clustered cells of VLo, and thus, little doubt was left that pallidal and cerebellar projections differ from each other with respect to their distribution in VLo and VLc (see, for example, the 8·1 level in Fig. 2). Some questions remained concerning the apparent absence of pallidal projections to 'area X' of VL, and to VAmc, both of which receive cerebellar fibers. CARPENTER and STROMINGER,[35] however, reported a similarly restricted distribution of pallido-thalamic fibers.

As indicated in Fig. 2, the pallido-thalamic connection also involves the nucleus centrum medianum (CM), but cerebellar projections to CM, suggested by findings in earlier studies by the Marchi method in the monkey[36] and man,[28] could not be confirmed in silver studies in either primate form. The afferent and efferent connections of CM were the subject of a recent review[37] that included new data supplementing RIOCH's[38] earlier note on the centre median nucleus of Luys.

The distribution of pallido-thalamic connections to cytoarchitecturally distinct sub-divisions of both the VL and the VA nucleus demonstrated a pattern of thalamic organization considerably different from that previously thought to exist. Instead of distributing to separate regions of the thalamus, the thalamic projections of these two major afferent systems apparently *converge*. For a more detailed accounting of the pertinent evidence, the reader is referred to NAUTA and MEHLER's[34] review, more recently updated by several further reports.[39-42] The current data, coupled with the discovery of fibers ascending from the substantia nigra to the VLm and VAmc suggest a need for thorough re-evaluation of the functional mosaic of the ventral nuclear complex.

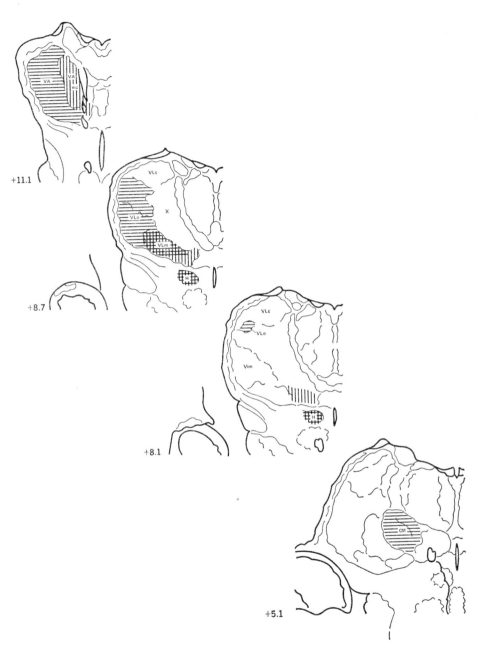

FIG. 2. Pallido-thalamic (horizontal lines) and nigro-thalamic connections (vertical lines) in the monkey.

NIGRO-THALAMIC CONNECTIONS

Nigro-thalamic connections ascending to the pars medialis (VLm) of the nucleus ventralis lateralis and to the medial, magnocellular district (VAmc) of the nucleus ventralis anterior in the Rhesus monkey (Fig. 2), and to corresponding ventro-medial thalamic regions in the cat, were first described by COLE *et al.*[43] By the use of Nauta silver methods, AFIFI and KAELBER[44] and CARPENTER and STROMINGER[35] confirmed and extended these findings in the cat and monkey respectively. FAULL and CARMAN[45] demonstrated a comparable nigro-thalamic connection in the rat.

The question has been raised whether these fibers are actually of nigral origin. To rule out error, all of the experiments leading to the identification of a nigro-thalamic connection have been assiduously controlled by such means as varying the insertion angle of the stereotaxic electrode, and the placing of lesions near, but not involving, the substantia nigra. FAULL and CARMAN,[45] especially, describe many of their control cases in detail.

An overlapping of the nigro-thalamic projection by cerebellar connections has been demonstrated in all of the three species of laboratory animals under consideration. The conspicuous lack of pallido-thalamic efferents distributed to the medially situated VL and VA cell groups projected upon by the substantia nigra, however, thus far has been noted only in the monkey. A re-study of our original cat material[46] has produced little if any evidence of fibers from the entopeduncular nucleus (i.e. the feline homologue of the medial segment of the primate globus pallidus) distributing in the nucleus ventralis medialis (VM), the chief nigro-thalamic fiber terminus in the cat, but it has revealed a considerable overlap of nigro- and pallidothalamic fibers in the medial VA region (VAmc). It is uncertain whether this difference between cat and monkey reflects an actual neurological species difference, or merely the unavoidable involvement of internal-capsule fibers in lesions of the ento-peduncular nucleus. These apparent connectional differences, as also certain interspecific cytoarchitectural variations in the thalamic nuclei in question, will require further clarification. Moreover, the question whether comparable 'pallido-thalamic' connections originate from the entopeduncular nucleus in the rat awaits careful investigation. However, despite these remaining uncertainties it can be said that the ascending course of the nigral fibers through the H-fields and their distribution chiefly to ventral and medial larger-celled regions of the thalamus are remarkably similar in the three species that have been studied.

Recent retrograde cell degeneration studies in the monkey have led METTLER[47] to question the existence of a nigro-thalamic connection and to reiterate earlier conclusions favoring nigro-pallidal and nigro-striatal connections. It is not our intention to review all of the old and new controversies concerning the polarity of the axonal projections of the substantia nigra or their sites of termination, but we would like to comment briefly upon Mettler's report for the reason that it challenges the recent description of nigro-thalamic connections incorporated in our present schema of thalamic organization. On the basis of a study of the reaction of the substantia nigra to a variety of chronic lesions of the cortex, striatum, globus pallidus or thalamus, Mettler has concluded that it is lesions of the pars externa of the globus pallidus that most consistently produce demonstrable retrograde cell changes

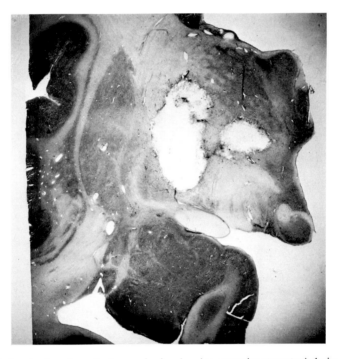

FIG. 3.   Nissl-stained section of a human brain, showing extensive stereotaxic lesions involving both thalamus and globus pallidus.

in the pars compacta of the substantia nigra, and striatal lesions that so affect the pars reticulata. According to Mettler's observations, medial thalamic lesions, destroying apparently most of the VLm and VAmc regions, elicit no retrograde cell changes in the nigra.

We would concur with the latter of Mettler's findings on the basis of some observations in cases of therapeutic thalamotomy. In two cases with lesions in the medial and basal 'VL' region, no cell loss was evident in either part of the nigra. The duration of postoperative survival times (two and three weeks, respectively) in these cases, however, while long enough for anterograde fiber-degeneration studies, may have been too short to provide conclusive evidence of retrograde cell changes. HASSLER[48] who examined comparable clinical thalamotomy cases, presumably of longer survival, also has questioned the existence of a nigro-thalamic connection in man.

In the same category of observations it is appropriate to mention another thalamotomy case that we have studied. In this case, the thalamotomy was coupled with a partial pallidectomy (Fig. 3). Despite the substantial dual lesion, nigral cell changes such as described by Mettler were lacking. As in the other two cases mentioned above, the post-operative survival of 21 days may have been too brief to have allowed the development of unambiguous histological changes in the substantianigra. However, even if the negative evidence from the three cases in question be considered conclusive, it should be kept in mind that the failure to produce retrograde nigral cell changes by thalamic lesion might be due to the existence of 'sustaining collateral' connections established by the nigro-thalamic fibers in the course of their ascent through the subthalamic region. Further experimental and clinico-anatomical studies of thalamotomy cases of longer standing, especially such with lesions involving field H of Forel, are needed to settle this question.

A further unanswered question is to what degree the degeneration of the substantia nigra following lesions of the corpus striatum is transneuronal rather than retrograde in nature. Because of the strong convergence of striato-nigral fibers in their course through the pallidal segments, even small lesions of the globus pallidus must interrupt a very much larger part of the massive striato-nigral projection than would be affected by lesions of similar size in the caudate nucleus or putamen. It is therefore interesting that COWAN and POWELL[49] noted more extensive gliosis in the pars reticulata of the substantia nigra following pallidal lesions than following striatal lesions. It is unknown, however, whether massive striato-nigral deafferentations alone are capable of eliciting cell changes in the substantia nigra. The main uncertainty in dealing with this problem concerns the trajectory followed by the reciprocating nigro-striatal fibers, and hence, the question to what extent lesions of the globus pallidus involve both striato-nigral and nigro-striatal fibers.

BÉDARD et al.,[50] for instance, have concluded that although both the origins and the terminal regions of the reciprocal connections between the striatum and the nigra are topologically equivalent, their respective descending and ascending pathways differ. These authors acknowledge the fact that the striato-nigral fibers follow a transpeduncular course, forming a major part of the 'comb system' but they believe that the ascending nigro-striatal pathway is incoporated in the medial forebrain bundle. The same authors confirm METTLER'S[47] observation that thalamic lesions elicit no nigral cell changes, and add the finding that such lesions do not alter dopamine concentrations in the striatum.

CORTICO-THALAMIC AND THALAMO-CORTICAL RELATIONSHIPS

The ventral tier of the thalamus labelled VL is, by functional definition, the thalamic nucleus dependent on cortical area 4, the 'precentral motor cortex'. Except for larger cells in the pars oralis (VLo) and smaller, more spindle-shaped cells in the pars medialis (VLm), the subdivisions of VL in the monkey are distinguished mostly on the basis of topographic criteria. The area designated 'X' by OLSZEWSKI[9] is apparently more closely related to area 6, the 'premotor cortex'.[51,52] Area X, like the VL and VA nuclei, receives cerebellar connections, but no pallidal projections and few if any nigro-thalamic fibers terminate in this less cellular, paralamellar region medial to the main VL complex. Another region that might be considered part of VL is the area redesignated V.im., or ventralis intermedius, in Fig. 1. Included in the VPLo by OLSZEWSKI,[9] this area of transition between the ventral posterior and VL complexes has been recognized as a separate cytoarchitectural entity on the basis of having some especially large cells among its neuronal population.[26,53] Marchi studies (monkey) led CROUCH and THOMPSON,[53] as it had caused CÉCILE VOGT[26] earlier, to conclude that V.im. was the principal terminus of the brachium conjunctivum. KRUGER and PORTER[51] concluded that V.im. probably is associated with the cortical area 3 in the depths of the central sulcus but is not part of the somesthetic complex. HASSLER[29] also subscribes to the notion that V.im. in man is cortically dependent on area 3a. As Fig. 1 indicates, V.im. in the monkey receives cerebellar efferents, but we have also observed that some spinal and lemniscal fibers terminate in this zone of cellular transition. There appears to be more overlap of ascending afferent systems in V.im. than was formerly realized. Actually, THOMAS et al.[30] originally reported cerebellar projections to a rostral VPL region in the cat, and we,[23] on the basis of too literal an interpretation of OLSZEWSKI's[9] atlas, likewise identified VPLo as a site of cerebellar fiber termination. In patients with parkinsonian dyskinesia, rhythmic discharges synchronous with the tremor were recorded from V.im.,[55] and this electrical sign has become a valuable neuro-physiological criterion identifying V.im. in the course of stereotaxic neurosurgery.

There is little question now that VLo and VA are the principal thalamic convergence areas of cerebellar and pallidal afferent fiber projections, while VLc, VAmc and 'area X' receive cerebellar connections but are avoided by pallido-thalamic fibers. As noted, VLc and VLo both degenerate after removal of the precentral cortex.[9] Functional differences between caudal and oral parts of VL, comparable to those identified by POGGIO and MOUNTCASTLE[56] in the somesthetic VPL region, have not been demonstrated in the monkey. The observations of NARABAYASHI and KUBOTA[57] and others in man, however, suggest that the caudal VL zone, now generally referred to as V.im., is more especially involved in the tremorogenic mechanisms of parkinsonian dyskinesia, and the oral VL region in the phenomenon of parkinsonian rigidity. HASSLER,[32] on the basis of a large series of clinical observations, concluded that functional differences exist between the anterior and posterior parts of the ventro-oral nucleus (i.e. V.o.a. and V.o.p. of HASSLER's[29] terminology). The latter nuclear subdivisions appear to be anatomically equivalent to VLc and VLo, but more data are needed to correlate the homologous nature of these areas in monkey and man.

VA projects chiefly to area 6. This is the consensus based upon retrograde cell degeneration studies in primates.[58,59,29] However, frequent reports of failure of VA cells to undergo retrograde degeneration subsequent to ablations of premotor regions led to notions that the cell group should be included among the non-specific thalamic nuclei. This is especially true of VAmc, stimulation of which frequently elicits electrophysiological recruitment phenomena in the EEG (see AJMONE MARSAN[4]). Based upon the evidence that all regions of VL and VA receive cerebellar afferents (Fig. 1), and that pallido-thalamic and nigro-thalamic connections converge on lateral and medial subdivisions of VL and VA respectively (Fig. 2) one might agree with KUHLENBECK'S[15] suggestion that VA is merely a rostral extension of the VL complex. On the other hand, the apparent division into lateral pallidal, and medial nigral regions suggests that the functional differences between medial and lateral parts of the ventral thalamic nucleus may be even more important than the usually emphasized functional differences between anterior (VA) and posterior (VL) subdivisions of the complex. Histochemical studies may eventually reveal some significant and hitherto undisclosed metabolic relationship supporting one or another of the current notions with respect to this problem.

Reports of anterograde fiber degeneration studies[60] have not as yet confirmed the existence of projections from area 6 to the VA region reciprocating the thalamo-cortical projection suggested by cell degeneration studies. SAKAI[61] makes no mention of such connections in her report on cortico-thalamic fiber connections originating from the precentral cortex, but concludes that the cortical region occupied by the precentral dimple, usually considered area 6, projects chiefly to VLo.

CARPENTER,[39] in an excellent review of the ventral tier thalamic nuclei, called attention to the confusion revolving around the connections of the VA region. CARMEL,[62] working in Carpenter's laboratory, undertook a re-examination of this problem in monkeys with cortical ablations or small intra-thalamic VA or VAmc lesions. His observations on retrograde cell changes in VA and VAmc confirm the results of earlier studies. In adult animals surviving extensive frontal lobe ablations for three months or less, Carmel found two-thirds of the cells in the VA region remaining. On the basis of the fiber degeneration observed in monkeys with lesions in VA, Carmel concluded that the major efferent connections of VA and VAmc are with other thalamic nuclei rather than with the cortex. According to Carmel, neither subdivision of VA appears to have connections with the striatum. In his experiments, only VAmc lesions consistently elicited degeneration of a well-defined group of thalamo-cortical fibers that could be traced to the lateral orbital gyrus. Ablation of this part of the orbital cortex, however, produced no cell changes in the VA region. Recognizing that numerous cortifugal fibers from the prefrontal and precentral areas traverse various regions of the VA complex, Carmel nonetheless argues in favor of descending intrathalamic connections originating from VA and VAmc. It appears that his argument is based mainly on his finding of a large number of unaffected cells in the VA region after cortical ablation, on some more or less tenuous Golgi evidence, and on neurophysiological data suggesting that VAmc and/or VA belong to the category of 'nonspecific' thalamic nuclei.

CARMEL'S[62] observation that large cortical ablations are needed to produce observable cell loss in the VA nucleus undoubtedly supports his conclusion that the thalamo-cortical fibers originating from VA are widely distributed and characterized by a great number of sustaining collaterals, rather than forming a projection of tight topographic organization. His evidence that VA does not project to either the caudate nucleus or putamen contradicts the generally accepted notion that 'non-specific' thalamic nuclei have at least collateral connections with the striatum. These new findings need verification and further elaboration. For example, a study of the fiber degeneration caused by VA lesions in animals with long-standing destruction of the nucleus medialis dorsalis might rule out the possibility that the thalamocortical fibers to the orbitofrontal cortex originated in the latter nucleus rather than in the VA proper. Lesions of VA, as also electrical stimulation within the nucleus, must affect not only VA neurons but also large numbers of fibers passing through the VA region to or from other thalamic nuclei.

SUMMARY

Experimental neuroanatomical studies by the aid of the Nauta method have demonstrated that ascending projections from the cerebellum form the most widely distributed single subcortical afferent system impinging on the thalamus in the primate brain.[23,24] Cerebello-thalamic fibers terminate throughout all subdivisions of the ventral lateral (VL) and ventral anterior (VA) nuclei, and in addition, compose the most massive of the known afferent connections of the intralaminar nucleus centralis lateralis[18,20,23] (Fig. 1). Pallido-thalamic[34,46] and nigro-thalamic[43] projections have a more restricted distribution in the VA-VL complex (Fig. 2). These two fiber systems show only slight mutual overlap in their distribution, but each has a unique well-defined area of convergence with the cerebello-thalamic projection. From a consideration of these data in the context of a brief literature review dealing with cortico-thalamic interrelationships, a new mosaic of thalamic organization emerges.

ABBREVIATIONS

AM	nuc. anterior medialis.
AV	nuc. anterior ventralis.
Cl	nuc. centralis lateralis.
CM	nuc. centrum medianum.
Csl	nuc. centralis superior lateralis.
D	nuc. Darkschewitsch.
H	nuc. campus Foreli.
In	nuc. interstitialis (Cajal).
LD	nuc. lateralis dorsalis.
LP	nuc. lateralis posterior.
MD	nuc. medialis dorsalis; mc, pars magnocellularis; mf, pars multiformis; pc, pars parvocellularis.
NR	nuc. ruber; mc, pars magnocellularis; pc, pars parvocellularis.
pc	pars parvocellularis of VPM.
Pcn	nuc. paracentralis.
Pf	nuc. parafascicularis.
Re	nuc. reuniens.
S	nuc. subthalamicus.
SN	substantia nigra.
VA	nuc. ventralis anterior; mc, pars magnocellularis.
Vim	nuc. ventralis intermedius.
VL	nuc. ventralis lateralis; c, pars caudalis; m, pars medialis; o, pars oralis; ps, pars postrema.

VPi   nuc. ventralis posterior inferior.
VPLo   nuc. ventralis posterior lateralis, pars oralis.
VPM   nuc. ventralis posterior medialis.
X   area X of Olszewski.
Zi   zona incerta.

REFERENCES

1. BELL, C. *Idea of a New Anatomy of the Brain*. Strehan & Preston, London, 1811.
2. CLARK, W. E. L. The structure and connections of the thalamus. *Brain* **55**, 406, 1932.
3. WALKER, A. E. *The Primate Thalamus*. University of Chicago Press, Chicago, 1938.
4. AJMONE MARSAN, C. The thalamus. Data on its functional anatomy and on some aspects of thalamo-cortical integration. *Archs ital. Biol.* **103**, 847, 1965.
5. SPIEGEL, E. A., WYCIS, H. T., MARKS, M. and LEE, A. J. Stereotaxic apparatus for operations on the human brain. *Science* **106**, 349, 1947.
6. GLEES, P. Terminal degeneration within the central nervous system as studied by a new silver method. *J. Neuropath. exp. Neurol.* **5**, 54, 1946.
7. NAUTA, W. J. H. Über die sogennante terminale Degeneration im Zentralnervensystem und ihre Darstellung durch Silberimprägnation. *Arch. Neurol. Neurochir. Psychiat.* Schweiz **66**, 353, 1950.
8. NAUTA, W. J. H. Silver impregnation of degenerating axons. In: *New Research Techniques of Neuroanatomy*, Windle, W. F. (Ed.), p. 17. C. C. Thomas, Springfield, Illinois, 1957.
9. OLSZEWSKI, J. *The Thalamus of the Macaca Mulatta*. S. Karger, Basel, 1952.
10. WALKER, A. E. Internal structure and afferent-efferent relations of the thalamus. In: *The Thalamus*, PURPURA, D. P. and YAHR, M. D. (Eds.), p. 1. Columbia University Press, New York, 1966.
11. RIOCH, D. McK. Studies on the diencephalon of carnivora. Part I. *J. comp. Neurol.* **49**, 1, 1929.
12. RIOCH, D. McK. Studies on the diencephalon of carnivora. Part II. *J. comp. Neurol.* **49**, 121, 1929.
13. RIOCH, D. McK. Studies on the diencephalon of carnivora. Part III. *J. comp. Neurol.* **53**, 319, 1931.
14. RIOCH, D. McK., WISLOCKI, G. B. and O'LEARY, J. L. A précis of preoptic, hypothalamic and hypophysial terminology with atlas. *Res. Publs. Ass. Res. nerv. ment. Dis.* **20**, 3, 1940.
15. KUHLENBECK, H. The human diencephalon. *Confinia neurol.* **14**, (Suppl.), 1, 1954.
16. FOREL, A. Untersuchungen über die Haubenregion und ihre oberen Verknüpfungen im Gehirne des Menschen und der Sägethiere, mit Beiträgen zu den Methoden der Gerhinforschung. *Arch. Psychiat.* **7**, 393, 1877.
17. CLARK, W. E. L. Immediate problems of the anatomy of the thalamus. In: *Proceedings, 4th International Neurologic Congress*, Vol. 1, p. 49. Masson Cie, Paris, 1949.
18. MEHLER, W. R., FEFERMAN, M. E. and NAUTA, W. J. H. Ascending axon degeneration following antero-lateral cordotomy. *Brain* **83**, 718, 1960.
19. MEHLER, W. R. Some observations on secondary ascending afferent systems in the central nervous system. In: *International Symposium on Pain, Henry Ford Hospital*, KNIGHTON, R. S. (Ed.), p. 11. Little, Brown, Boston, 1966.
20. MEHLER, W. R. Some neurological species differences—*a posteriori*. *Ann. N.Y. Acad. Sci.* **167**, 424, 1969.
21. KRIEG, W, J. S. The hypothalamus of the albino rat. *J. comp. Neurol.* **55**, 18, 1932.
22. KRIEG, W. J. S. A reconstruction of the diencephalic nuclei of Macacus rhesus. *J. comp. Neurol.* **88**, 1, 1948.
23. MEHLER, W. R., VERNIER, V. G. and NAUTA, W. J. H. Efferent projections from the dentate and interpositus nuclei in primates. *Anat. Rec.* **130**, 430, 1958.
24. MEHLER, W. R. A comparison of cerebellar projections to vestibular, reticular and diencephalic nuclei in the monkey, cat and rat. *VIIIth Int. Congr. Anat.*, Wiesbaden, Germany, 1965.
25. MEHLER, W. R. Double descending pathways originating from the superior cerebellar penduncle. *Anat. Rec.* **157**, 374, 1967.
26. VOGT, C. Le myéloarchitecture du thalamus du cercopithèque. *J. Psychol. Neurol.*, Lpz. **12**, 285, 1909.
27. HASSLER, R. Über Kleinhirnprojektionen zum Mittelhirn und Thalamus beim Menschen. *Dt. Z. NervHeilk.* **163**, 629, 1950.
28. HASSLER, R. Über die afferenten Bahnen und Thalamuskerne des motorischen Systems des Grosshirns. I and II. *Arch. Psychiat. NervKrankh.* **182**, 759, 1949.

D

29. HASSLER, R. Anatomy of the thalamus. In: *Introduction to Stereotaxis with an Atlas of the Human Brain*, SCHALTENBRAND, G. and BAILEY, P. (Eds.), p. 230. Grune & Stratton, New York, 1959.

30. THOMAS, D. M., KAUFMAN, R. P., SPRAGUE, J. M. and CHAMBERS, W. W. Experimental studies of the vermal cerebellar projections in the brain stem of the cat (fastigiobulbar tract). *J. Anat.* **90**, 371, 1956.

31. NASHOLD, B. S. and SLAUGHTER, D. G. Effects of stimulating or destroying the deep cerebellar regions in man. *J. Neurosurg.* **31**, 172, 1969.

32. HASSLER, R. Thalamic regulation of muscle tone and the speed of movements. In: *The Thalamus*, PURPURA and YAHR (Eds.), p. 418. Columbia University Press, New York, 1966.

33. TARLOV, E. The rostral projections of the primate vestibular nuclei: an experimental study in macaque, baboon and chimpanzee. *J. comp. Neurol.* **135**, 27, 1969.

34. NAUTA, W. J. H. and MEHLER, W. R. Projections of the lentiform nucleus in the monkey. *Brain Res.* **1**, 3, 1966.

35. CARPENTER, M. B. and STROMINGER, N. L. Efferent fibers of the subthalamic nucleus in the monkey. A comparison of the efferent projections of the subthalamic nucleus, substantia nigra and globus pallidus. *Am. J. Anat.* **121**, 41, 1967.

36. CARPENTER, M. B, Lesions of the fastigial nuclei in the rhesus monkey. *Am. J. Anat.* **104**, 1, 1959.

37. MEHLER, W. R. Further notes on the centre median nucleus of Luys. In: *The Thalamus*, PURPURA and YAHR (Eds.), p. 109. Columbia University Press, New York, 1966.

38. RIOCH, D. McK. A note on the centre median nucleus of Luys. *J. Anat.* **65**, 324, 1931.

39. CARPENTER, M. B. Ventral tier thalamic nuclei. In: *Modern Trends in Neurology* 4, WILLIAMS, D. (Ed.), p. 1. Butterworths, London, 1967.

40. CARMAN, J. B. Anatomic basis of surgical treatment of Parkinson's disease. *New Engl. J. Med.* **279**, 919, 1968.

41. HAYMAKER, W., MEHLER, W. R. and SCHILLER, F. Extrapyramidal motor disorders. In: *Bing's Local Diagnosis in Neurological Diseases*, 15th Ed., HAYMAKER, W. (Ed.), p. 404. C. V. Mosby, St. Louis, 1969.

42. NAUTA, W. J. H. and MEHLER, W. R. Fiber connections of the basal ganglia. In: *Psychotrophic Drugs and Dysfunctions of the Basal Ganglia*, USPHS Pub. 1938, CRANE, G. E. and GARDNER, R., JR. (Eds.), p. 68. U.S. Government Printing Office, Washington, 1969.

43. COLE, M., NAUTA, W. J. H. and MEHLER, W. R. The ascending efferent projections of the substantia nigra. *Trans. Am. neurol. Ass.* **89**, 74, 1964.

44. AFIFI, A. and KAELBER, W. W. Efferent connections of the substantia nigra in the cat. *Expl Neurol.* **11**, 474, 1965.

45. FAULL, R. L. M. and CARMAN, J. B. Ascending projections of substantia nigra in rat. *J. comp Neurol.* **132**, 73, 1968.

46. NAUTA, W. J. H. and MEHLER, W. R. Some efferent connections of the lentiform nuclei in the monkey and cat. *Anat. Rec.* **139**, 260, 1961.

47. METTLER, F. A. Nigrofugal connections in the primate brain. *J. comp. Neurol.* **138**, 291, 1970.

48. HASSLER, R. Substantia nigra regulation of muscle tone and movement. In: *Substantia Nigra and Sensorimotor Activities*, FRIGYESI, T. L. (Ed.) Newark, New Jersey, 1969.

49. COWAN, W. M. and POWELL, T. P. S. Strio-pallidal projection in the monkey. *J. Neurol. Neurosurg. Psychiat.* **29**, 426, 1966.

50. BÉDARD, P., LAROCHELLE, L., PARENT, A. and POIRIER, J. L. The nigrostriatal pathway: a correlative study based on neuroanatomical and neurochemical criteria in the cat and the monkey. *Expl Neurol.* **25**, 365, 1969.

51. KRUGER, L and PORTER, P. A behavioral study of the functions of the rolandic cortex in the monkey. *J. comp. Neurol.* **109**, 439, 1958.

52. GOLDMAN, P. S. and ROSVOLD, H. E. Localization of function within the dorsolateral prefrontal cortex of the rhesus monkey. *Expl Neurol.* **27**, 291, 1970.

53. CROUCH, R. L. The nuclear configuration of the thalamus of macacas thesus. *J. comp. Neurol* **59**, 451, 1934.

54. CROUCH, R. L. and THOMPSON, J. K. Termination of the brachium conjunctivum in the thalamus of the macaque monkey. *J. comp. Neurol.* **69**, 449, 1938.

55. ALBE-FESSARD, D., ARFEL, G. and GUIOT, G. Activités électriques caractéristiques de quelques structures cérébrales chez l'homme. *Annls Chir.* **17**, 1185, 1963.

56. POGGIO, G. F. and MOUNTCASTLE, V. B. The functional properties of ventrobasal thalamic neurons studied in unanesthetized monkeys. *J. Neurophysiol.* **26**, 775, 1963.

57. NARABAYASHI, H. and KUBOTA, K. Reconsideration of ventrolateral thalamotomy for hyperkinesis. *Prog. Brain. Res.* **21B,** 339, 1966.

58. CLARK, W. E. L. and BOGGON, R. H. The thalamic connections of the parietal and frontal lobes of the brain in the monkey. *Phil. Trans. R. Soc. Ser. B.* **224,** 313, 1935.

59. CHOW, K. L. and PRIBRAM, K. H. Cortical projection of the thalamic ventrolateral nuclear group in monkeys. *J. comp. Neurol.* **104,** 57, 1956.

60. PETRAS, J. M. Fiber degeneration in the basal ganglia and diencephalon following lesions in the precentral and postcentral cortex of the monkey (Macaca mulatta); with additional observations in the chimpanzee. *VIIIth Internat. Congr. Anat.,* Wiesbaden, Germany, 1965.

61. SAKAI, S. Some observations of the cortico-thalamic fiber connections in the monkey. *Proc. Japan Acad.* **43,** 822, 1967.

62. CARMEL, P. W. Efferent projections of the ventral anterior nucleus of the thalamus in the monkey. *Am. J. Anat.* **128,** 159, 1970.

J. psychiat. Res., 1971, Vol. 8, pp. 219–224. Pergamon Press. Printed in Great Britain.

THE GLIA-NEURONAL INTERACTION:
SOME OBSERVATIONS

ROBERT GALAMBOS

Department of Neurosciences, University of California at San Diego, La Jolla, California

UNTIL some 10 years ago, the functions performed by glial cells in the brain and peripheral nerves lay almost entirely in the realm of speculation. As an example, CAJAL, in an early paper entitled "Anatomical Mechanisms of Thought, Association and Attention"[1] attributed two different roles to the cortical glia, each dependent upon the motility of glial processes which his extensive microscopic examinations of stained material seemed to him to support. He supposed, on the one hand, that glial processes might insinuate themselves between pre- and post-synaptic elements and by impeding the flow of 'nervous currents' there produce mental relaxation and natural or induced sleep. Retraction of the neuroglial pseudopods would allow reestablishment of the synapse and "the brain would pass from the relaxed to the active stage." These glial contractions, which might occur "automatically or by an act of will" in his scheme, could direct associative processes in specific directions. "The unpredictable turns that associations sometimes take—the fading away of ideas and words, the momentary halting of speech, the obsessive persistence of memory, the repression of an idea or experience as well as all types of erroneous motor reactions and other psychological phenomena can be understood . . . by supposing the neuroglia of the gray matter serve as an insulating and switching mechanism for nervous currents, permitting connections when they are active, and acting as insulators during repose."

His second hypothesis holds that when the perivascular astrocytes contracted, their endfeet attached to the walls of brain capillaries would pull on the wall of the vessel, enlarge its lumen, and thus increase local blood flow. To explain attention, he hypothesized that such contractions were voluntarily initiated in the cortical zone appropriate for the perceptions or recollections in order to produce and sustain the increased metabolism there.

Apparently these ideas soon lost their appeal for CAJAL since he does not mention them in the two volumes on neuroanatomy that insure for him a permanent place in the history of science.[2] Though SCHLEICH[3] restates the glial switchboard idea in a fanciful way, neither of Cajal's ideas seems to have received much currency nor, to my knowledge has either of them been directly tested experimentally. This despite Cajal's statement about them at the end of his paper: "Needless to point out, a hypothesis represents a new path, opened up by experiments and observations, and even if it does not immediately reveal the truth, it always leads to investigations and criticisms that bring us nearer to it. Our future investigations may not confirm these hypotheses, but their outcomes will provide valuable information. Negative findings will limit the number of tenable hypotheses and reduce the possibility of making unproductive investigations in the future."

As of 10 years ago, the glial were generally supposed to function as nutritive and supportive cells in the normal brain, and to proliferate to repair it after damage. Recent solid data about glia morphology and glia physiology generally support these ideas and put them in a realistic framework (see, for example, FRIEDE,[4] KUFFLER.[5]) These data include biochemical, microscopic and electrophysiological information that clarifies both the specialized features of the cells themselves and the interactions that presumably go on among them, and between them and the neurons with which they are so intimately associated. The remainder of this paper will examine a few of these new facts.

In a review as brief as this, the developing body of information on macromolecular synthetic activities of glia must be given short shrift. The pioneer, and still the principal student of this problem, is Holger Hyden. Using micro techniques developed for the assay of quantities of material contained in a few nerve or glia cells, he has developed a picture of the ebb and flow of RNA, enzyme and protein synthesis in these cells during functional activities of animals such as rats and rabbits. Evidence for altered synthesis in glia has, for instance, been correlated with disease in man in a study of the glia from patients with basal ganglia disorders (GOMIRATO and HYDEN[6]), with sleep in the rabbit (HAMBERGER et al.[7]), and with learning in the rat (HYDEN and EGYHAZI[8]). From similar analyses made upon the neurons associated with these glia, some details of the active chemical interactions going on in what he calls the glia-neuron functional unit are beginning to emerge (HYDEN[9,10]). In an otherwise excellent review (KUFFLER and NICHOLLS[11]), Hyden's attempts to map out the special biochemical properties of glia in the functioning brain receive, in this writer's opinion, unnecessarily harsh treatment.

At the light microscope level direct evidence for an active proliferation of glial cells during function has been provided by several studies. For example, both ALTMAN and DAS[12] and DIAMOND et al.[13] count more glial nuclei in the somewhat thicker cortex of rats raised communally in enriched, challenging environments than in the cortex of littermate controls raised alone under conditions where there is little for them to do and experience. The implication of these studies, that a relationship exists between glial multiplication and the functional requirements of nerve cells, has been tested in other kinds of experiments. MURRAY,[14] for instance reports that dehydration in the rat stimulates hypothalamic glial proliferation only in the supraoptic nucleus (100 per cent in two weeks) and in the posterior pituitary (about 25 per cent), which is to say, in precisely the regions predicted from other evidence to be stimulated into activity by dehydration. From such studies one can assert that, in some cases at least, one result of the glial-neuronal interactions taking place during increased functional activity is the stimulation of glial mitoses. Why more neuronal activity should require the increased glial metabolism implied by an increase in cell number is an unanswered question (but see FRIEDE[4]).

Thanks to the electron microscope the cytoplasmic characteristics of the different types of glia and the varied contacts their membranes make with one another and with the neurons they attend have been greatly clarified (e.g. GRAY,[15] MUGNAINI and WALBERG[16] and others). It is by now an old story pictured in the textbooks that peripheral Schwann cells and central oligodendroglia invest their axons and create the myelin sheath around them (see SMITH[17] for a discussion of this biosynthetic event). Without this sheath the rapid saltatory conduction upon which central integration depends is impossible, as is so evident in a disease like multiple sclerosis where the sheath is abnormal or absent. The increased transverse resistance offered by the myelin sheath provides the basis for this saltatory conduction, namely, depolarization at the nodes only. Here at least is a clear case where the two cells must work together to produce a functionally important end product.

Not all axons are myelinated, however, and the ones with and without myelin both display extensive glia–neuron membrane contacts where functional interactions might occur. What transpires across the membrane of an unmyelinated peripheral nerve fiber which is everywhere surrounded by the membrane of a Schwann cell (CAUSEY[18])? Myelinated axons possess this same intimate membrane-to-membrane contact, and therefore, if an interesting interaction takes place in the unmyelinated fiber it may do so in the myelinated form as well. Other curious details to which no functional significance has yet been attached include the complete absence of glial cytoplasm at central nodes and its presence in peripheral ones, and the investment of some cell bodies in the CNS by astrocytic processes and of others by oligodendroglial membrane (PALAY[19]).

Turning now to the contacts between glial cells (gliapses; GALAMBOS[20]), it is clear that specialized regions called gap junctions abound in the nervous systems of many animals (MUGNAINI and WALBERG,[16] BRIGHTMAN and REESE[21]). Gap junctions differ from synaptic, desmosomal and tight junctions in being limited to glial membranes, in having five layers with a space of 20–30Å intervening between the middle pair, and in providing the most likely anatomical substratum for the low-resistance pathway needed to explain the easy passage of electrical currents between one glial cell and its neighbor. If these gap junctions should indeed be areas through which ions pass freely, their number and distribution in a particular volume of brain would determine how much, and in what direction, any currents generated by neuronal activity would flow. We shall return to this matter shortly.

Another morphological specialization of glia is revealed after serial reconstructions of electron microscopic pictures of such regions as the lateral geniculate (COLONNIER and GUILLERY[22]) and the granular layer of the cerebellum (ECCLES et al.[23]). In these structures, limited collections of pre- and post-synaptic elements turn out to be completely invested by sheets of glial membrane. Such synaptic regions may lie tightly packed beside one another, each wrapped into a kind of package by the thin glial processes. It has been speculated that this glial covering, like the shell of an egg, protects what is inside from undesirable outside influences or, like the walls of a stove, prevents what goes on inside from spreading into the surroundings.

The many important electrophysiological observations upon glia made by the group associated with Kuffler are summarized in the review already cited (KUFFLER and NICHOLLS[11]). Using microelectrode methods on the leech and mudpuppies—forms with especially large cells that simplify intracellular recording—they have shown the properties of glial membranes to differ from those of neurons in four ways important for understanding the reciprocal interactions between the two cell types. First, glial membranes show graded depolarizations, never spikes. Second, their resting potential (regularly 90 mV as opposed to 70 in the neurons) is remarkably sensitive to external K^+ concentration, responding to increases by depolarizing in a manner almost exactly predicted for a K^+ electrode by the Nernst equation. Third, the glial membrane depolarizes as impulses traverse adjacent axons in just the manner, and to the degree that would be predicted by the release of K^+ from the neuron during the impulse. Fourth, experimentally injected current passes freely from one glial cell to the next, presumably by way of the gap junctions already discussed. These facts, derived from a series of elegant experiments that is still in progress (e.g. NICHOLLS and BAYLOR[24]), have led to the following important new generalization about glia. During normal neuronal activity, the K^+ released by neuronal activity into the extracellular space produces a drop in glial membrane potential (proportional to log K^+ concentration) at that site. Current then flows to this region from undisturbed membranes via the extracellular space and the glial cytoplasm until the K^+ concentration returns to its resting level. The time course, as well as the metabolic and electrical consequences of this dynamic interaction are questions for which answers are being sought in several laboratories.

For instance, electrical currents generated by such glial depolarizations should produce recordable potentials at a distance from the site of their initiation. Evidence that the well-known negative afterpotential recorded from the surface of mixed nerves originates from this source has in fact been assembled (ORKAND et al.[25]). The question of whether some unknown fraction of the voltages recorded from the surface of the brain arises in a similar manner has been raised, (ORKAND,[26] POLLEN[27]) and recordings made from the so-called idle or silent cells in cat cortex contribute to the answer. These silent cells, identified by dye-marking as glia, resemble the glia or lower forms in several ways: their membrane resting potentials range up to 90 mV; they are electrically inexcitable; and they depolarize when neurons are active nearby. Reasonable values for the speed, magnitude and extent of K^+ movement across their membranes in cat cortex have been established and interpreted as showing the glia to regulate K^+ concentration at synaptic regions there (TRACHTENBERG and POLLEN[28]) as they do in invertebrate ganglia (NICHOLLS and BAYLOR[24]). If such regulation of K^+ in the synaptic environment is indeed a major function of the glia, then the glia found in cortical scars might be unable to perform this function; POLLEN and TRACHTENBERG[29] have suggested the essential lesion of focal epilepsy in man to be just this failure to buffer extracellular K^+ concentration normally.

Depolarizations in the cortical silent cells accompany spontaneous brainwave spindles as well as the neuronal activity evoked by either thalamic or direct cortical stimulation. These responses seem in all important ways analogous to the glial responses of lower forms. Several experimental observations have provided information on the possible contribution of these glial depolarizations to the slow waves recordable with large electrodes from brain and elsewhere. The most recent of them (CASTELLUCCI and GOLDRING[30]) calls attention to the striking resemblance between the silent-cell depolarizations and certain steady potential shifts recorded from the cortical surface during seizure discharge and brain stimulation. The authors suggest " . . . that glia lying closest to a focus of neuronal activity in the cerebral cortex become depolarized by local release of K^+ and draw current from neighbouring 'source' glia to which electrical linkage occurs in all directions." It seems likely that the possibility of a glial contribution to all the various spontaneous and evoked electrical responses recordable from nervous tissue will in time be directly tested. It has already been claimed that the b-wave of the electroretinogram, an event long considered to be a manifestation of neuronal acitivity, is due solely to depolarization of the Müller fiber, a glial cell in the retina (MILLER and DOWLING[31]).

The experiments of WALKER and HILD[32] on mammalian brain cells in culture show low-resistance junctions to exist via glia over distances up to 200 μm. Surprisingly, a similar electrical coupling seems to exist between these glia and certain neurons in the culture which are incapable of action potentials and in still other ways display glia-like properties. Such studies with cultured cells also provide opportunities for verifying and testing the variety of current hypotheses of glial function. It has been shown, for instance, that the impedance of glial clumps is altered by pharmacologically active molecules in the bath (WALKER and TAKENAKA[33]), that enzyme activity increases in astrocytes after Na^+ (but not K^+) additions to the medium (FRIEDE[34]), and that O_2 consumption of glial clumps, but not of nerve cells, declines rapidly in Na^+-free medium and rises two or three-fold when K^+ is added (HERTZ[35]). Such experiments validate evidence available from the electrophysiologists on the sensitivity of glia to K^+ ions, suggest the wide range of metabolic activities that could be initiated in glia by activity of adjacent neurons, and point to the possibility that glia may respond selectively to biologically important molecules. On this last point, ROITBAK,[36] working with cat cortex, has shown that morphine and other analgesics reduce or abolish potentials that seem to originate in glial depolarizations; he hypothesizes on the basis of this evidence that the glia are related to the mechanism of pain since drugs that relieve pain act upon them.

The studies epitomized above illustrate some of the new hypotheses about glia and new experiments upon them which Cajal encouraged 75 years ago. These ideas and experiments have their origins in the inclusive biochemical generalizations, insights into fine structure provided by the electron microscope, and electrophysiological data that have developed during David Rioch's lifetime of devotion to the nervous system. He has seen the view of nervous system function shift from that of all-or-nothing, purely neuronal interactions to the current conception where neurons and glia cooperate to store and deliver the variety of actions which nervous systems produce. If, like Cajal, he applauds what is heuristic in hypothesis, he may well accept the glia-neuron hypothesis, for it has already led to many new and surprising observations on the nervous system.

REFERENCES

1. CAJAL, S. R. Algunas conjeturas sobre el mecanismo anatomico de la idecion asociacion y atencion. *Revta Med. Cirug. práct.* **36**, 497, 1895.
2. CAJAL, S. R. *Histologie du Systeme Nerveux de l'Homme et des Vertebres*, Maloine, Paris, 2 vols. 1909, 1911. Reprinted, Madrid: Consejo Superior de Investigaciones Cientificas, Vol. 1—1952, Vol. II—1955.
3. SCHLEICH, C. L. *Vom Schaltwerk der Gedanken*. S. Fischer Verlag, Berlin, 1918.
4. FRIEDE, R. L. Enzyme histochemistry of neuroglia. In: *Progress In Brain Research, Biology of Neuroglia*, DE ROBERTIS, E. D. and CARREA, R. (Eds.), Vol. 15, p. 35, 1965.
5. KUFFLER, S. W. Neuroglial cells: physiological properties and a potassium mediated effect of neuronal activity on the glial membrane potential. *Proc. R. Soc.* B. **168**, 1, 1967.
6. GOMIRATO, G. and HYDEN, H. A biochemical glia error in the Parkinson disease. *Brain* **86**, 773, 1963.

7. HAMBERGER, A., HYDEN, H. and LANG, P. W. Enzyme changes in neurons and glia during barbiturate sleep. *Science* **151**, 1394, 1966.
8. HYDEN, H. and EGYHAZI, E. Glial RNA changes during a learning experiment in rats. *Proc. natn. Acad. Sci. U.S.A.* **49**, 618, 1963.
9. HYDEN, H. Biochemical changes accompanying learning. In: *The Neurosciences*, QUARTON, G. C., MELNECHUK, T., SCHMITT, F. O. (Eds.), p. 765. The Rockerfeller University Press, New York, 1967.
10. HYDEN, H. RNA in brain cells. In: *The Neurosciences*, QUARTON, G. C., MELNECHUK, T., SCHMITT, F. O. (Eds.), p. 248. The Rockefeller University Press, New York, 1967.
11. KUFFLER, S. W. and NICHOLLS, J. G. The Physiology of Neuroglial Cells. *Ergebn. Physiol.* **57**, 1, 1966.
12. ALTMAN, J. and DAS, G. D. Autoradiographic examination of the effects of enriched environment on the rate of glial multiplication in the adult rat brain. *Nature* **204**, 1161, 1964.
13. DIAMOND, M. C., LAW, F., RHODES, H., LINDNER, B., ROZENSWEIG, M. R., KRECH, D., and BENNETT E. L. Increases in cortical depth and glia numbers in rats subjected to enriched environment. *J. comp. Neurol.* **128**, 117, 1966.
14. MURRAY, M. Effects of dehydration on the rate of proliferation of hypothalamic neuroglia cells. *Expl. Neurol.* **20**, 460, 1968.
15. GRAY, E. G. Ultra-Structure of synapses of the cerebral cortex and of certain specializations of neuroglial membranes. In: *Electron Microscopy In Anatomy*, BOYD, J. D., JOHNSON, F. R., LEVER, J. D. (Eds.), p. 54. Edward Arnold, London, 1961.
16. MUGNAINI, E. and WALBERG, F. Ultrastructure of Neuroglia. *Ergebn. Anat. EntwGesch.* **37**, 194, 1964.
17. SMITH, M. E. The metabolism of myelin lipids. *Adv. Lipid Res.* **5**, 241, 1967.
18. CAUSEY, G. *The Cell of Schwann*. E. & S. Livingston, Edinburgh and London, 1960.
19. PALAY, S. L. Morphology of neuroglial cells. In: *Basic Mechanisms of the Epilepsies*, JASPER, H. H., WARD, A. A. and POPE, A. (Eds.), p. 747. Little, Brown, Boston, 1969.
20. GALAMBOS, R. A glia-neural theory of brain function. *Proc. natn. Acad. Sci. U.S.A.* **47**, 129, 1961.
21. BRIGHTMAN, M. W. and REESE, T. S. Junctions between intimately apposed cell membranes in the vertebrate brain. *J. Cell Biol.* **40**, 648, 1969.
22. COLONNIER, M. and GUILLERY, R. W. Synaptic Organization in the Lateral Geniculate Nucleus of the Monkey. *Z. Zellforsch. mikrosk. Anat.* **62**, 333, 1964.
23. ECCLES, J. C., ITO, M. and SZENTÁGOTHAI, J. *The Cerebellum as a Neuronal Machine*. Springer–Verlag, New York, 1967.
24. NICHOLLS, J. G. and BAYLOR, D. A. Long lasting hyperpolarization after activity of neurons in leech central nervous system. *Science* **162**, 279, 1968.
25. ORKAND, R. K., NICHOLLS, J. G. and KUFFLER, S. W. Effect of nerve impulses on the membrane potential of glial cells in the central nervous system of amphibia. *J. Neurophysiol.* **29**, 788, 1966.
26. ORKAND, R. K. Neuroglial-neuronal interactions. In: *Basic Mechanisms of the Epilepsies*, JASPER, H. H., WARD, A. A. and POPE, A. (Eds.), p. 737. Little, Brown, Boston, 1969.
27. POLLEN, D. A. Discussion on the generation of neocortical potentials. In: *Basic Mechanisms of the Epilepsies*, JASPER, H. H., WARD, A. A. and POPE, A. (Eds.), p. 411. Little, Brown, Boston, 1969.
28. TRACHTENBERG, M. C. and POLLEN, D. A. Neuroglia: biophysical properties and physiologic function. *Science* **167**, 1248, 1970.
29. POLLEN, D. A. and TRACHTENBERG, M. C. Neuroglia: gliosis and focal epilepsy. *Science* **167**, 1252, 1970.
30. CASTELLUCCI, V. F. and GOLDRING, S. Contribution to steady potential shifts of slow depolarization in cells presumed to be glia. *Electroenceph. clin. Neurophysiol.* **28**, 109, 1970.
31. MILLER, R. F. and DOWLING, J. E. Intracellular responses of the Müller (glial) cells of mudpuppy retina: their relation to b-wave of the electroretinogram. *J. Neurophysiol.* **33**, 323, 1970.
32. WALKER, F. and HILD, W. J. Neuroglia electrically coupled to neurons. *Science* **165**, 602, 1969.
33. WALKER, F. D. and TAKENAKA, T. Electric impedance of neuroglia in vitro. *Expl. Neurol.* **11**, 277, 1965.
34. FRIEDE, R. L. The enzymatic response of astrocytes to various ions in vitro. *J. Cell Biol.* **20**, 5, 1964.
35. HERTZ, L. Neuroglial localization of potassium and sodium effects on respiration in brain. *J. Neurochem.* **13**, 1373, 1966.
36. ROITBAK, A. I. Further analysis of slow surface-negative potentials of the cortex: action of X-rays and analgesics. *Acta Biol. exp., Vars.* **29**, 125, 1969.

J. psychiat. Res., 1971, Vol. 8, pp. 225–235. Pergamon Press. Printed in Great Britain.

RECEPTOR CHARACTERISTICS AND CONDUCTION VELOCITIES IN BLADDER AFFERENTS

DAVID L. WINTER

Department of Neurophysiology, Division of Neuropsychiatry, Walter Reed Army Institute of Research, Washington, D.C.

INTRODUCTION

A CLASSIC problem in the neurophysiology of sensory systems has been the correlation of structure with function in peripheral nerves. The physiologic characterization of sensory receptors and the measurement of the fiber diameters and/or conduction velocities of these afferents form the basis for this approach. Conduction velocities have been determined for sensory fibers whose terminations respond to touch,[1-3] hair displacement,[3,4] muscle stretch,[5,6] nociceptive stimuli[7,8] and temperature changes.[9]

In contrast to this relative wealth of information about exteroceptive and proprioceptive inputs, far less is known about structure–function relationships of interoceptive inputs. With the exception of studies on the vagus nerve (reviewed by PAINTAL[10]), there have been few attempts to relate the physiological characteristics of visceral receptors to the conduction velocities or fiber diameters of their parent fibers in other abdominal nerves.[11-13] The present work is an attempt to establish such relationships for sensory receptors in the bladder which send afferents centrally via the sacral plexus and hypogastric nerves.

METHODS

Experiments were carried out in 24 adult cats under pentobarbital sodium (Nembutal) anesthesia. Respiratory rate, EKG, blood pressure, and rectal temperature were monitored by standard transducers. The bladder was routinely exposed by a midline suprapubic incision and the uretha canulated at the bladder neck. Retrograde filling was done through this canula either by hand or at various constant rates by a perfusion pump. Pressure records were obtained through an additional canula in the bladder dome.

Filaments of the pelvic or hypogastric nerve were identified on the bladder surface and followed centrally where they were dissected and cut. Recordings of afferent activity were made from the cut end of the peripheral portion. Conduction velocity studies were made on nerve filaments dissected as far away as possible from the bladder. Recordings were

made from the cut end and electrical stimulation performed on the same filaments adjacent
to the bladder.

Successive division of filaments was carried out until one or a few afferents were clearly
identified as responding to physiological stimulation. Monopolar recordings were made
from platinum electrodes, a high-impedance negative-capacitance electrometer (BAK) and
standard recording equipment. Neuronal activity and pressure recordings were taped and
analyzed later, although certain analyses were done on-line. Data analysis was performed
by a system which consisted of a window-discriminator and a special purpose digital
computer. Single unit identification was determined on the basis of amplitude and
configuration. Computer output for on-line analysis of afferent discharge (total events per
unit time) was recorded on a polygraph.

RESULTS

Afferents responding to three types of physiological stimulation were found. The
adequate stimuli were: (a) stretch or displacement of the detrusor musculature, (b) light
mechanical displacement of the mucosa-submucosa, and (c) very slight displacement or
vibration of the perivesicular tissue.

Detrusor afferents

Over 90 per cent of the units studied responded to stretch of the detrusor musculature.
Adequate stimuli which produced tension changes and neuronal discharge were: filling the
intact bladder with fluids, spontaneous and evoked bladder contractions, and mechanical
distortion of the bladder wall.

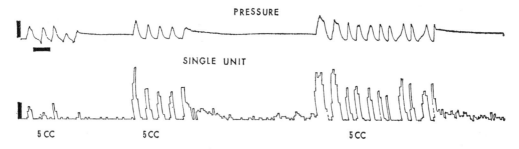

FIG. 1. Response of single detrusor-afferent to rapid filling and emptying of the bladder.
Top line: bladder pressure, calibration 0–20 mm Hg. Bottom line: single-unit firing rate in
spikes/sec, calibration 0–10 spikes. In this and subsequent figures afferent discharges are
presented as total events per sec. Time calibration—10 sec.

Detrusor receptors were silent in the empty bladder and fired in a uniform manner
following tension changes. Figure 1 shows the response of a single unit to filling and
emptying the bladder. In this experiment successive 5cm³ increments were introduced into
and withdrawn from the bladder. The first stimulus was delivered to an empty bladder,

the second and third with 5 and 10cm³ of saline in the bladder, respectively. In this experiment a total of 4 units were identified. The responses of all 4 units are plotted in Fig. 2. Filling, indicated by the solid lines, and emptying, indicated by the various dashed lines, evoked different responses, even though identical pressures were recorded.

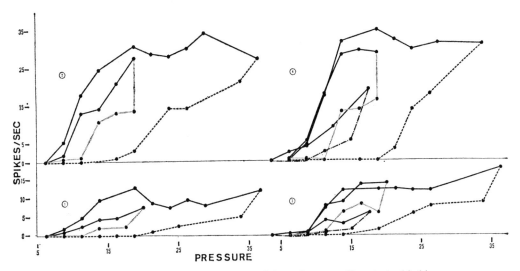

FIG. 2.   Relation of afferent discharge rate of four detrusor-afferents to bladder pressure. Units recorded simultaneously during successive filling and emptying of the bladder. Details in text. Pressure in mm Hg.

Threshold differences are evident for the separate receptors. Units 1 and 2 responded only to the last two fillings while units 3 and 4 responded to all 3 fillings. Each unit responded to the successive filling conditions with an increase in firing rate until a maximum rate was reached. Firing continued at that level in spite of an increase in developing pressure. This maximum firing rate and the pressure level at which it was reached was different for each unit. While the pressure level is not the exclusive stimulus for unit firing, it is referred to here because it was the variable measured. It was not possible to obtain true tension measurements under these conditions.

Detrusor receptors behaved in a similar fashion during spontaneous contractions of the bladder. Figure 3 shows the relationship between pressure and firing rate in a single unit during spontaneous contractions when the bladder contained three different amounts of saline. Again, firing during the increase and decrease of developing pressure is dissociated. This unit was silent between contractions even though the resting pressure level had increased almost ten-fold. When the bladder was filled and emptied by hand, as in Fig. 1, it responded in a manner similar to that observed during spontaneous contractions. This response is indicated by the large filled circles and the left-hand scale. Detrusor receptors, therefore, appear to behave similarly to natural contractions or to an artificial stimulus, differing only in degree.

DAVID L. WINTER

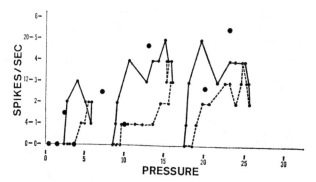

FIG. 3. Relation of afferent discharge rate of single detrusor-afferent to bladder pressure during spontaneous contractions and during experimental filling and emptying. Pressure in mm Hg. Spikes/sec scale on the right for spontaneous contractions, scale on the left for experimental filling and emptying.

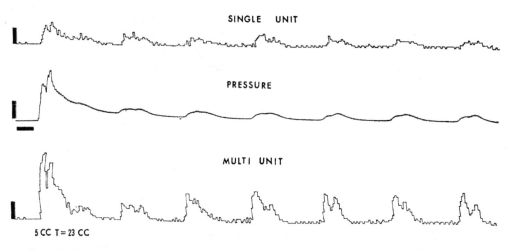

FIG. 4. Response of detrusor afferents to bladder-filling. Top record: single unit response, calibration 0–10 spikes/sec. Middle record: bladder pressure, calibration 0–20 mm Hg. Bottom trace: total response of these units, calibration 0–10 spikes/sec. Time calibration—10 sec.

Responses to filling and spontaneous contractions are shown in Fig. 4. Three different units were recorded simultaneously and the total firing rate of all three is compared to that of one of the three. While the single unit followed the pressure curve rather closely, the multiunit record shows an even more detailed following. All the small changes in the pressure curve are clearly mirrored by variations in the total firing rate. In this example the single unit shown (top line) had the lowest threshold and contributed most to the multiunit record. The other two units fired at higher pressure levels and added detail to the total record. This type of display shows the value of combined single and multiunit analysis in the study of afferent systems.

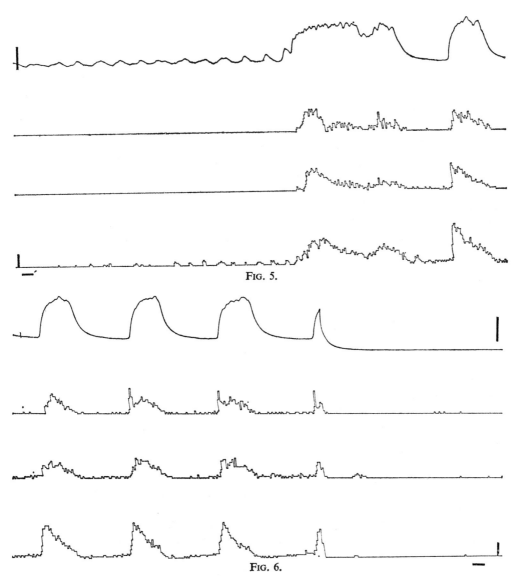

FIG. 5.

FIG. 6.

FIGS. 5 and 6.   Response of three detrusor-afferents to slow filling of the bladder. Top line: bladder pressure, calibration 0–30 mm Hg. Bottom three lines: firing rate of three single units simultaneously recorded; calibration, 0–10 spikes/sec. Time calibration—10 sec, records continuous.

Responses to slow filling

It is important to recognize that hand or machine filling of the bladder under the conditions described above is a highly artificial situation. While stimuli such as these give useful information about how the detrusor receptors *can* respond, they in no way resemble actual conditions that occur in the normal physiological state. To approximate more closely the actual conditions of urine accumulation in the bladder, very slow filling of the bladder was carried out. A vol. of 15–20 cm³ of saline was injected at constant rates over one-half to one hour and the afferent discharges were followed. Figures 5 and 6 illustrate an example of one such experiment.

The typical bladder response was characterized by a series of contractions which slowly increased in amplitude. These contractions gradually became more regular and synchronized, and developed from a slowly rising baseline. Individual units fired, at first irregularly, then on the rising phase of the contractions and finally, as resting pressures became high, in a more tonic fashion with phasic bursts during contractions.

Units with different thresholds were successively activated. Each one followed the same firing pattern sequence but was at a different point in relation to its maximal activation. Bladder contractions varied somewhat from animal to animal and reflected to some degree the depth of anesthesia. There was a tendency towards large prolonged contractions with longer relaxation periods in the animals which, by clinical observations, were more deeply anesthetized. However, the afferent responses bore the same relationship to the contractions, regardless of the nature of these contractions.

Conduction velocities

Conduction velocities were determined on 77 fibers in the sacral plexus and 55 fibers in the hypogastric nerve which responded to bladder filling. All units were initially identified by their response to bladder filling. Electrical stimulation of the nerve filaments as they left the bladder was then carried out, the units were matched and the distance between stimulation and recording electrodes measured. Figure 7 is an example of two such determinations. A shows the response to electrical stimulation while B and C show the same units responding to physiological stimulation. D and E show the response of different units to graded electrical stimulation and F demonstrates their activation by bladder filling. A small unit noted in the center of traces D and E was not clearly identifiable in any of the traces following physiological stimulation.

This technique is successful if the filaments are very small. Since both afferents and efferents are activated by electrical stimulation some confusion can exist when matching units which fire both to bladder filling and to electrical activation unless there are only a few units in the filament.

The histograms of the conduction velocities from both afferent pathways are shown in Fig. 8. Although the hypogastric fibers tend to have slightly lower conduction velocities, the shape of the histograms is rather similar. A few fibers in the sacral plexus, however, were considerably faster than any seen in the hypogastric nerve.

Since the conduction velocities of the fibers had been determined, it was possible to attempt a correlation between spike amplitude and conduction velocity for these afferent fibers. No firm correlation was found. As seen in the two examples of Fig. 7, the large unit in the left-hand column has a higher conduction velocity than the smaller unit, while in the right-hand column, the reverse is true. It is also noted that, in this latter case, the smaller-amplitude unit had a lower electrical threshold than the large amplitude unit. Figure 9 shows other samples in which no firm correlation could be observed between conduction velocity and spike amplitude. An analysis of all units was made, both

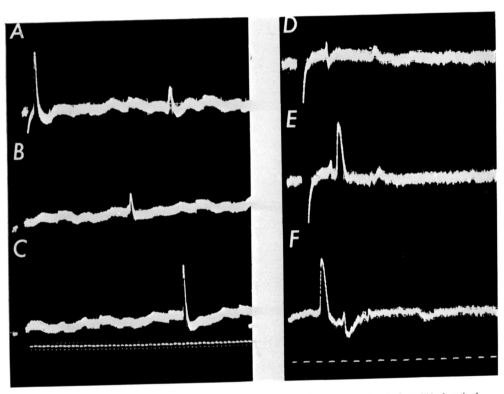

FIG. 7. Response of detrusor afferents to physiological and electrical stimulation. (A) electrical excitation of two afferents. (B) and (C) physiologic excitation of the same units. (D) and (E) electrical excitation of three units with increasing stimulus strength. (F) physiologic excitation of two detrusor afferents. Time calibration—1000 Hz.

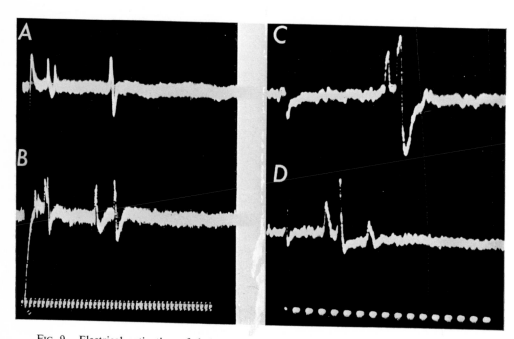

FIG. 9. Electrical activation of detrusor afferents. Four examples in which no correlation between spike amplitude and conduction velocity was found. Time calibration—1000 Hz.

individually, and in groups of two, three or four, depending upon the number observed in the particular filament. There was no statistical significance in a relationship between spike amplitude and conduction velocity either between groups or within a single group. It must be pointed out, however, that the range of conduction velocities under study was rather limited, and one cannot confidently generalize from this narrow range to the situation that may exist when fibers of much higher velocities are considered.

A lack of correlation was also noted between spike amplitude and threshold of afferents responding to bladder filling.

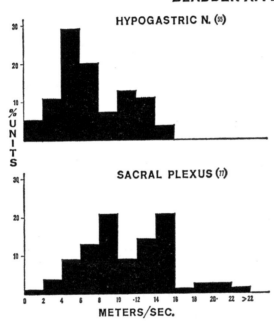

FIG. 8. Conduction velocities of individual detrusor-afferents in the sacral plexus and hypogastric nerve.

Afferents from the mucosa

Light mechanical displacement of the mucosa-submucosa activated a small number of afferent fibers. The usual response of these normally silent fibers was a short burst discharge which rapidly adapted. Various manipulations of stimulus presentations confirmed that the receptive fields were very small, averaging 1–8 mm². While the receptive fields of afferents from the sacral plexus were located throughout the bladder, the largest number were observed in the trigone area. Receptive fields of afferents in the hypogastric nerve were primarily located in the trigone. No outstanding differences in receptive field sizes were noted between the two afferent pathways.

E

The identification of these receptors necessitated opening the bladder. Accordingly, we have no information about the participation of these afferents during bladder filling or contractions.

Conduction velocity measurements were obtained for six such units located in the sacral plexus. Values ranged from 18–22 m/sec.

Afferents from the perivesicular tissue

Occasional units were found which responded to bladder filling but had unusual firing characteristics. After careful search and manipulation, it was found that these units were located in the perivesicular tissue, and were extremely sensitive mechanoreceptors. They generally appeared as tonically firing units which responded strongly to bladder filling but not to sustained pressure within the bladder. Figure 10 is an example of one such unit.

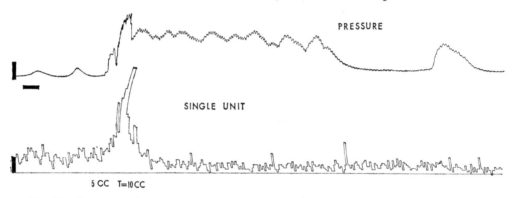

Fig. 10.   Response of perivesicular afferent to bladder-filling. Top line—bladder pressure, calibration 0–20 mm Hg. Bottom line—discharge of single afferent. Note phasic response to filling but lack of response to sustained pressure and spontaneous bladder contraction. Calibration 0–10 spikes/sec. Time calibration—10 sec.

The most characteristic feature of these units was their lack of response to spontaneous contractions of the bladder. The extreme sensitivity of these units could be demonstrated by their response to vibration of the animal by tuning fork or tap, and to blowing air gently over the exposed viscera. In some cases, tapping the recording table was sufficient to excite these extremely sensitive units.

Five such units were encountered during the conduction-velocity studies. They were all located in sacral-plexus filaments and conducted at rates from 25–40 m/sec. None of these units was noted in the hypogastric nerve sample.

It is suggested that these receptors are mechanoreceptors, probably Pacinian corpuscles, which are incidentally stimulated by movement of the bladder itself or movement transmitted through other tissues.

Responses to other, less sensitive mechanoreceptors were observed in hypogastric-nerve filaments. These receptors responded to tissue distension, and the receptive fields of these units were located in the descending colon, the uterus, fallopian tubes, and in connective tissue and fat in the lower abdominal cavity. These receptors were not studied in any detail once their location outside the bladder was established. They were clearly different from those described above in the sacral plexus sample.

DISCUSSION

The great majority of bladder afferents was found to respond to tension changes of the detrusor musculature. As previously demonstrated by TALAAT[14] and IGGO,[15] both active contraction and passive distention are adequate stimuli for the activation of detrusor afferents. There is essentially no receptor activity in the empty bladder. However, with bladder filling and the subsequent development of small spontaneous contractions, afferent activity appears in some units. As filling continues and contractions increase in magnitude, additional afferents are activated as their thresholds are exceeded.

The firing pattern of any single detrusor afferent, in general, follows the pattern of developed pressure within the bladder. However, the combined activity pattern of multiple detrusor afferents very closely follows this pressure record. In all the individual units studied, firing frequency reached some maximum level which was not exceeded in spite of an increase in developing pressure. The multiunit records indicate that the afferent system does not saturate but can transmit information over a very wide range of pressure conditions. This information appears to be very precise as to minor fluctuations in developed pressure. This afferent mechanism is apparently a reflection of the successive recruitment of detrusor receptors with different thresholds which operate over different pressure ranges. This is the same type of mechanism that is seen in the baroceptor system of the carotid sinus.

The conduction-velocity data indicate that most detrusor afferents conduct impulses at rates below 16 m/sec. Although there were no marked differences in conduction velocities between the hypogastric and sacral plexus populations, the hypogastric fibers did conduct more slowly. Considering the differences in length of conduction paths to the spinal cord for these two inputs, the conduction-velocity differences may have some physiological importance. The majority of these conduction velocities fall within the Aδ range (small myelinated fibers), and a few in the C range (unmyelinated fibers). These findings differ from those of IGGO,[16] who, in his studies on cat gastric tension receptors, found conduction velocities primarily in the C range. Although it is difficult to record slowly conducting C fiber potentials, a large number were found in the efferent supply to the bladder under identical recording conditions (Winter, in preparation). It is suspected, therefore, that the afferent conduction velocities presented above are representative of the range of detrusor tension afferents in the cat. These values are similar to those found by LEEK[17] in studies of tension receptors in the sheep rumen. Units which projected centrally via the vagus nerve averaged about 14 and 16 m/sec for the dorsal and ventral vagal trunks respectively.

No relationship was found between conduction velocity and receptor threshold, as estimated by pressure recordings. In multiunit preparations, firing sequences of three, four and five individually identifiable units were studied. There was no correlation between activation sequence and conduction velocity within these groups of units.

Rapidly adapting receptors which responded to gentle mechanical displacement of the mucosa were found throughout the bladder, but most frequently in the trigone. Although care was taken to limit mechanical stimulation to the mucosal-submucosal layers only, the possibility does exist that the stimulus activated receptors lying deeper in the musculature. In the body and fundus of the bladder superficial afferents were infrequent, although detrusor afferents could readily be activated by strong mechanical stimuli. The greatest number of mucosal afferents was found in the trigone region, and these afferents traveled centrally through both the pelvic and hypogastric nerves.

Conduction-velocity measurements were difficult to obtain for the receptors because of technical problems which arose from opening and everting the bladder. Values for the units successfully studied ranged from 18–22 m/sec.

A source of some confusion in the early experiments was the observation of an occasional afferent which exhibited 'spontaneous' activity, increased firing during bladder-filling, and a high conduction velocity. Further study indicated that these receptors were not located in the bladder but in the perivesicular tissue. The essential points in making this distinction were the extreme sensitivity to vibration of the bladder and surrounding tissue and the absence of increased firing during spontaneous contractions. These receptors are probably Pacinian corpuscles which were inadvertently stimulated by bladder filling. The conduction velocities of these units (25–40 m/sec) support this point.

Thus, a spectrum of conduction velocities was found in the afferent nerves of the bladder. There was a tendency for the slowest conducting fibers to be associated with detrusor tension receptors, an overlapping but slightly faster group to be associated with mucosal-submucosal receptors, and the fastest conducting group to be associated with receptors located in the perivesicular tissue. If these conduction velocities are converted into fiber diameters, considering the special case of small myelinated fibers,[13] one can rather closely reconstruct the distribution of myelinated afferent-fiber diameters described for the pelvic nerve.[18]

SUMMARY

A correlation between receptor function and conduction velocity was made for bladder afferents in the anesthetized cat (24). Single-unit recordings were used to identify primary afferents which were activated by physiological and electrical stimulation. Three types of afferents were identified: Detrusor afferents which responded to tension changes in the detrusor musculature; afferents which responded to mechanical distention of the mucosal-submucosal surface; and mechanoreceptors which were located in the perivesicular tissue. Detrusor afferents conducted below 16 m/sec, mucosal afferents between 18 and 22 m/sec, and perivesicular afferents between 25 and 40 m/sec.

Acknowledgement—I wish to thank Mr. Calvin Henson for his superb technical help in carrying out these experiments, Dr. Carl F. Tyner for his critical reading of the manuscript, and Mrs. Catherine Anderson for her patience in the typing of this manuscript.

REFERENCES

1. HUNT, C. C. and McINTYRE, A. K. An analysis of fibre diameter and receptor characteristics of myelinated cutaneous afferent fibres in cat. *J. Physiol., Lond.* **153**, 99, 1960.

2. WERNER, G. and MOUNTCASTLE, V. B. Neural activity in mechanoreceptor cutaneous afferents: Stimulus-response relations, Weber functions, and information transmission. *J. Neurophysiol.* **28**, 359, 1965.
3. JÄNIG, W., SCHMIDT, R. F. and ZIMMERMANN, M. Single unit responses and the total afferent outflow from the cat's footpad upon mechanical stimulation, *Expl Brain Res.* **6**, 100, 1968.
4. BROWN, A. G. and IGGO, A. A quantitative study of cutaneous receptors and afferent fibres in the cat and rabbit. *J. Physiol., Lond.* **193**, 707, 1967.
5. HUNT, C. C. Relation of function to diameter in afferent fibers of muscle nerves. *J. gen. Physiol.* **38**, 117, 1954.
6. FUKAMI, Y. Tonic and phasic muscle spindles in snake. *J. Neurophysiol.* **33**, 28, 1970.
7. PERL, E. R. Myelinated afferent fibres innervating the primate skin and their response to noxious stimuli. *J. Physiol., Lond.* **197**, 593, 1968.
8. BESSOU, P. and PERL, E. R. Response of cutaneous sensory units with unmyelinated fibers to noxious stimuli. *J. Neurophysiol.* **32**, 1025, 1969.
9. HENSEL, H., IGGO, A. and WITT, I. A quantitative study of sensitive cutaneous thermoreceptors with C afferent fibres. *J. Physiol., Lond.*, **153**, 113, 1960.
10. PAINTAL, A. S. Vagal afferent fibres. *Ergebn. Physiol.* **52**, 74, 1963.
11. NIIJIMA, A. The afferent innervation of the kidney and testis of toad. *Jap. J. Physiol.* **9**, 239, 1959.
12. NIIJIMA, A. Afferent impulses from single myelinated fibers in splanchnic nerves, elicited by mechanical stimulation of toads' viscera. *Jap. J. Physiol.* **10**, 42, 1960.
13. BESSOU, P. and PERL, E. R. A movement receptor of the small intestine. *J. Physiol., Lond.* **182**, 404, 1966.
14. TOLAAT, M. Afferent impulses in the nerves supplying the urinary bladder. *J. Physiol., Lond.* **89**, 1, 1937.
15. IGGO, A. Tension receptors in the stomach and the urinary bladder. *J. Physiol., Lond.* **128**, 593, 1955.
16. IGGO, A. The electrophysiological identification of single nerve fibres, with particular reference to the slowest-conducting vagal afferent fibres in the cat. *J. Physiol., Lond.* **142**, 110, 1958.
17. LEEK, B. F. Reticulo-ruminal mechanoreceptors in sheep. *J. Physiol., Lond.* **202**, 585, 1969.
18. PATTON, H. D. Taste Olfaction and Visceral Sensation. In: *Physiology and Biophysics*, RUCH, T. C. and PATTON, H. D. (Eds), p. 372. W. B. Saunders, Philadelphia, 1965.

J. psychiat. Res., 1971, Vol. 8, pp. 237–257. Pergamon Press. Printed in Great Britain.

THE CELLULAR BASIS OF BEHAVIOR IN *APLYSIA*

FELIX STRUMWASSER

Division of Biology, California Institute of Technology, Pasadena, California

HISTORICAL INTRODUCTION

TEN YEARS ago, in June of 1960, I started work on the nervous system of the sea hare, *Aplysia californica*, while spending 6 weeks at the MBL, Woods Hole, as a guest in the laboratory of I. Tasaki and C. Spyropoulos. Those 6 weeks at Woods Hole terminated my official duties with the NIH and started me off in an association with the Department of Neurophysiology at the Walter Reed Army Institute of Research for which, in looking back, I have only fond memories.

The first shipment ever of *Aplysia californica* to cross this country came in a jet to Boston and was packed in Venice, California, by Dr. Rimmon C. Fay.* Both he and I have learned a great deal since those early experiences. In the first shipment, *Aplysia* had been packed with moist sea weed and it took me a few days to appreciate that the sea hares which I had transferred to sea water were not sessile animals but were dead or dying. The peculiar odor that was only apparent on dissection turned out not to be a characteristic of the living *Aplysia*, this fact being determined by the second shipment. Present day shipments of *Aplysia* are made by Dr. Fay in sealed plastic bags filled with sea water and expanded with air to provide oxygen and minimize crushing.

I had come to Woods Hole to receive instruction from Angelique Arvanitaki and her husband Nick Chalazonitis in the methodology of electrophysiological work on the nervous system of *Aplysia*. In 1955, ARVANITAKI and CHALAZONITIS[1] and quite independently, TAUC,[2] had performed the first intracellular recordings from the large neurons of *Aplysia*. Arvanitaki's and Chalazonitis' early interests were in the photoexcitability of certain of the neurons and are well summarized in a 1960 publication.[3] They were late in arriving at Woods Hole and this gave me the opportunity to learn in an inefficient, but creative way, by making mistakes.

I must confess that it was one lecture given at the NIH, some months before, by Arvanitaki, that made me decide then and there that there was nothing more that I wanted to do than to work on the nerve cells of the sea hare. Arvanitaki's presentation, at the lecture, was slow and halting because English is not her native language. This allowed much time for me to observe her beautiful pictures, presented during the lecture, of what

---

* Pacific Bio-Marine Supply Co., P.O. Box 536, Venice, Calif. 90291.

the nerve cells in the parieto-visceral ganglion looked like. If I could be said to have been hypnotized at any time of my life, it was certainly then. In the next few days, while Arvanitaki and Chalazonitis were at the NIH, I remember remaining excited about the possible advantages of the preparation for neurophysiological and behavioral experiments and recall hurried arrangements to collaborate with them in Woods Hole while both they and I were guests of Tasaki and Spyropoulos.

Because of the limited time I had to stay at Woods Hole and because of Arvanitaki's and Chalazonitis' late arrival, I never received the benefits of their instruction, but still filled with excitement I returned to Washington, D.C., and my new home in the Division of Neuropsychiatry at Walter Reed. A significant factor in my being able to work productively on the nervous system of *Aplysia* was the complete and enthusiastic support by Bob Galambos and David Rioch. I remember, only too well, an excited telephone call which I placed, from a public telephone booth on the main street at Woods Hole, to Galambos at his home. As I described my enthusiasm for the preparation and my desire to continue work on it, I received warm and encouraging responses. It is important for senior investigators like Galambos and scientific administrators such as Rioch to realize the importance of their acceptance and flexibility in the management of the young investigator. I owe my greatest debt, during my postdoctoral research period, to Dave Rioch and Bob Galambos for making it so easy for me to think of science instead of how to financially support my research. In all truthfulness, I find my position to be different as a professor at a university—the protected days are clearly over.

THE UTILITY OF STUDYING SIMPLE NERVOUS SYSTEMS

In the remainder of this review I want to outline briefly the major findings from research on *Aplysia* that gives us some insights into the cellular basis of behavior. In addition, I would like to emphasize that studies of invertebrate nervous systems are likely to give us insights into the organization of behavior directly applicable to vertebrates, including man.

An argument can be made that neurons are basically conservative elements. Whether we consider conduction of an impulse or chemical synaptic transmission, the two most commonly studied properties of neurons, the mechanisms have been found to be similar in invertebrate and vertebrate neurons. Sodium and/or calcium ions have been found universally to be responsible for the inward current and subsequent depolarization during a normal action potential, while potassium carries the outward current responsible for repolarization in most systems. The conservative nature of the membrane mechanism can be appreciated when one is reminded that tetrodotoxin blocks the electrically excitable membrane channel that passes sodium in all invertebrate[4] and vertebrate[5] neurons so far examined.

There is a fundamental similarity and simplicity in the range of transmitters that are synthesized by neurons from diverse animal species. Acetylcholine is of course a well established transmitter between nerve and skeletal muscle in the vertebrates. In the invertebrate, *Aplysia*, acetylcholine is a natural transmitter between certain neurons; activation of the postsynaptic membrane receptor by this agent is also blocked by curare,[6] as in vertebrates. The enzyme that synthesizes acetylcholine from acetyl CoA and choline, choline acetyltransferase, is extractable from both systems.[7] Of course there are many other fairly well-established transmitters—GABA, norepinephrine, glycine, serotonin (5-hydroxy-tryptamine), and glutamate. The neuromuscular junction of crustaceans utilizes glutamate for excitation[8] and GABA for inhibition[9,10] while the basket cell inhibition of Purkinje neurons in the vertebrate cerebellum appears to be induced by GABA[11]. It is only a matter of a short time before we will know whether the postsynaptic membrane receptors of invertebrate and vertebrate neurons are pharmacologically identical,* but all the present evidence indicates that they are quite similar in most cases.[12,13] The ability to generalize about the principles, and even details of mechanism, of nervous action between invertebrates and vertebrates should give us hope that similar principles concerning the neural basis of behavior can be discovered from the invertebrates.

THE SEA HARE, *APLYSIA*

The sea hare, *Aplysia*, an opisthobranch mollusk, has a distributed nervous system. There are eight discrete ganglia which are interconnected by commissures or connectives. These eight ganglia together probably contain a total of 10–20,000 neurons. The number of peripheral neurons, which includes at least sensory and motor elements (for example in the gill[14]) and perhaps even interneurons, is unknown. However, a reasonable guess would bring the total number of neurons in this organism to around 50,000 at a minimum. That number represents one quarter of the total number of motoneurons estimated for man.[15] With these 50,000 neurons the sea hare finds particular plant foods in its marine environment,[16] evades predators, sleeps and wakes with a circadian cycle similar to our own, mates with other *Aplysia* but only during summer and fall, can perform a variety of learned tasks[17,18] and probably migrates.

REPRODUCTIVE BEHAVIOR

Two symmetrical clusters of neurosecretory neurons (termed bag cells[19]) have been shown by KUPFERMANN[20] and my laboratory[21,22] to produce a product which when injected into recipients causes egg-laying with correlated behavior. The product has been shown by two of my students, TOEVS and BRACKENBURY,[23] to be a polypeptide with a molecular weight about 6000.[24] Within the first 15 min after injection of a crude sea-water extract of the parieto-visceral (abdominal) ganglion into an adult sea hare, the active recipient usually climbs a vertical wall and becomes quiet. Within an hour from this phase, the sea hare begins to extrude eggs, in the form of an egg-string, along the spermatic groove (an external channel on the right side of its body), and winds the eggs with its mouth onto the surface of the tank (Fig. 1). Recently, ARCH,[25] in my laboratory, has demonstrated the release of

---

* This means that the *active sites* on the receptor molecule are similar enough, between different animal groups, to be blocked by the same pharmacological agents.

radioactively labeled polypeptide from the isolated PVG upon potassium- or electrically-induced depolarization of the entire ganglion or bag cell clusters. The polypeptide is not released in the absence of calcium in the perfusion fluid which is in agreement with the general principles of excitation–secretion coupling.[26] Since the released labeled polypeptide runs, on electrophoresis, in a position identical with the bag-cell specific polypeptide, the evidence is now excellent that this is the major product of these cells and that the neurosecretion functions to induce egg-laying.

In spite of a great deal of past controversy, neurosecretion is now an accepted phenomenon even for vertebrates. The neurons of the vertebrate supraoptic nucleus synthesize vasopressin (antidiuretic hormone) which is a polypeptide and those of the paraventricular nucleus probably synthesize oxytocin which is also a polypeptide.[27] While these neurohormones are entirely peripheral and metabolic or neuromuscular, as far as site and mechanism of action, it is not unlikely that the egg-laying neurohormone induces the behavioral phase of egg-laying (termination of locomotor activity or quiescence) by a direct action on key central neurons.

SLEEP AND WAKING

Sleep,* as a behavioral phenomenon, clearly occurs in *Aplysia*. (This was demonstrated with a time lapse movie during the symposium.) The California sea hare, under laboratory conditions, is day active (or diurnal),[28–30] typically rising around dawn when it becomes very active in search of food. By dusk it stops locomoting, contracts, goes to sleep, and exhibits head and tentacle movements during the night. Such night movements may be the evolutionary precursors of the so-called REM (rapid eye movement) sleep in mammals.†
Time lapse movies demonstrate that the sea hare will return to a particular location in the marine tank to sleep and will check a food dish on rising, even when there is no food, providing that it had been exposed to food in that dish recently. I suspect that sleep in *Aplysia* may be controlled, as is egg-laying, by a neurosecretory product for there is a circadian rhythm of impulse activity in an identifiable neurosecretory cell (the parabolic burster), a discovery which I first made while at Walter Reed[31] and which has been confirmed by one of my past associates, LICKEY.[32]

Studies of the locomotor behavior of the sea hare were conducted together with Mr. CARY LU in 1965–1966.[28] In these studies, continuous time lapse movies were taken of one or two sea hares in a divided 100 gal tank of flowing, temperature-controlled sea water. The sea hares were studied in isolation from each other. Pictures were taken with a 35 mm kymograph camera at automatic framing rates of 1 per 1·5 min or 1 per 3 min. The sea

---

* The term 'sleep' is used in this paper as a convenient short hand expression for a continuous state of relatively motionless behavior. It is realized that tests are needed to determine whether a state of decreased sensitivity to sensory input also exists in this organism, as it appears to exist in mammals during their sleep.

† We have so little knowledge of the phenomenology of sleep in lower vertebrates and particularly in the invertebrates, that while we should be cautious about making such analogies, we should be equally reserved about the notion that REM during mammalian sleep, and its implications, are unique phenomena to organisms with a cerebral cortex.

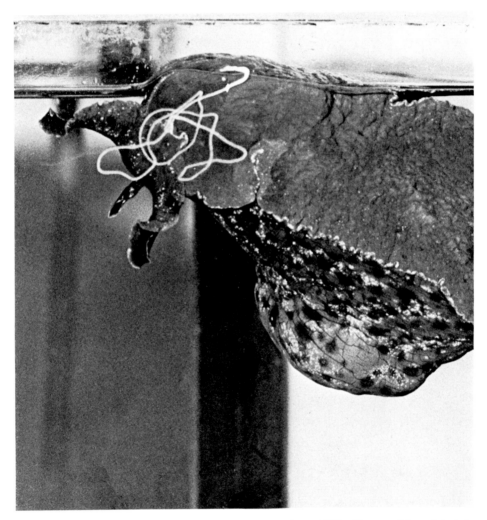

FIG. 1.   Egg-laying induced by a sea water extract of two intact PVGs. The material was injected into the haemocoel through the anterior third of the foot of the recipient. The sea hare is on the vertical glass wall of an aquarium and was photographed 60 min after the injection. Egg-laying had started 10 min prior to the photograph. (From STRUMWASSER, JACKLET and ALVAREZ, 1969.[22])

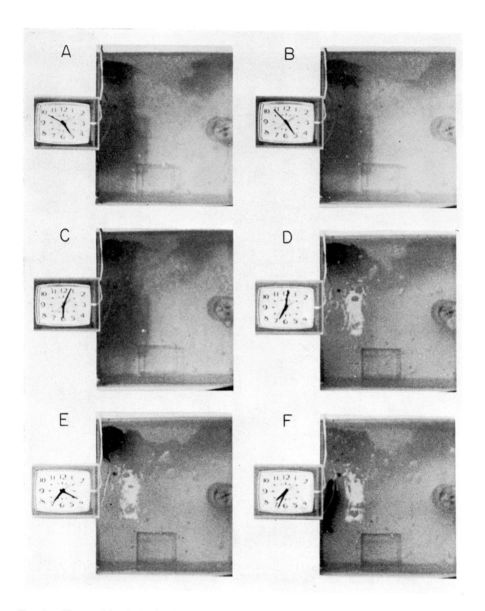

FIG. 2. Sleep-waking behavior in the sea hare, *Aplysia californica*. Six frames from a time lapse movie, all taken between 4.50–7.34 a.m. The sea hare was under light-dark entrainment; lights were on from 7 a.m. to 7 p.m. A, B and C were obtained during the dark period, while D, E and F were obtained during the light period. (See text for further details.)

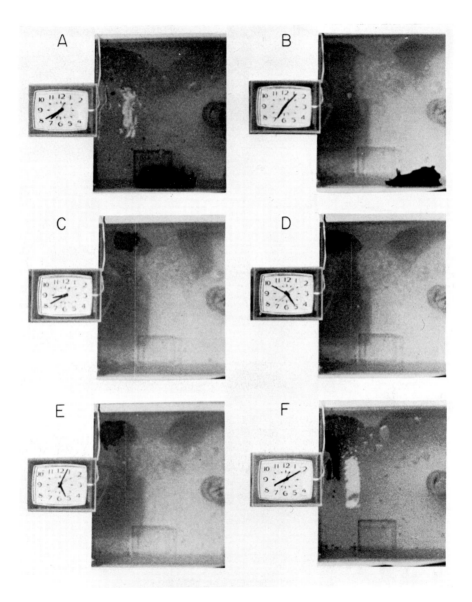

Fɪɢ. 3. Sleep-waking behavior in the sea hare, *Aplysia californica*. These six frames are a continuation, using the same animal, from Fig. 2. Frames A to F were obtained between 6.40 p.m. and 8.10 a.m. of the next day. B through E were taken during the artificial night, while A and F were taken during the artificial day. (See text for further details.)

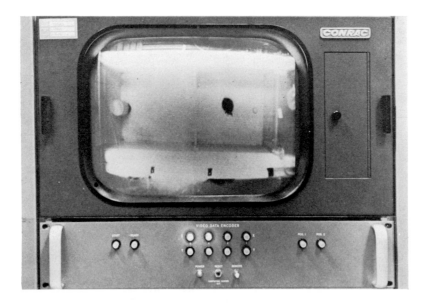

FIG. 4a. Top view (taken by TV camera) of 100 gal tank with animal (*Aplysia californica*) in right compartment. The video data encoder is immediately below monitor.

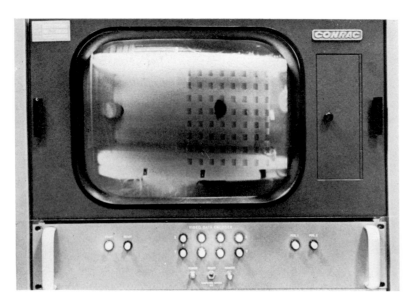

FIG. 4b. Encoder determines position of animal as $x = 7$, $y = 6$. 15 × 15 matrix allows operator to confirm reading and alignment.

days in vitro

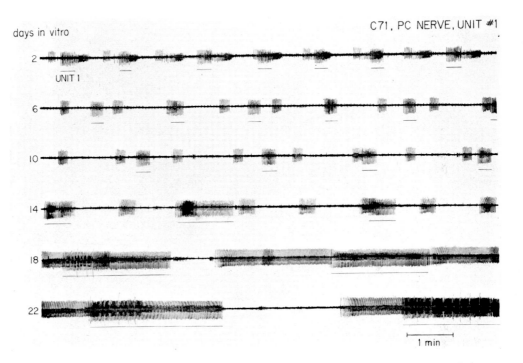

FIG. 13. Long-term extracellular recordings of axonal (unit) discharges from the PVG in organ culture. The isolated PVG was cultured in Eagle's Minimum Essential Medium made up in sea water containing 20 per cent *Aplysia* blood.[37] Polygraph records were obtained continuously over a 42 day period from the pericardial nerve by means of a nerve cuff (see text for further details). Each line is a 10 min sample taken around midnight of the day *in vitro* indicated in the left column. Unit No. 1 is identified by a line just below each of its bursts. Temperature was maintained at $13°C \pm 1°$.

water was kept at 14°C and the room was artificially lighted by 'warm white' fluorescent lights for 12 hr followed by 12 hr of darkness. Each time the shutter of the camera was opened a strobe flashed regardless of whether it was artificial night or day. A clock in the center of the tank allowed time identification of each frame. Since the sea hares became inactive during the artificial night, it appears as if the bright flash of the strobe, at least at rates of 1 flash every 1·5 min, did not significantly alter the animal's interpretation of night.

Figures 2 and 3 illustrate 12 frames of a 2-day period during which the artificial day extended from 7 a.m. to 7 p.m. Frame A (Fig. 2) taken at 4.50 a.m. shows the animal (upper left corner) contracted in the typical sleeping position. The very next frame (B), taken 3 min later, reveals one of the head movements which intermittently occurs during sleep. At 6.04 a.m. (C), as well as at 7 a.m. (D), when the room lights have come on, the animal is still asleep. The first stretch, associated with awakening, takes place 20 min after the onset of light (frame E). Some sea hares are systematic late risers, such as this one; others systematically anticipate dawn (see Fig. 5). Some 14 min after the first stretch (34 min after light onset), the animal is clearly moving away from the sleeping area (frame F).

A few minutes later (Fig. 3A), the animal has reached the feeding bowl area (for the first time since awakening) and is shown passing above it. The animal remains active, by circumnavigating the tank, for more than 12 hrs. At 7.07 p.m., just after the start of the artificial night, the animal is still actively moving around (frame B). The animal arrived at the regular sleeping area at 7.55 p.m. and is shown in the typical contracted position of sleep at 8.40 p.m. (frame C). Frames D and E show the animal still asleep at 4.50 a.m. and 5.04 a.m., respectively, and another example of a head movement during sleep is shown in the latter frame. The first movement away from the sleeping area occurs at 8.10 a.m., some 36 min later than the previous day.

These studies of sleep-waking behavior have allowed us to conclude that sleep is a regular and continuous phenomenon in the sea hare as in the more complex vertebrates, that there are periodic head and tentacle movements during sleep, perhaps equivalent to the REM phase of mammalian sleep, and that sleep is entrainable to photoperiod.

NEWER METHODS IN THE STUDY OF SLEEP

More recent studies of sleep and locomotor behavior have been performed by an automated system developed together with Mr. James Elliott of the CIT Computing Center. A television camera is used to obtain an electrical analog signal of the animal in the tank. A special device, a video encoder, analyzes the line-by-line signal making up a TV frame. When a sufficient number of contiguous scanning lines of the TV frame have voltage information above an adjustable threshold, the co-ordinates are stored and are used to determine the location of the animal. The transit time of the line sweep, until criterion is met, gives the X co-ordinate. The Y co-ordinate is proportional to the center line number of the set of lines that include the animal. In actual practice the field of the tank over which one animal moves is divided into a 15×15 co-ordinate grid.

Figure 4a shows the view taken by the TV camera. The video data encoder is immediately below the TV monitor. Figure 4b shows the electronically superimposed grid which allows the experimenter to confirm a reading. In this figure the position of the animal has been determined by the encoder as $X = 7$, $Y = 6$. In normal operation, the video encoder reports the position co-ordinates once every minute to a digital computer and a program in the computer stores the data for later processing. Programs are available to print out, automatically, position data and to compute smoothed velocities from the data matrix. Plots of movement as a function of time are produced by a digital plotter controlled by the computer.

A biological question that arises concerning sleep–waking behavior in the sea hare is the extent to which the movements of the animal during the day are a direct response to the onset and presence of light. Figure 5 clearly shows that the onset of light (or darkness) does not produce (or inhibit) the animal's movements in a simple reflex manner. After several days of light/dark entrainment (12 hr on, 12 hr off), of which the last 2 days are shown (calendar days 61 and 62), the lights are not turned off at the end of the light period for day 62 (at the arrow). Although the lights were not turned off, the animal sleeps or rests during the projected night as is evident by the virtually zero movement during the first part of day 63. It is interesting that the animal anticipates dawn much earlier than usual and that this behavior carried over into days 64 and 65. For the first three days of con-tinuous light the animal wakes up with a *free-running period* of approximately 20 hr. This finding indicates that the sleep-waking cycle is driven by a circadian oscillator of endogenous origin.

After these three days, the animal becomes virtually continuously active (calendar day 66). At this stage one would predict that if the animal were simply responding to light as a stimulus in a reflex way, that turning off the light (to restart DL cycles) would im-mediately stop the locomotor activity. However, as the recording of day 66 shows, turning off the light at the projected night onset (arrow) does not inhibit the locomotor movements which continue for several hours. Within the $\frac{1}{2}$ cycle of the first new night, the animal is able to anticipate slightly the onset of the new dawn. However, it is extremely interesting that active locomotion persists during the second new night (day 68) and requires at least two or three more entrainment cycles before it is dissipated.

The response of the sleep-waking system to 3 days of continuous light is to first produce an acceleration in the *free-running period* which culminates in essentially continuous activity. The slow build-up of the system, requiring three days before continuous activity emerges, suggests a humoral coupling somewhere between the reception of light and the locomotor output. This argument can also account for the fact that several nights are required before night locomotion is extinguished after reintroduction of the old photoperiod.

A CIRCADIAN RHYTHM IN THE EYE OF *APLYSIA*

The suggestion made above of a humoral coupling between the reception of light and the locomotor output brings up the question of the nature of light reception in *Aplysia*. The sea hare has two small eyes, each located slightly anterior to the rhinophore on either

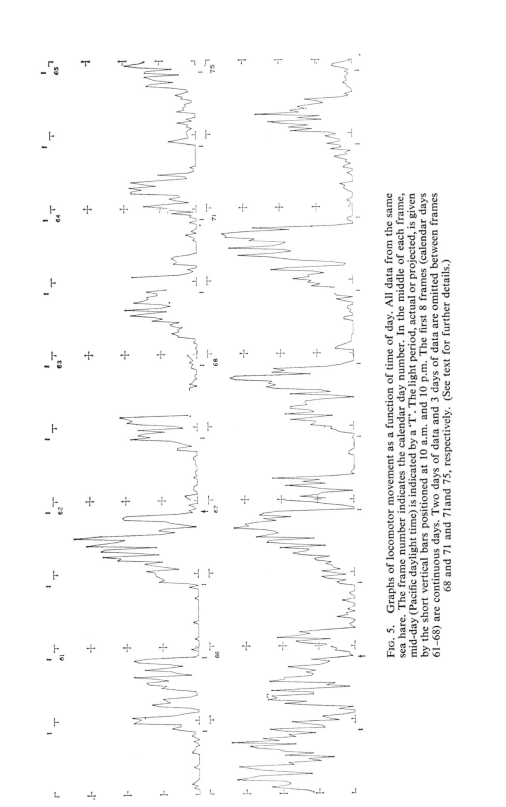

Fig. 5. Graphs of locomotor movement as a function of time of day. All data from the same sea hare. The frame number indicates the calendar day number. In the middle of each frame, mid-day (Pacific daylight time) is indicated by a 'T'. The light period, actual or projected, is given by the short vertical bars positioned at 10 a.m. and 10 p.m. The first 8 frames (calendar days 61–68) are continuous days. Two days of data and 3 days of data are omitted between frames 68 and 71 and 71and 75, respectively. (See text for further details.)

side of the body. The eye is connected via the optic nerve to the cerebral ganglion. JACKLET,[33] working in my laboratory, demonstrated that the output spikes recorded from the optic nerve of the eye, are in the form of compound action potentials, that is, the output elements are normally synchronized when they discharge. The spectral sensitivity of the sea hare's eye has been measured by WASER,[34] using the compound spikes in the optic nerve. He found that while sensitivity fell markedly at wavelengths above 600 mμ, it extended all the way down to the near u.v. There are at least three types of neurons of functional interest in the eye. The photoreceptor is of the microvillous type and while it is depolarized by light in a graded fashion, there is no convincing evidence that it can support an action potential.[33] There are second order elements in the eye classifiable according to the usual permutations of responses to light: excited at ON, inhibited at ON, excited at OFF, possibly inhibited at OFF, and certain combinations of these. Certain of these second order neurons have spikes, that correlate with the compound action potentials of the optic nerve, which occur either spontaneously in darkness or in response to a light stimulus. Some of the second order elements in the eye contain neurosecretory granules, based on electronmicroscopic criteria.[33] The situation remains unclear as to what proportion of the second order neurons project in the optic nerve to the cerebral ganglion and as to whether the neurosecretory neurons release their neurosecretion within the eye and/or within the cerebral ganglion.

Interest in the eye exists not only because it is a light receptor and can therefore act as a mediator of photoperiodic entrainment of the sleep-waking cycle, but also because it possesses a circadian rhythm. JACKLET[35] showed that there was a large circadian rhythm in the rate of optic nerve compound action potentials from the isolated eye under conditions of constant darkness. If the eyes had been isolated from sea hares entrained to a light/dark cycle, then the onset of spiking anticipated the *projected* onset of day and this activity declined before the *projected* onset of night. This important finding correlates with the diurnal behavior of the sea hare's arousal from sleep and subsequent locomotion. It also correlates with the circadian activity cycle of the parabolic burster, a neurosecretory neuron in the parieto-visceral ganglion that will be discussed later. This was the first demonstration that a sense organ, in isolation from light input and controls from the rest of the organism, possesses a marked circadian rhythm. A function of the circadian rhythm may be to arouse the animal in an anticipatory fashion (prior to the normal day) through a direct neural connection or an indirect neurosecretory mediation.

There are a number of unresolved questions concerning the neural relations between the eyes, the cerebral ganglion and the rest of the central nervous system in the sea hare. The precise projection of visual information within the cerebral ganglion and the rest of the nervous system remains unknown. Recent experiments, in my laboratory, by ESKIN[36] and AUDESIRK indicate that there is a centrifugal, inhibitory influence from the cerebral ganglion to the eye. In preparations where the eye is connected to the cerebral ganglion, the centripetal optic nerve compound action potentials have a certain amount of irregularity which disappears on cooling the cerebral ganglion. Cooling causes the disappearance of the centrifugal spikes emanating from the cerebral ganglion. These spikes are small and, at normal temperatures, can still be recorded after the eye has been disconnected.

Since a circadian rhythm of optic nerve impulses occurs in the isolated *Aplysia* eye, it was important to establish whether entrainment to photoperiods could occur *in vitro*.

ESKIN,[36] has demonstrated that eyes can be maintained in a healthy state in an organ culture medium[37] for 9 or more days (Fig. 6). The right and left eyes were dissected from a group of sea hares that had been entrained to a LD cycle (12:12 hr). Each eye was independently organ-cultured and exposed to a photoperiod. Certain eyes were exposed to

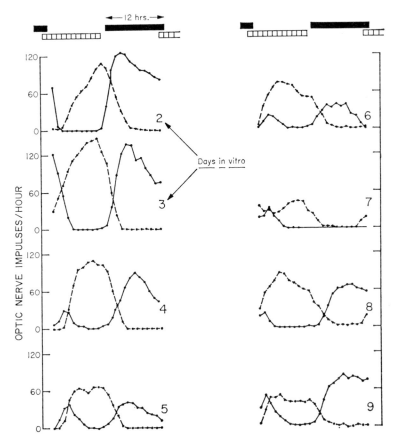

FIG. 6. *In vitro* entrainment of the circadian rhythm of optic nerve impulses in the isolated eye of *Aplysia californica*. Eyes were removed on day 1 from intact sea hares that had been exposed to an LD schedule shown as the solid black rectangles (black rectangle = lights on). Half the group were maintained on this schedule *in vitro* (control group, solid line graph). The remainder of the eyes were exposed to an LD schedule 13 hr out of phase with respect to the onset of light (dash line represents the graph for this group and sectioned rectangle indicates period of lights on). (From ESKIN, 1971.[36])

the old photoperiod, while the contralateral eyes were exposed to a photoperiod 13 hr out of phase with respect to light onset. A pair of eyes from the same donor, one right and one left, were removed from organ culture daily and recordings of the optic nerve impulses were made under constant dark conditions using suction electrodes. Eskin found that after one cycle of the new photoperiod, eyes had already phase-shifted somewhat from the old schedule (dashed curve, day 2). Two or three more days of entrainment were required before the phase advance reached a steady state. These results clearly indicate that the mechanism of entrainment, as well as the circadian rhythm itself, are contained within the eye.

A CIRCADIAN RHYTHM IN A SINGLE NEUROSECRETORY NEURON

I demonstrated, while working at the Walter Reed, that an identifiable neurosecretory neuron in the isolated parieto-visceral ganglion (PVG) produced a circadian rhythm of impulse activity. This neuron, when active, produces groups or bursts of impulses separated by silent periods. Since the successive intervals between impulses during a burst formed a parabola (convex down) as a function of time, I called this neuron the parabolic burster (PB)*. When the PB is studied by means of intracellular recording in an isolated PVG, maximum impulse activity is correlated with projected dawn if the donor sea hare had been exposed to light/dark cycles. When these findings were published in 1965,[31] there was some question as to whether the circadian rhythm was truly endogenous to this neuron. Phase-shifting experiments had been performed to demonstrate that the faster microcycle of bursting was indeed endogenous to the neuron. In these experiments it had been demonstrated that suppression of a burst, by transmembrane hyperpolarization, phase-advanced the onset of the subsequent burst. However, the only evidence that the circadian cycle was also endogenous to this neuron was the observation that phase-shifts could be produced by intracellular injection of Actinomycin D, an inhibitor of DNA-dependent RNA synthesis.

The ideal experiment to test whether the circadian rhythm is endogenous to the cell would be the total isolation, by dissection, of the PB from the ganglion. Negative evidence would not be convincing since in such a procedure the neurite emerging from the cell would have to be severed and the trauma may inhibit the response. In addition, it would be very difficult, perhaps impossible, to remove all of the glia covering the soma and neurite because they invaginate the surface of this neuron.

However, it is possible to isolate a neuron pharmacologically by blocking synaptic transmission and by blocking impulse activity in all of the cells of the ganglion.[39] I have used tetrodotoxin (TTX) to block the sodium-dependent impulses and used an artificial zero calcium sea water to block synaptic transmission and the calcium-dependent impulses,[40] in the ganglion. The combination of TTX and zero calcium are highly effective in blocking interneuronal transmitter-mediated and electrically-coupled activity as is evidenced by the total suppression of all impulse activity in the various nerve trunks. An intracellular recording from the PB, under these pharmacological conditions, reveals approximately 30 mV membrane potential oscillations with a period similar to that of the bursting cycle before pharmacological manipulation (Fig. 7). These self-sustained oscillations of membrane potential must be the driving force producing the pattern of impulse output. The impulses then appear to be a very secondary type of process.

---

* R15 of FRAZIER et al.[38]

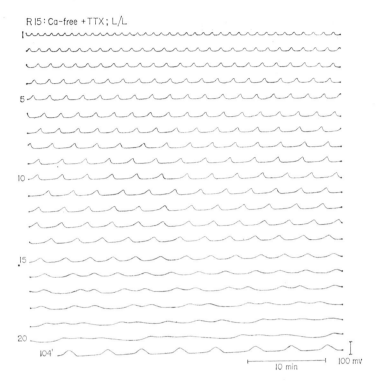

R 15 : Ca-free + TTX ; L/L

10 min   100 mv

FIG. 7. Continuous intracellular recording from the parabolic burster in the presence of calcium-free artificial sea water and tetrodotoxin (25 μg/ml.). The parieto-visceral ganglion, in which the parabolic burster is located, was obtained from a sea hare, *Aplysia californica*, that had been kept in constant light for about 1 week. Record reads from top to bottom; Nos. 1–20 on left are line numbers; each line is 40 min long. 104 min are skipped between line 20 and the last line. The last line shows that the oscillations can be restored in amplitude by moderately hyperpolarizing the membrane. 100 mV calibration applies to all lines. Chamber temperature was 14°C.

The self-sustained membrane potential oscillations of the PB (under the pharmacological conditions of TTX and calcium-free artificial sea water) run continuously, but slowly decrease in frequency as is evident from the 16 hr intracellular recording illustrated in Fig. 7. Such recordings are typical of PBs whose ganglia have been obtained from sea hares kept in constant light. In contrast, intracellular recordings from PBs in isolated PVGs, obtained from sea hares kept under entrainment by light/dark cycles, show a cycle consisting of long periods of silence followed by self-sustained oscillations and then another period of silence as in Fig. 8. As is evident from Fig. 8, the activity of the PB is more complicated (than when measured from an LL sea hare) in that it can produce self-sustained oscillations or silence, the timing of which depends on the past environmental photoperiod. In addition, the record of Fig. 8 shows many square step-like oscillations which are not as simple to

F

account for, in terms of mechanism, as are the continuous oscillations. TTX and the calcium-free artificial sea water produce a significant phase shift as to the onset of activity. In the record of Fig. 8, the onset of activity (self-sustained oscillations) occurs at the projected offset of day or with a 180° phase shift from normal. The nature of this phase shift needs to be worked out.

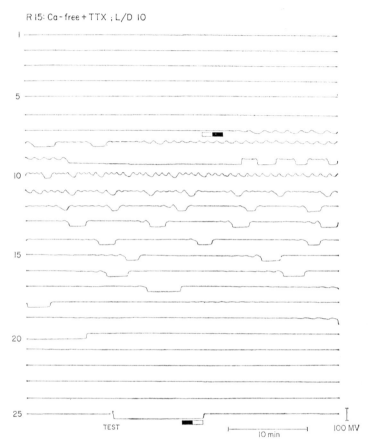

FIG. 8. Continuous intracellular recording from the parabolic burster in the presence of calcium-free artificial sea water and tetrodotoxin (25 μg/ml.). The ganglion was obtained from a sea hare that had been kept in LD cycles (12:12) for 10 days. Projected LD cycle indicated on lines 7 (lights out) and 25 (lights on). Record reads from top to bottom; Nos 1–25 on left are line numbers; each line is 40 min long. The last line shows that although oscillations of the membrane potential have stopped, initiation of a step to a hyperpolarized state can still be induced by application of a short depolarizing current at 'TEST' (see STRUMWASSER, 1967[42]). 100 mV calibration applies to all lines. Chamber temperature was 14°C.

Cells that do not normally produce endogenous activity (such as the giant cell, R2), do not produce any self-sustained oscillations under the conditions of TTX and calcium-free artificial sea water (Fig. 9). However, other neurons in the PVG, producing endogenous impulse bursts, produce self-sustained oscillations under these pharmacological conditions. The waveform of these oscillations, as in L4, may be quite different from that of the PB.

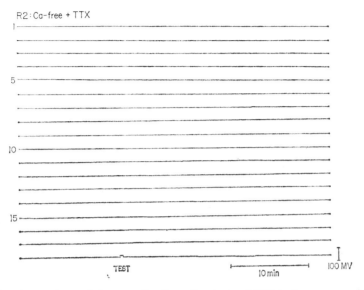

FIG. 9. Continuous intracellular recording from the giant cell (R2) in the presence of calcium-free artificial sea water and tetrodotoxin (25 μg/ml.). Record reads from top to bottom; Nos. 1–18 on left are line numbers; each line is 40 min long. The last line shows that the application of a short depolarizing current at 'TEST' does not induce a step to a hyperpolarized state as in the PB (see Fig. 8). 100 mV calibration applies to all lines. Chamber temperature was 14°C.

Some information has been obtained concerning the nature of the self-sustained oscillations in the PB.[41] A reduction of the sodium in artificial sea water by 40 per cent is sufficient to block these oscillations (Strumwasser and Kim, unpublished). The oscillations also depend on chloride since substitution with impermeant anions, such as acetate or propionate, also blocks oscillations.[41,42] The endogenous oscillations are also blocked by Ouabain at 10^{-4}M concentration, this effect only being reversible within the first 10–15 min.[41] Applied hyperpolarizing current increases the amplitude and decreases the frequency of such endogenous oscillations while applied depolarizing current has the opposite effect.[39]

STRUMWASSER and KIM[39] have produced a model that can quantitatively account for the endogenous oscillations. The model assumes that the PB neuron has a high resting sodium conductance (g_{Na}) and that an electrogenic sodium pump extrudes sodium from within the cell. In order to account for the dependency of the oscillations on external chloride, the model further assumes that internal sodium (Na) can only be pumped out in combination with, or dependent on, the presence of internal chloride. The model has three essential components: (1) a standard nerve membrane with separate channels for Na and K, however with g_{Na} and g_K fixed (electrically inexcitable) but adjusted to give a V_M of -30 mV; (2) a Na-Cl hyperpolarizing electrogenic pump which is activated by [Na$^+$] at the inner membrane surface (*im*). Pump rate as a function of [Na$^+$]$_{im}$ was assigned counterclockwise asymmetrical hysteresis and first-order kinetics was assumed; (3) $[Na^+]_{im}$ was calculated from considerations of diffusion and its dynamics was approximated by a fourth-order ordinary differential equation. The three components and their coupling are illustrated by transfer function notation in Fig. 10. According to the model the existence of oscillations is critically dependent on the slope of the hysteresis curve and the amplitude and the frequency of the oscillations are a function of the hysteresis interval.

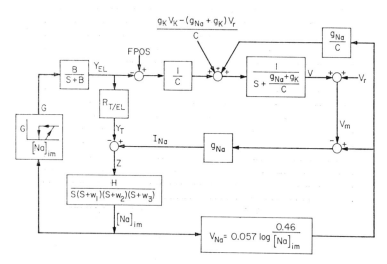

Fig. 10. Block diagram of the quantitative model accounting for endogenous pacemaker oscillations. The diagram follows the conventions of transfer function notation where S is the Laplacian operator, the boxes are the multiplier functions, and the circles are summing points. V_r and V_m are the initial and running values of the nerve membrane potential, respectively. V_{Na} and V_K are the equilibrium potentials for sodium and potassium across the membrane. C is the membrane capacitance and g_{Na} and g_K are the membrane conductances for sodium and potassium, respectively. $[Na]_{im}$ is the internal sodium concentration at the inner membrane surface. G is the value of the Na-Cl coupled electrogenic pump current. B is a rate constant for activation of the electrogenic pump. Y_T represents the rate of total sodium moved across the membrane, whereas Y_{EL} represents that portion of the sodium that is electrogenic (uncoupled to chloride). W_1, W_2, and W_3 are coefficients of the fourth-order ordinary differential equation.

H depends on cell diameter, and with a cell of 150 μ dia., $\dfrac{H}{W_1 \cdot W_2 \cdot W_3}$ has a value of 5860 molar/coulomb. FPOS is the applied current. (From STRUMWASSER and KIM, unpublished.)

The self-sustained oscillations, as generated by the model, are shown in Fig. 11. By adjusting parameters to physiologically reasonable values, the membrane potential is found to oscillate with an amplitude and period similar to that observed in actual experiments on the PB. As the cell radius is decreased in the simulation, the frequency of oscillations increases and below a 60 μ radius the amplitude decreases. The results from the model tell us that if an average sized cell has a high resting sodium conductance and an electrogenic sodium pump, oscillations can be expected. This will occur providing that the cell is not too small and providing that the dependence of the pump rate on $[Na]_{im}$ has a certain critical slope. In other words, from the results of the model, none of the complexity of the electrically excitable membrane (such as the voltage and time dependent g_{Na} and g_K utilized in producing the spike) is essential to produce pacemaker oscillations.

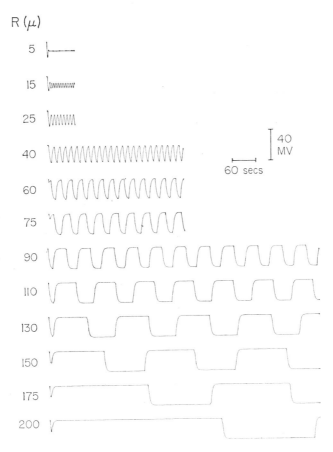

FIG. 11. Computed membrane potential oscillations as a function of time and cell radius. Calculations performed by a program written for a digital computer (IBM 360/75) using the model illustrated in Fig. 10. In these computations the lumped membrane conductance was left fixed at 3×10^{-7} mho, regardless of the cell size. (See text for further details.) (From STRUMWASSER and KIM, unpublished).

The quantitative model does not attempt to account for the circadian rhythm in the PB. However, our work on the model has suggested at least two possible mechanisms for starting (or stopping) endogenous oscillations. If the resting sodium conductance is not sufficiently high, then oscillations do not occur. One mechanism for this type of control would be to allow the resting sodium conductance of the membrane to be under dynamic control *from within the cell*, for example, through a small molecule that can block or unblock g_{Na}. Another suggestion, from work on the model, as to suppressing oscillations is the translation of the pump rate/$[Na]_{im}$ function along the abscissa so that the control curve is to the right of the normal range of $[Na]_{im}$. Again, an internal control could account for such a mechanism by the clock-coupled selective biosynthesis of a molecule which binds with and alters the properties of the membrane ATPase[43] associated with the pump.

THE RELEVANCE OF INTRACELLULAR NEURONAL CONTROLS

The presence of a circadian rhythm in a system of neurons, such as the eye, or in a single neurosecretory neuron of the parieto-visceral ganglion, such as the parabolic burster, provides the possible basis for the temporal organization and continuity of behavior, a problem not evidently answered by our current neurophysiological concepts. Because cellular neurophysiology has overemphasized the membrane of the nerve cell as the site of 'where the (interesting) action is', the inside of the nerve cell has been, by comparison, badly neglected. However, we should remember that synaptic activity is a very transient phenomenon, lasting usually some tens of milliseconds, and that the propagated impulses which result are even more fleeting since they usually last (for vertebrates) 1 or 2 msec. The membrane of the nerve cell merely serves as a passive and active cable which can have no memory, and from this argument, memory must be an inside-the-nerve-cell process. When the isolated eye, or the single neuron, such as the parabolic burster, produce activity correlated with yesterday's dawn, they exhibit a form of memory which we would like to understand and which may give us insights into more complex forms of memory.

It seems likely that the membrane of a nerve cell must couple to intracellular processes within the cell in a reciprocal way.[30] That is to say, that significant patterns of synaptic input arriving on particular parts of the postsynaptic membrane might change the pattern of macromolecular synthesis which in turn may change the mood of that cell for hours or perhaps days. Toward that understanding, DAVID WILSON,[44] in my laboratory, has demonstrated that the spectrum of proteins synthesized within identifiable neurons of the parieto-visceral ganglion systematically differs in particular cells. In these experiments single nerve cells, which have been allowed to incorporate H^3-leucine into protein while part of the ganglion, are dissected, homogenized, and the extract electrophoresed on miniature SDS polyacrylamide gels which separate proteins according to molecular weight. Three neurons of the parieto-visceral ganglion, all endogenously active cells, R 14, R 15 (the PB), and L 11 synthesize much protein around 12,000 mol. wt. (Fig. 12). In contrast, two non-pacemaker cells, R 2 and its symmetrical mate—the left pleural giant neuron, synthesize an excess of higher mol. wt. protein. It is already known that synaptic activation of R 2 increases RNA synthesis.[45-50] What then remains to be demonstrated is the functional significance of these macromolecules for neuronal behavior and this is going to be very difficult.

PROSPECTS FOR THE FUTURE

Our knowledge of the long-term physiology of nerve cells is quite limited. This is due to the fact that it is technically difficult to record the activity of the single neuron, in the intact animal, over long periods of time with assurance that the same neuron is being

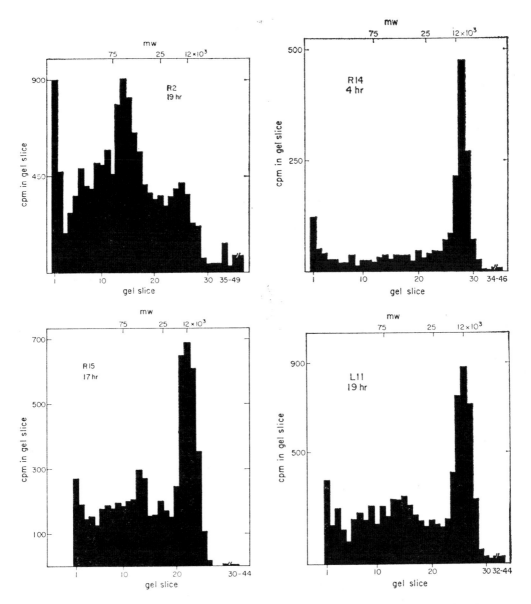

FIG. 12. Gel labeling patterns from pacemaker (R 14, R 15, and L 11) and non-pacemaker (R 2) neurons of the PVG of *Aplysia californica*. Isolated ganglia were incubated in H^3-leucine containing medium for the number of hours indicated in each frame. The single cells were dissected and extracts were electrophoresed on SDS-polyacrylamide gels which sieve proteins according to molecular weight. Protein molecular weight calibration, as determined by migration of standards relative to the bromophenol blue tracking dye, is indicated on each abscissa. A gel slice is $1\frac{1}{4}$ mm in length. A portion of the gels, in front of the tracking dye, was extruded and counted as a single piece; its length is indicated by the inclusive gel slice numbers. Forty-five counts/min background was subtracted. 8.5×10^6 counts/min = 1 μg L-leucine. (R 14 and L 11 gel labeling patterns from Fig. 7 of WILSON, 1971;[44] R 2 and R 15 from Fig. 2 and Fig. 6 of WILSON.[44])

monitored continuously. Attempts have been made to perform such measurements in unrestrained mammals[48,49] and in crayfish,[50] with partial success at least over periods of days. Using intact preparations, the number of variables which cannot be controlled by the experimenter is large and this becomes problematical for insightful interpretation of results. Furthermore, attempts to manipulate the chemical environment of neurons in such preparations, that are being recorded from over a long period of time, are fraught with technical and interpretive difficulties.

The ability to maintain the abdominal ganglion of *Aplysia* in organ culture,[30,37] over a 6 week period, offers the experimenter distinct advantages for the analysis of long-term physiological and biochemical neuronal processes. By using a special sterilizable chamber containing indwelling recording electrodes, it is possible to record the discharges of single neurons from the nerve trunks of the abdominal ganglion continuously over several weeks. This special chamber manufactured of Silastic rubber and Kel-F plastic contains several nerve cuffs (or tunnels) through which a nerve may be pulled easily and in which are located a pair of circular platinum-iridium electrodes. Since the nerve is stabilized in the tunnel and the tunnel is insulated from the surrounding organ culture medium by the Silastic rubber, stable long-term records of the firing of several units can be easily obtained from each of the six major nerves of the ganglion.

A typical record obtained from the pericardial nerve of the organ-cultured PVG is shown in Fig. 13. Data was collected simultaneously and continuously from the pericardial and the genital nerves of this preparation for 42 days by low speed polygraph recording. Ten minute samples of the pericardial nerve activity are shown for days 2, 6, 10, 14, 18, and 22 *in vitro*, around midnight. Two independent large units are easily observed and close inspection of the continuous record reveals three smaller, but discrete units. As is obvious from the record, the two larger units are burster-type neurons whose bursts become markedly prolonged between days 14 and 18 in organ culture. These records demonstrate the feasibility of continuous, stable, long-term recording in the organ-cultured ganglion by monitoring the multi-unit discharges in any of the six major trunks of the PVG.

A careful analysis of the burst frequency of unit 1 was performed by Suzy Bower for the 42 days of continuous recording. The mean daily burst frequency computed as bursts/30 min and the standard deviations of the mean are graphed in Fig. 14. It is clear that 'spontaneous' bursting is maintained throughout the entire 42 day period, but slowly declines over the first 17 days until a stable rate is achieved and maintained for the next 8 days. When the organ culture medium is refreshed on day 26, the mean burst frequency is clearly elevated and remains in this state for the next 17 days until the experiment is terminated.

The time is now ripe, since the techniques of such long-term maintenance and recording have been highly successful, to ask significant biological questions of this type of preparation. An important question will be to determine whether the procedure of uncoupling synaptic transmission within the ganglion for several days will alter the subsequent neural organization upon re-establishment of synaptic transmission. Another way of stating the basic question is to determine to what extent patterned neural and coupled organization is dependent on maintained electrical and transmitter activity of synapses. We are presently developing computer programs to handle the massive data that can be obtained in such long-term recordings from the organ-cultured ganglion.

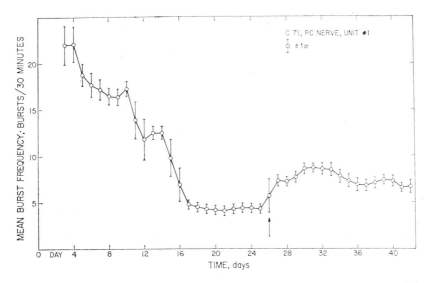

FIG. 14. The mean burst frequency per day of a spontaneously active neuron, recorded over 42 days from the organ cultured PVG. Same preparation as in Fig. 13. The burst frequency of Unit No. 1 was counted by hand for 30 min intervals throughout each day and the mean burst frequency/day and its standard deviation (σ) computed from these counts. At the arrow (day 26) the old culture medium was drained from the chamber and fresh culture medium was added.

SUMMARY

This essay includes some of the more important findings of our continuing research on the nervous system of the sea hare, *Aplysia*. My associates and I have tried and are trying to understand the temporal organization of behavior in terms of cellular processes and macromolecular metabolism which can be readily studied in the large and identifiable neurons of *Aplysia*. The long-term cyclic processes which we have discovered in some of these neurons may underlie behaviors such as sleep and waking, reproductive cycles, and periodic feeding. In view of the conservative nature of neuronal physiology, as reviewed earlier, it would be surprising if our investigations of these processes in *Aplysia* did not have relevance for the vertebrates including man.

Acknowledgements—I am particularly grateful to Drs. Stephen Arch, Arnold Eskin, and David Wilson for their helpful comments on this paper. I owe a special debt of gratitude to Mr. James J. Gilliam who patiently and creatively designs and constructs all the clever gadgets that we use in my laboratory. Thanks are due also to Mr. Floyd Schlechte who wrote many of the programs to analyze the locomotor activity of the sea hare. This work has been supported by grants from the NIH (NS 07071), NASA (NGR 05-002-031), and the American Heart Association.

REFERENCES

1. ARVANITAKI, A. and CHALAZONITIS, N. Les potentiels bioélectriques endocytaires du neurone géant d'*Aplysia* en activité autorhythmique. *C. r. Acad. Sci. Belles-lett. Arts Clermont-Ferrand.* **240**, 349, 1955.

2. TAUC, L. Réponse de la cellule nerveuse du ganglion abdominal d'*Aplysia depilans* à la stimulation directe intracellulaire. *C. r. Acad. Sci. Belles-lett. Arts Clermont-Ferrand.* **239**, 1537, 1954.

3. ARVANITAKI, A. and CHALAZONITIS, N. Photopotentiels d'excitation et d'inhibition de différents somata identifiables (*Aplysia*). *Bull. Inst. océanogr. Monaco* **57**, 1, 1960.

4. NARAHASHI, T., MOORE, J. W. and SCOTT, W. R. Tetrodotoxin blockage of sodium conductance increase in lobster giant axons. *J. gen. Physiol.* **47**, 965, 1964.

5. HILLE, B. Pharmacological modifications of the sodium channels of frog nerve. *J. gen. Physiol.* **51**, 199, 1968.

6. TAUC, L. and GERSCHENFELD, H. M. A cholinergic mechanism of inhibitory synaptic transmission in a molluscan nervous system. *J. Neurophysiol.* **25**, 236, 1962.

7. GILLER, E. JR. and SCHWARTZ, J. H. Choline acetyltransferase: regional distribution in the abdominal ganglion of *Aplysia*. *Science* **161**, 908, 1968.

8. TAKEUCHI, A. and TAKEUCHI, N. The effect on crayfish muscle of iontophoretically applied glutamate. *J. Physiol.* **170**, 296, 1964.

9. OTSUKA, M., IVERSEN, L. L., HALL, Z. W. and KRAVITZ, E. A. Release of gamma-aminobutyric acid from inhibitory nerves of lobster. *Proc. natn. Acad. Sci. U.S.A.* **56**, 1110, 1966.

10. TAKEUCHI, A. and TAKEUCHI, N. Localized action of gamma-aminobutyric acid on the crayfish muscle. *J. Physiol.* **177**, 225, 1965.

11. CURTIS, D. R., DUGGAN, A. W., FELIX, D. and JOHNSTON, G. A. R. Bicuculline and central GABA receptors. *Nature, Lond.* **228**, 676, 1970.

12. WALKER, R. J. Certain aspects of the pharmacology of *Helix* and *Hirudo* neurons. In: *Neurobiology of Invertebrates*, SALÁNKI, J. (Ed.), p. 227. Plenum Press, New York, 1968.

13. McLENNAN, H. Bicuculline and inhibition of crayfish stretch receptor neurones. *Nature, Lond.* **228**, 674, 1970.

14. PERETZ, B. Habituation and dishabituation in the absence of a central nervous system. *Science* **169**, 379, 1970.

15. YOUNG, J. Z. *A Model of the Brain.* Clarendon Press, Oxford, 1964.

16. FRINGS, H. and FRINGS, C. Chemosensory bases of food-finding and feeding in *Aplysia juliana* (Mollusca, Opisthobranchia). *Biol. Bull. mar. biol. Lab., Woods Hole* **128**, 211, 1965.

17. LICKEY, M. E. Learned behavior in *Aplysia vaccaria*. *J. comp. physiol. Psychol.* **66**, 712, 1968.

18. LEE, R. M. *Aplysia* behavior: Effects of contingent water-level variation. *Comm. behav. Biol.* **4**, 157, 1969.

19. COGGESHALL, R. E., KANDEL, E. R., KUPFERMANN, I. and WAZIRI, R. A morphological and functional study of a cluster of neurosecretory cells in the abdominal ganglion of *Aplysia californica*. *J. Cell. Biol.* **31**, 363, 1966.

20. KUPFERMANN, I. Stimulation of egg-laying: Possible neuroendocrine function of bag cells of abdominal ganglion of *Aplysia californica*. *Nature, Lond.* **216**, 814, 1967.

21. STRUMWASSER, F., JACKLET, J. W. and ALVAREZ, R. Behavioral egg-laying induced by extracts of various portions of the parieto-visceral ganglion in *Aplysia*. *Proc. int. Un. physiol. Sci.* **7**, Washington, D.C., 420, 1968.

22. STRUMWASSER, F., JACKLET, J. W. and ALVAREZ, R. A seasonal rhythm in the neural extract induction of behavioral egg-laying in *Aplysia*. *Comp. Biochem. Physiol.* **29**, 197, 1969.

23. TOEVS, L. and BRACKENBURY, R. W. Bag-cell specific proteins and the humoral control of egg-laying in *Aplysia californica*. *Comp. Biochem. Physiol.* **29**, 207, 1969.

24. TOEVS, L. Identification and characterization of the bag-cell hormone from the neurosecretory bag-cells of *Aplysia*. Ph.D. thesis, California Institute of Technology, 1970.

25. ARCH, S. W. Polypeptide secretion from the isolated parieto-visceral ganglion of *Aplysia californica*. *J. gen. Physiol.* (Submitted), 1971.

26. RUBIN, R. P. The role of calcium in the release of neurotransmitter substances and hormones. *Pharmac. Rev.* **22**, 389, 1970.

27. BISSET, G. W., HILTON, S. M. and POISNER, A. M. Hypothalamic pathways for independent release of vasopressin and oxytocin. *Proc. R. Soc. Lond. Ser. B.* **166**, 422, 1967.

28. KUPFERMANN, I. A circadian locomotor rhythm in *Aplysia californica*. *Physiol. Behav.* **3**, 179, 1968.

29. STRUMWASSER, F., LU, C. and GILLIAM, J. J. Quantitative studies of the circadian locomotor system in *Aplysia*. Calif. Instit. of Tech. *Biol. Ann. Rep.* **153**, 1966.

30. STRUMWASSER, F. Neurophysiological aspects of rhythms. In: *The Neurosciences: An Intensive Study Program*, QUARTON, G. C., MELNECHUK, T. and SCHMITT, F. O. (Eds), p. 516. Rockefeller University Press, New York, 1967.

31. STRUMWASSER, F. The demonstration and manipulation of a circadian rhythm in a single neuron. *Circadian Clocks*, ASCHOFF, J. (Ed.), p. 442, North-Holland Publishing, Amsterdam, 1965.

32. LICKEY, M. Seasonal modulation and non-twenty-four hour entrainment of a circadian rhythm in a single neuron. *J. comp. physiol. Psych.* **68**, 9, 1969.

33. JACKLET, J. W. Electrophysiological organization of the eye of *Aplysia. J. gen. Physiol.* **53**, 21, 1969.

34. WASER, P. M. The spectral sensitivity of the eye of *Aplysia californica. Comp. Biochem. Physiol.* **27**, 339, 1968.

35. JACKLET, J. W. A circadian rhythm of optic nerve impulses recorded in darkness from the isolated eye of *Aplysia. Science* **164**, 562, 1969.

36. ESKIN, A. Properties of the *Aplysia* visual system: *in vitro* entrainment of the circadian rhythm and centrifugal regulation of the eye. *Zeit. vergl. Physiol.* (Submitted), 1971.

37. STRUMWASSER, F. and BAHR, R. Prolonged *in vitro* culture and autoradiographic studies of neurons in *Aplysia. Fedn Proc. Fedn Am. Socs exp. Biol.* **25**, 512, 1966.

38. FRAZIER, W. T., KANDEL, E. R., KUPFERMANN, I., WAZIRI, R. and COGGESHALL, R. E. Morphological and functional properties of identified neurons in the adbominal ganglion of *Aplysia californica. J. Neurophysiol.* **30**, 1288, 1967.

39. STRUMWASSER, F. and KIM, M. Experimental studies of a neuron with an endogenous oscillator and a quantitative model of its mechanism. *Physiol.* **12**, 367, 1969.

40. GEDULDIG, D. and JUNGE, D. Sodium and calcium components of action potentials in the *Aplysia* giant neurone. *J. Physiol.* **199**, 347, 1968.

41. STRUMWASSER, F. Membrane and intracellular mechanisms governing endogenous activity in neurons. In: *Physiological and Biochemical Aspects of Nervous Integration*, CARLSON, F. D. (Ed.), p. 329. Prentice-Hall, New Jersey, 1968.

42. STRUMWASSER, F. Tetrodotoxin reveals two stable states of the resting potential in a neuron generating endogenous bursts. *Physiol.* **10**, 318, 1967.

43. DUNHAM, P. B. and HOFFMAN, J. F. Partial purification of the Ouabain-binding component and of the Na, K-ATPase from human red cell plasma membranes. *Proc. natn. Acad. Sci.* **66**, 936, 1970.

44. WILSON, D. L. Molecular weight distribution of proteins synthesized in single, identified neurons of *Aplysia. J. gen. Physiol.* **57**, 26, 1971.

45. BERRY, R. W. Ribonucleic acid metabolism of a single neuron: correlation with electrical activity. *Science* **166**, 1021, 1969.

46. PETERSON, R. P. and KERNELL, D. Effects of nerve stimulation on the metabolism of ribonucleic acid in a molluscan giant neurone. *J. Neurochem.* **17**, 1075, 1970.

47. KERNELL, D. and PETERSON, R. P. The effect of spike activity versus synaptic activation on the metabolism of ribonucleic acid in a molluscan giant neurone. *J. Neurochem.* **17**, 1087, 1970.

48. STRUMWASSER, F. Long-term recording from single neurons in brain of unrestrained mammals. *Science* **127**, 469, 1958.

49, OLDS, J., MINK, W. D. and BEST, P. Single unit patterns during anticipatory behavior. *Electroenceph. clin. Neurophysiol.* **26**, 144, 1969.

50. ARÉCHIGA, H. and WIERSMA, C. A. G. Circadian rhythm of responsiveness in crayfish visual units. *J. Neurobiol.* **1**, 71, 1969.

J. psychiat. Res., 1971, Vol. 8, pp. 259–272. Pergamon Press. Printed in Great Britain.

THE VESTIBULAR NUCLEI AND SPINAL MOTOR ACTIVITY

VICTOR J. WILSON*

The Rockefeller University, New York, N.Y. 10021

INTRODUCTION

NUMEROUS supraspinal components of the central nervous system participate in regulation of spinal motoneuron activity, among them the vestibular nuclei located in the lower brain stem. The cells making up these nuclei are themselves under the influence of inputs from several sources, particularly the labyrinth and cerebellum, and the efferent pathways to which they give rise act as relays for impulses arising in these regions. The vestibular nuclei exert a fairly direct influence on the spinal cord by means of two pathways: the lateral vestibulospinal tract originating in Deiters' nucleus and the medial vestibulospinal tract originating in the medial and, to a lesser extent, the descending vestibular nuclei.[1,2] The excitatory influence of the lateral tract on limb extensor muscles has been recognized for some time,[1] while the role of the medial vestibulospinal tract has remained obscure. In recent years, the synaptic actions that both tracts exert on spinal motoneurons have been studied in several laboratories including ours. One aspect of our work has been a comparison of the effects that vestibulospinal fibers exert on motoneurons located at different segmental levels, and controlling different muscle groups. This has led to electrophysiological confirmation of the long known fact that the labyrinth and vestibular nuclei are related particularly closely to the neck musculature. In general, all the investigations have shown that the two vestibulospinal tracts exert short-latency actions on many alpha motoneurons at all levels of the cord, and I will review these findings. The two tracts will be considered sequentially, and in each case the discussion of recent electrophysiological experiments will be preceded by a brief description of the anatomical background.

FULTON, LIDDELL and RIOCH[3] are among those who determined the effect that Deiters' nucleus exerts on the musculature. It is a real pleasure for me, as I now discuss the vestibulospinal system of the cat, to return to an area of neurophysiology to which Dr. Rioch made a contribution so long ago.

THE LATERAL VESTIBULOSPINAL TRACT

Many cells in Deiters' nucleus project to the ipsilateral spinal cord, and their axons end at all levels from upper cervical to sacral. Anatomical investigations have indicated that

---

* Work in the author's laboratory supported in part by N.I.H. grants NS 02619 and NS 05463.

the nucleus is somatotopically organized and that cells projecting to the cervical cord are located mainly in its rostroventral part, while cells projecting to the lumbrosacral cord tend to be located dorsocaudally.[1] This arrangement is confirmed by electrophysiological observations. Cells whose level of projection is determined by antidromic stimulation of the vestibulospinal tract can later be located quite accurately within the nucleus by means of dye marks deposited during recording.[4] This approach has shown that the dorsocaudal part of the nucleus does contain mainly cells whose axons extend to the lumbosacral cord; in the ventral part of the nucleus various cell types are intermingled, with cells projecting to the forelimb and thoracic region somewhat outnumbering more caudally projecting neurons. This somatotopic arrangement, blurred though it may be, is of interest because of the distribution of the labyrinthine input within Deiters' nucleus. Degeneration studies clearly show that vestibular afferent fibers end mainly in the rostroventral part of the nucleus,[5,6] and this is where cells driven monosynaptically by labyrinthine stimulation are found.[4,7,8] As a result of this pattern of termination far more Deiters' cells projecting to cervical and thoracic segments of the cord are activated monosynaptically by labyrinthine stimulation than are Deiters' cells projecting to lumbrosacral segments. Deiters' nucleus is therefore better suited to relay labyrinthine information to the rostral than to the caudal segments of the spinal cord. How the lateral vestibulospinal fibers influence motoneurons is not completely clear from anatomical findings. The fibers apparently do not end on motoneuron somata, except perhaps in thoracic segments.[9,10] Their effects are therefore exerted either by axodendritic monosynaptic linkage, or polysynaptically.

With this background in mind we turn to the effects produced in individual spinal motoneurons by activation of Deiters' nucleus. Such effects have been produced experimentally in anesthetized cats by electrical stimulation of the nucleus by means of fine metal electrodes. Attempts at localized stimulation within the central nervous system encounter many difficulties. In the lower brain stem, as elsewhere, different cell groups are present in close proximity and are often traversed by fiber bundles: stimulation of structures other than that meant to be stimulated is always a possibility, and precautions must be taken to guard against this. In our experiments[11] an array of electrodes was inserted into the brain stem so that one or two of these electrodes were placed in Deiters' nucleus, while others were in the other regions of the vestibular nuclei and in the medial longitudinal fasciculus (MLF). The nature and threshold of the synaptic actions produced by stimulation at these various locations could then be compared, and those originating in Deiters' nucleus identified. In the same experiments electrodes were also implanted into the labyrinth; the results of stimulating the sense organ and higher order vestibular neurons could then be compared.

LUND and POMPEIANO[12] were the first to show that some hindlimb alpha motoneurons could be facilitated monosynaptically by Deiters' stimulation. Subsequently the connections between the nucleus and motoneurons at different levels of the spinal cord have been studied in great detail.

Neck motoneurons

The labyrinth exerts an important effect on the neck musculature.[13,14] Because of its connections, Deiters' nucleus is well suited to be a link in the pathway mediating this effect, and lateral vestibulospinal fibers may be expected to represent an important input to neck motoneurons. WILSON and YOSHIDA[11] have studied this input in a population of alpha motoneurons located in C2 and C3 segments. The motoneurons were identified by antidromic stimulation, and consisted of cells innervating the splenius muscle and cells with axons in the remainder of the dorsal rami of the spinal nerves, supplying principally the complexus and biventer cervicis muscles. All of these motoneurons act as extensors of the head. Stimulation of Deiters' nucleus with single shocks produced excitatory postsynaptic potentials (EPSPs) in many of these motoneurons with a latency

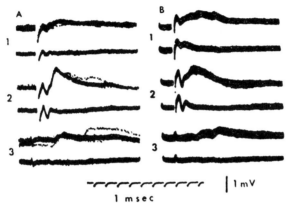

FIG. 1.   EPSPs evoked in neck extensor motoneurons by stimulation of Deiters' nucleus, MLF and labrynth. (A) EPSP produced in C3 splenius motoneuron by stimulation of Deiters' (1) and MLF (2), with a pulse of 10V (0·33 mA). Response in (3) was evoked by stimulation of ipsilateral labyrinth with stimulus of 0·4V (3·1 × N1 threshold). (B) EPSPs seen in mononeuron with axon in C3 dorsal rami. Stimulus of 8·3V (0·28 mA) was applied to Deiters' (1) and MLF (2). EPSP in (3) was evoked by stimulation of ipsilateral labyrinth with 0·9V pulse (1·5 × N1 threshold). Lower records of each pair show field potentials recorded juxtacellularly. Each record consists of several superimposed sweeps. Upward deflection positive in this and other figures. From: WILSON, V. J. and YOSHIDA, M. Comparison of the effects of stimulation of Deiters' nucleus and the medial longitudinal fasciculus on neck, forelimb and hindlimb motoneurons. *J. Neurophysiol.* **32**, 743, 1969.

of 0·9–1·5 msec (Fig. 1). The vestibulospinal volley arrived at the segmental level of the motoneurons at 0·4–0·7 msec, depending on the level of recording and the size of the animal, and the time remaining for segmental delay makes it clear that the Deiters'-evoked EPSPs were monosynaptic. The amplitude of the EPSPs was small (mean 0·8 mV), but because of recording conditions it is likely that the measurements somewhat underestimated the true size of the potentials. Monosynaptic potentials of vestibulospinal origin were seen in 54/92 motoneurons. An even greater fraction of motoneurons received a monosynaptic input from fibers in the MLF, many presumably reticulospinal fibers. The latency of these EPSPs ranged from 0·8–1·3 msec, suggesting, in agreement with other observations, that the conduction velocity of reticulospinal fibers is somewhat higher than that of vestibulospinal fibers. The large number of motoneurons receiving an input from both Deiters' and MLF suggests that, despite the relativity small size of the potentials recorded, these two structures are an important source of excitation for neck extensor motoneurons.

In a substantial number of motoneurons, EPSPs were evoked by stimulation of the ipsilateral labyrinth, and latency measurements indicated that many were disynaptic. In general, these EPSPs resembled EPSPs evoked by Deiters' stimulation (Fig. 1), and it is reasonable to assume that most were produced by a pathway starting in the labyrinth and relaying in this nucleus.

Limb motoneurons

Both hindlimb and forelimb alpha motoneurons have been investigated. Whereas initial investigations suggested that the lateral vestibulospinal tract monosynaptically activates hindlimb extensors in general,[12] more recent experiments have shown that the pattern of vestibulospinal excitation is more specific. Monosynaptic EPSPs, similar in appearance to, and of the same order of magnitude as, EPSPs observed in neck motoneurons, are often found in the ankle and knee extensors gastrocnemius and quadriceps, but not in other extensors or in flexors.[11,15] Monosynaptic activation by fibers in the MLF is observed in many hindlimb flexor cells, as well as in extensors. Unlike the situation in the neck segments however, extensor motoneurons have not been observed to receive a monosynaptic input from both Deiters' and MLF: the two inputs seem to be distributed reciprocally.[11,16]

Whereas a monosynaptic input from Deiters' nucleus is found in some types of hindlimb extensor cells, it has not been found at all in a sample of forelimb motoneurons that included cells innervating the elbow extensors lateral and long heads of triceps; the elbow flexor biceps; and various muscles of the wrist and digits.[11] Although the number of motor nuclei tested was small, and the possibility of monosynaptic contact with some cells in these or other nuclei is not excluded, such contact is obviously not a prominent feature in the relation between Deiters' nucleus and forelimb motoneurons. On the contrary, just as in the neck and hindlimb motor nuclei already described, the fiber systems descending in the MLF do make monosynaptic contact with many extensor and flexor cells.[11]

When Deiters' nucleus is stimulated with short trains of high frequency stimuli, poly-synaptic potentials, resembling the potential in Fig. 2a, are commonly seen in most extensor, and even some flexor, limb motoneurons.[11,15] Even in animals under barbiturate anesthesia these polysynaptic potentials reach much greater amplitudes (several millivolts) than the monosynaptic potentials described above. In addition to this excitatory effect trains of stimuli, and occasionally single shocks, evoke inhibitory potentials (IPSPs) in a number of motoneurons, usually flexor but sometimes extensor.[11,15] These potentials are apparently produced by pathways at least disynaptic, although some questions about the nature of the pathway are raised by experiments that will be described in connection with the medial vestibulospinal system.

One difference, then, between the lateral vestibulospinal input to neck motoneurons on the one hand and limb motoneurons on the other, is that in the former case monosynaptic connections are prominent whereas in the latter polysynaptic connections dominate. There is another difference. As we described above, stimulation of the labyrinth often evokes disynaptic potentials in neck motoneurons and it appears that in the case of these moto-neurons one important function of Deiters' nucleus is to act as a relay for impulses of labyrinthine origin. This is not the situation with respect to limb motoneurons. In animals prepared and anesthetized in a manner similar to the animals used for experiments on the neck segments of the spinal cord, stimulation of the labyrinth did not evoke synaptic potentials in any limb motoneurons.[11] Certainly this does not mean that there are no pathways linking the labyrinth to the motor centers of the limbs. An anatomical substrate for such pathways to both forelimb and hindlimb segments exists;[4] and in some types of preparations, for example in animals that are decerebrate or anesthetized with chloralose, stimulation of the labyrinth can evoke both discharge in lower cervical, or lumbosacral, ventral roots and muscular contraction.[17-20] The result does indicate that pathways between labyrinth and neck are more powerful and more direct than pathways between labyrinth and limbs. It also confirms the view that in exerting a clear excitatory influence on limb muscles, Deiters' nucleus is acting as a relay for impulses from many sources of which the labyrinth is not the most important.[1,13]

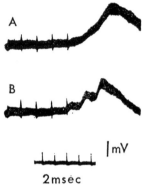

FIG. 2. Polysynpatic and monosynpatic EPSPs in flexor digitorum longus motoneuron. (A) polysynaptic EPSP evoked by four shocks to Deiters' at 6·4V. (B) steplike monosynaptic EPSPs evoked by four shocks to MLF at 6·4V. Smooth rising phase of Deiters'-evoked potential contrasts with steplike response to MLF stimulus. From: WILSON, V. J. and YOSHIDA, M. Comparison of the effects of stimulation of Deiters' nucleus and the medial longitudinal fasciculus on neck, forelimb and hindlimb motoneurons. *J. Neurophysiol.* **32**, 743, 1969.

Back motoneurons

It might be expected on anatomical grounds (i.e. the termination of lateral vestibulospinal fibers medially in the spinal cord)[21] and on functional grounds (i.e. they are axial motoneurons like neck motoneurons) that back extensor motoneurons should receive a direct input from Deiters' nucleus and a disynaptic input from the labyrinth. We have therefore, recently studied the effect of stimulation of Deiters' nucleus and other regions of the brain stem on a group of motoneurons innervating extensors of the vertebral column, located in the Th 1 to Th 10 segments.[22,23] In a number of these motoneurons, including those supplying the longissimus dorsi muscle and some whose projection could not be identified, monosynaptic EPSPs were produced by Deiters' stimulation and disynaptic EPSPs by ipsilateral labyrinthine stimulation. Because in some motoneurons potentials were evoked from the labyrinth but not from Deiters', it is apparent that another brain stem relay is also involved in this pathway, and the descending vestibular nucleus has been suggested as a possibility.[23]

Comment

The lateral vestibulospinal tract is an excitatory pathway, as all monosynaptic connections it makes with motoneurons or interneurons are excitatory.[11,15,24] The results described above show that, whereas the vestibulospinal fibers extend as far as the lumbosacral cord and whereas in general their effect is excitatory on extensor motoneurons and inhibitory on flexors, the segmental pathways by which these actions are exerted are not the same in all regions of the cord. A simplified statement is that excitatory monosynaptic pathways are the predominant link between Deiters' nucleus and axial extensor motoneurons (neck, back), while polysynaptic pathways are the more important link between Deiters' and limb extensors (forelimb, hindlimb). The difference between these two types of linkage is not really a quantitative one: the polysynaptic action can be strong or stronger than the monosynaptic. The important difference is one of security of transmission. The presence of segmental interneurons in the polysynaptic pathway exposes it to regulation (inhibition or enhancement) by a variety of peripheral or descending inputs.

We have seen that the labyrinth has greater access to neck and back than to limb motoneurons. This follows both from the anatomical organization of Deiters' nucleus, and from the prevalence of monosynaptic vestibulospinal connections with axial motoneurons.[11] An important role for the Deitersian projection to axial motoneurons is therefore to act as a relay for labyrinthine impulses. The projection to limb, and especially hindlimb, segments is not controlled by the labyrinthine input to the same degree, and is more dominated by the input from the cerebellar vermis, known to be inhibitory and to terminate mainly in the dorsal region of Deiters' nucleus.[25,26]

In this summary of the influence of the lateral vestibulospinal tract on motor activity, the emphasis has been on the direct and reasonably direct pathways impinging on alpha motoneurons. The tract, however, can modify segmental activity by other means. For example, the lateral vestibulospinal tract also activates gamma motoneurons, some monosynaptically,[24,27] and this represents another route for excitation of alpha motoneurons. Second, the tract can influence spinal activity by termination on interneurons present in various reflex pathways.[28,29] All of these possibilities must be taken into account when the function of the lateral vestibulospinal system is considered.

THE MEDIAL VESTIBULOSPINAL TRACT

This tract, originating mainly in the medial vestibular nucleus, is found in the MLF in the lower brain stem, and bilaterally in the medial part of the ventral funiculus in the spinal cord. Consisting of small to medium caliber fibers, it is distributed most abundantly in the upper cervical segments, but according to anatomists extends as far as the cervical enlargement or even midthoracic segments.[30-32] Electrophysiological evidence suggests that some fibers may even reach the lumbar cord.[33] The descending fibers end in the medial part of the ventral horn, where terminations are seen on large and small cells but not on motoneuron somata.[32] The termination sites, however, do not seem to have been studied in the most rostral cervical segments.

Inputs from various sources can excite medial nucleus neurons, but the labyrinth is especially effective: 80 per cent of the cells with axons reaching the spinal cord can be fired monosynaptically by stimulation of the labyrinth.[34] The nucleus and medial vestibulospinal tract therefore can act to relay a labyrinthine inflow to the spinal cord, particularly to its most rostral levels.

No positive evidence bearing on the functional significance of this descending pathway had been produced before our experiments. Most recently GERNANDT[35] reported that section of the MLF did not affect the motor outflow produced at forelimb or hindlimb levels by vestibular stimulation. This result is an excellent agreement with our findings, which suggest that the medial vestibulospinal tract is predominantly an inhibitory pathway and appears to have little effect on limb motoneurons.[36]

As in our investigations of the lateral vestibulospinal tract, we have studied synaptic potentials evoked in motoneurons by electrical stimulation of the labyrinth and brain stem, and the same experimental procedures were used. Often as many as thirteen stimulating electrodes were inserted into the brain stem in order to improve localization of zones from which the excitability of motoneurons could be influenced.

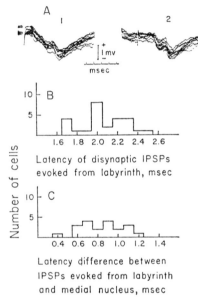

FIG. 3. Brain stem and labyrinthine IPSPs in motoneurons. (A) typical IPSP evoked in a motoneuron by stimulation of medial vestibular nucleus (1) and labyrinth (2). Medial nucleus stimulus was 6V, threshold 2·4V (0·14 mA). Labyrinthine stimulus was 1·1V, threshold was 1·4 × N1 threshold. (B) distribution of latencies of those IPSPs in C2 and C3 considered disynaptic. (C) latency differences between IPSPs evoked in the same cell by stimulation of of medial nucleus and labyrinth. From: WILSON, V. J. and YOSHIDA, M. Monosynaptic inhibition of neck motoneurons by the medial vestibular nucleus. *Exp. Brain. Res.* **9**, 365, 1969.

Most of the successful experiments have dealt with the population of neck extensor motoneurons described above. When such a cell was penetrated by a microelectrode and stimuli were applied sequentially at the various brain stem electrodes, inhibitory post-synaptic potentials were frequently observed (Fig. 3a). The latency of these IPSPs varied from 0·9 to 1·5 msec, that is, overlapped almost completely with the latency of vestibulo-spinal and reticulospinal EPSPs, produced by rapidly conducting fibers and already shown to be monosynaptic. In addition, stimuli that evoked IPSPs also produced a conducted descending tract potential that arrived in the vicinity of motoneurons 0·3–0·6 msec after the stimulus. Even if this is not the nerve volley evoking IPSPs, it is the earliest volley arriving in the segments investigated. The short delay (mean 0·6–0·7 msec) between the arrival of this volley and the start of IPSPs therefore demonstrates unequivocally that the latter are monosynaptic.

Monosynaptic IPSPs were evoked in many motoneurons by stimulation of the vestibular nuclei (40/61). In a number of cells longer-latency potentials were evoked by stimulation of the labyrinth (Fig. 3a, b). The appearance of IPSPs produced by stimulation at these two loci was similar and the latency difference was often just sufficient for one synaptic relay: the labyrinth-evoked IPSP was disynaptic (Fig. 3). Because in the medulla and pons vestibular afferent fibers end almost exclusively in the vestibular nuclei, this is evidence that the cells responsible for monosynaptic IPSPs in neck motoneurons are located in these nuclei.

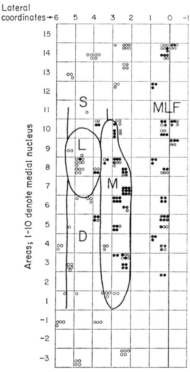

FIG. 4. Distribution of monosynaptic IPSP thresholds in the horizontal plane in medulla and pons. Results of several experiments pooled. Low thresholds (<100 arbitrary units, with 100 = 0·4 mA) represented by filled circles, intermediate thresholds (100–150 units) by dotted circles, high thresholds (>150 units) by circles. Grid of brain stem divided in 15 rostrocaudal areas of equal length in each experiment, with medial nucleus located between 1 and 10 inclusive; lateral coordinates in mm. Approximate outlines of medial and lateral nuclei have been drawn in. Abbreviations: D, descending nucleus; L, Deiters' nucleus; M, medial nucleus; S, superior nucleus; MLF, medial longitudinal fasciculus. From: Wilson, V. J. and Yoshida, M. Mono-synaptic inhibition of neck motoneurons by the medial vestibular nucleus. *Exp. Brain Res.* **9,** 365, 1969.

When a map, in the horizontal plane, of ipsilateral IPSP thresholds was prepared by pooling the values measured in many experiments, it became clear that low threshold points were present mainly in the medial vestibular nucleus and MLF (Fig. 4). This is consistent with the hypothesis that the cell bodies of the inhibitory neurons are located in this nucleus. Their axons can then be stimulated in the MLF not only at and caudal to the level of the nucleus but also rostral to it: some of the axons are known to dichotomize into an ascending and descending branch.[1,37]

The possibility that the stimulating electrode in the medial nucleus is really stimulating cells below the nucleus (either by activation of collaterals or by stimulus spread) must be eliminated. This was done by moving the stimulating array in the vertical plane and comparing IPSP thresholds at different depths (Fig. 5). Thresholds are lowest in the medial nucleus and rise with increasing depth. All of the evidence therefore points to the medial vestibular nucleus as a source of inhibition of spinal motoneurons in the C2 and C3 segments.

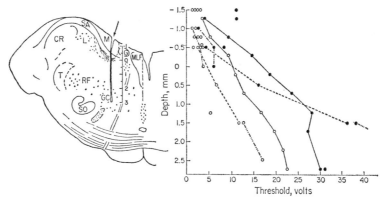

FIG. 5. Measurement of IPSP threshold in tranverse plane. Diagram on left shows transverse section of brain stem in rostral half of medial nucleus. Ventral part of diagram more rostral than dorsal part because of head flexion. Arrow shows beginning of electrode track through medial nucleus into reticular formation. Approximate limits of medial nucleus indicated by dashed line. Abbreviations: CR, restiform body; G, genu of facial nerve; GC, gigantocellular reticular formation; L, Deiters' nucleus; M, medial nucleus; MLF, medial longitudinal fasciculus; RF, reticular formation; SA, stria acustica; T, spinal tract of trigeminal. Scale alongside track is in mm and O represents bottom of medial nucleus. In graph on right, points represent thresholds measured in 18 cells at a different depth with respect to medial nucleus, whose ventral edge is again indicated by O. Negative values are within the nucleus, positive values below it. Hollow circles represent measurements with monopolar stimulation, filled circles measurements with bipolar stimulation between two electrodes at same depth and about 2·5 mm apart. Measurements are for different cells except where points are joined by lines. Similar lines (solid, dashed, etc.) are used to connect points obtained from same cell with mono- and bipolar stimulation. From: WILSON, V. J. and YOSHIDA, M. Monosynaptic inhibition of neck motoneurons by the medial vestibular nucleus. *Exp. Brain Res.* 9, 365, 1969.

Although stimulation of the brain stem or labyrinth with single shocks often produced short latency inhibitory potentials in neck motoneurons, we have not observed monosynaptic IPSPs in forelimb or hindlimb motoneurons (WILSON and YOSHIDA, unpublished observations). Occasionally, however, single shocks to the vestibular nuclei or MLF do produce IPSPs in limb motoneurons, but the apparent segmental delay is such that the potentials have been assumed to be disynaptic.[12,16,35] The experiments described in the next section raise some doubts about this assumption.

Inhibition of back motoneurons

We have already seen that lateral vestibulospinal fibers make monosynaptic contact with some back motoneurons after apparently bypassing forelimb motoneurons. A monosynaptic inhibitory pathway, that can be activated in the brain stem and that is itself activated with monosynaptic delay by labyrinthine afferents, displays the same pattern of termination. This pathway will be discussed here although the evidence that it is the medial vestibulospinal tract that produces inhibition of back motoneurons is indirect.

Stimulation of the MLF in the medulla with single shocks produces EPSPs and IPSPs in many back motoneurons.[22,23] The EPSPs are widespread, and are found in a majority of cells of the various motoneuron groups studied, both back extensors (interspinales, longissimus dorsi, spinalis dorsi) and unidentified motoneurons. From the short segmental delay between the earliest-arriving descending volleys and EPSP onset (mean 0·6–0·7 msec), it is obvious that the EPSP, presumably produced by reticulospinal fibers, is monosynaptic. More information about the excitatory pathway can be obtained by an analysis to which this population of motoneurons lends itself particularly well. Motoneurons receiving the same descending input are spread over a distance of approximately 100 mm between Th 1 and Th 10. Because of this, it is possible to do a linear regression analysis of synaptic potential latency versus distance and, by the use of relatively standard formulae, to calculate both the conduction velocity of the descending fibers and the time not used for conduction, which is made up principally of segmental delay.[22,23] A latency-distance plot for EPSPs is shown in Figure 6a. The slope of the line (the conduction velocity of the fibers producing EPSPs) is 107 msec (90 per cent confidence bounds 96·2–121·5 msec), while a more recent calculation including unidentified motoneurons gives a velocity of 127 msec.[23] Both values agree with the known rapid conduction velocity of reticulospinal fibers. The y-intercept, corresponding to the total of utilization time, segmental conduction and synaptic delay, is 0·9 msec, confirming the monosynaptic nature of the pathway.

For the excitatory pathway the analysis adds only conduction velocity to what we already knew, but it is far more revealing in the case of the inhibitory pathway. In response to single shocks to the MLF, IPSPs are observed in many back motoneurons; in most cases the delay between arrival of the earliest descending volleys and IPSP onset exceeds 1·2 msec, suggesting the potential is at least disynaptic. Preliminary analysis revealed that two motoneuron pools, interspinales and unidentified motoneurons, behaved homogeneously and linear regression analysis was applied to the IPSPs in these cells. The latency-distance plot for interspinales cells is shown in Fig. 6b. Calculations reveal that the conduction velocity of the inhibitory pathway is 65 msec (90 per cent confidence bounds 57·2–74·2 msec) and the mean y-intercept is 0·8 msec: IPSPs are produced monosynaptically by a pathway with a conduction velocity that is considerably slower than that of the excitatory pathway.

A threshold analysis similar to that illustrated in Fig. 4 demonstrates that the monosynaptic IPSPs do not originate in the ipsilateral medial nucleus.[22] Because disynaptic

IPSPs are often produced by stimulation of the contralateral labyrinth, it is certain that the inhibitory cells are in the contralateral vestibular nuclei, and of these, the medial nucleus is the most likely. The moderate conduction velocity of the fibers is consistent with the hypothesis that the medial vestibulospinal tract is the inhibitory pathway in this case.[23,36] In addition this tract is known to be bilateral, and it has already been shown that contralateral as well as ipsilateral disynaptic inhibition of labyrinthine origin is seen in neck motoneurons.[38]

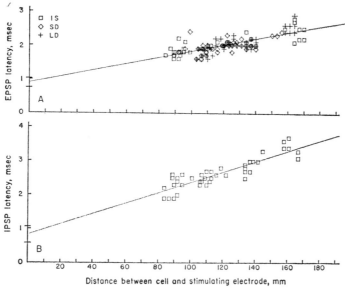

FIG. 6.   Relation between latency of synaptic potentials evoked in thoracic motoneurons by brain stem stimulation (ordinate), and distance of motoneurons from stimulating electrode (abcissa). EPSP latency plotted in A, IPSP latency in B. Some motoneurons are represented by more than one point: potentials were sometimes evoked by each of 2 or 3 electrodes, and the latency of each potential was plotted. Note marks denoting 90 per cent confidence bounds on each side of the *y*-intercept. From WILSON, V. J., YOSHIDA, M. and SCHOR, R. H. Monosynaptic excitation and inhibition of thoracic motoneurons by fibers in the medial longitudinal fasciculus. *Brain Res.* **18**, 181, 1970.

Comment

The evidence strongly suggests that the component of the medial vestibulospinal tract that originates in the medial nucleus is inhibitory, and therefore provides the first electrophysiologically defined example of a direct inhibitory pathway of supraspinal origin acting on the spinal cord in general and on motoneurons in particular. This postulated inhibitory function for cells in the medial nucleus is in keeping with other monosynaptic inhibitory actions ascribed to the nucleus: inhibition of cells in the contralateral medial nucleus;[39] and in the ipsilateral abducens nucleus.[40] Possibly the inhibitory fibers in these pathways consist in part of branches of dichotomizing fibers, the other branch descending to the spinal cord. Although the medial nucleus is involved in several inhibitory pathways, it does not necessarily consist only of inhibitory neurons. The nucleus contains a heterogeneous collection of neurons, and some may be excitatory. It is even possible that there are excitatory fibers among medial vestibulospinal axons originating in the medial nucleus, although it is simpler to begin with the hypothesis that this group of fibers is uniform in nature.

Just as there are secure, disynaptic excitatory pathways between labyrinthine receptors and axial motoneurons, there are similar inhibitory pathways. The excitatory lateral vestibulospinal tract, while connected to limb motoneurons by relatively scarce mono-synaptic links, does influence these motoneurons strongly via polysynaptic pathways. There is little information on the relation between the medial vestibulospinal tract and limb motoneurons. Presumably this tract does not reach the lumbosacral enlargement and therefore does not exert a direct influence on hindlimb motoneurons (but see Ref. 33). Apparently the tract also does not inhibit forelimb motoneurons monosynaptically. With the information now available on the conduction velocity of the inhibitory pathway, and on the presence of monosynaptic inhibition in neck and back motoneurons, it may be worthwhile to re-examine inputs to forelimb motoneurons.

CONCLUSIONS

Some aspects of the experimental findings have already been discussed together with description of the results themselves, but a few comments remain. Two are fairly general. First, it has been a common procedure to investigate the effects produced by some descending pathway on hindlimb motoneurons and, by implication or otherwise, to generalize the results to all motoneurons. The present description of two tracts having different relations with motoneurons at different cord levels, even though one tract at least descends the length of the spinal cord, shows that such generalization is not necessarily correct. Second, the population of thoracic motoneurons permits analysis of the properties of descending pathways that is not possible with motoneurons located in a more restricted region of the cord. Such analysis, employing either thoracic motoneurons or other populations sufficiently separated rostro-caudally, may be profitably extended to other descending tracts.

Some direct and secure pathways between labyrinth, vestibular nuclei and spinal motoneurons have been described in this review. Certainly in normal function other, more complex, pathways are superimposed on this simple framework. Nevertheless the mono- and polysynaptic effects that electrical activation of the lateral and medial vestibulospinal tracts produces in anesthetized cats do give an indication of the functions that these tracts can fulfill. One such function is to connect the labyrinth to axial motoneurons.

Many years ago SHERRINGTON[41] put forward the view that "labyrinthine proprioceptors are largely the equilibrators of the head". The bilateral disynaptic excitatory and inhibitory pathways between labyrinth and neck motoneurons,[38] presumably consisting in brain stem and spinal cord of the lateral and medial vestibulospinal tract respectively,[11,36] are ideally suited to carry out this equilibrating function. In fact they provide reciprocal innervation of the motoneurons controlling the neck musculature. SZENTAGOTHAI,[19] has shown that microstimulation of different receptor areas in the labyrinth results in contraction of different combinations of neck muscles. The pathways described in this summary provide the neural basis of these reflexes. Further analysis of the reflex connections requires both more localized stimulation of the labyrinth, and further subdivision of motoneuron pools, than employed in experiments to date.

REFERENCES

1. BRODAL A., POMPEIANO, O. and WALBERG, F. *The Vestibular Nuclei and their Connections, Anatomy and Functional Correlations.* Oliver & Boyd, Edinburgh, 1962.
2. NYBERG–HANSEN, R. Functional organization of descending supraspinal fibre systems to the spinal cord. Anatomical observations and physiological correlations. *Ergebnisse Anat.* **39**, (No. 2) 1, 1966.
3. FULTON, J. F., LIDDELL, E. G. T. and RIOCH, D. McK. The influence of unilateral destruction of the vestibular nuclei upon posture and the knee-jerk. *Brain* **53**, 327, 1930.
4 WILSON, V. J., KATO, M., PETERSON, B. W. and WYLIE, R. M. A single-unit analysis of the organization of Deiters' nucleus. *J. Neurophysiol.* **30**, 603, 1967.
5. MUGNAINI, E., WALBERG, F. and BRODAL, A. Mode of termination of primary vestibular fibres in the lateral vestibular nucleus. An experimental electron microscope study in the cat. *Expl Brain Res.* **4**, 186, 1967.
6. WALBERG, F., BOWSHER, D. and BRODAL, A. The termination of primary vestibular fibers in the vestibular nuclei of the cat. An experimental study with silver methods. *J. comp. Neurol.* **110**, 391, 1958.
7. ITO, M., HONGO, T. and OKADA, Y. Vestibular-evoked postysynaptic potentials in Deiter's neurons. *Expl Brain Res.* **7**, 214, 1969.
8. PETERSON, B. W. A single unit analysis of the properties and distribution of gravity responses in the vestibular nuclei of the cat. Doctoral thesis, Rockefeller University, 1969.
9. NYBERG–HANSEN, R. Do cat spinal motoneurones receive direct supraspinal fibre connections? A supplementary silver study. *Archs ital. Biol.* **107**, 67, 1969.
10. NYBERG–HANSEN, R. and MASCITTI, T. A. Sites and mode of termination of fibers of the vestibulospinal tract in the cat. An experimental study with silver impregnation methods. *J. comp. Neurol.* **122**, 369, 1964.
11. WILSON, V. J. and YOSHIDA, M. Comparison of the effects of stimulation of Deiters' nucleus and the medial longitudinal fasciculus on neck, forelimb and hindlimb motoneurons. *J. Neurophysiol.* **32**, 743, 1969.
12. LUND, S. and POMPEIANO, O. Monosynaptic excitation of alpha motoneurons from supraspinal structures in the cat. *Acta physiol. scand.* **73**, 1, 1968..
13. BATINI, C., MORUZZI, G. and POMPEIANO, O. Cerebellar release phenomena. *Archs ital. Biol.* **95**, 71, 1957.
14. MAGNUS, R. Some results of studies in the physiology of posture. *Lancet* **211**, 531, 585, 1926.
15. GRILLNER, S., HONGO, T. and LUND, S. The vestibulospinal tract. Effects on alpha-motoneurons in the lumbosacral spinal cord in the cat. *Expl Brain Res.* **10**, 94, 1970.
16. GRILLNER, S., HONGO, T. and LUND, S. Reciprocal effects between two descending bulbospinal systems with monosynaptic connections to spinal motoneurons. *Brain Res.* **10**, 477, 1968.
17. DIETE-SPIFF, K., CARLI, G. and POMPEIANO, O. Comparison of the effects of stimulation of the VIIIth cranial nerve, the vestibular nuclei or the reticular formation on the gastrocnemius muscle and its spindles. *Archs ital. Biol.* **105**, 243, 1967.
18. GERNANDT, BO. E. and GILMAN, S. Descending vestibular activity and its modulation by proprioceptive, cerebellar and reticular influences. *Expl Neurol.* **1**, 274, 1959.
19. SZENTAGOTHAI, J. *Die Rolle der einzelnen Labryinthrezeptoren bei der Orientation von Augen und Kopf im Raume.* Akademiai Kiado, Budapest, 1952.
20. YAMAUCHI, T. and KATO, M. The effects of electrical stimulation of vestibular nerve from lateral semicircular canal upon spinal cord. *Brain Res.* **14**, 227, 1969.
21. SCHIMERT, J. S. Die Endigungsweise des Tractus vestibulospinalis. *Z. Anat. Entw Gesch.* **108**, 761, 1938.
22. WILSON, V. J., YOSHIDA, M. and SCHOR, R. H. Monosynaptic excitation and inhibition of thoracic motoneurons by fibers in the medial longitudinal fasciculus. *Brain Res.* **18**, 181, 1970.

23. WILSON, V. J., YOSHIDA, M. and SCHOR, R. H. Supraspinal monosynaptic excitation and inhibition of thoracic back motoneurons. *Expl Brain Res.* **11**, 282, 1970.

24. GRILLNER, S., HONGO, T. and LUND, S. Descending monosynpatic and reflex control of gamma motoneurons. *Acta physiol. scand.* **75**, 592, 1969.

25. ECCLES, J. C., ITO, M. and SZENTAGOTHAI, J. *The Cerebellum as a Neuronal Machine.* Springer, New York, 1967.

26. ITO, M. and YOSHIDA, M. The origin of cerebellar-induced inhibition of Deiters' neurones— I. Monosynaptic initiation of the inhibitory postsynaptic potentials. *Expl Brain Res.* **2**, 330, 1966.

27. CARLI, G., DIETE-SPIFF, K. and POMPEIANO, O. Responses of the muscle spindles and of the extrafusal fibres in an extensor muscle to stimulation of the lateral vestibular nucleus in the cat. *Archs ital. Biol.* **105**, 209, 1967.

28. BRUGGENCATE, G. TEN., BURKE, R. E., LUNDBERG, A. and UDO, M. Interaction between the vestibulospinal tract and contralateral flexor reflex afferents. *Brain Res.* **14**, 529, 1969.

29. LUNDBERG, A. Intergration in the reflex pathway. *Muscular Afferents and Motor Control, Nobel Symposium 1*, GRANIT, R. (Ed.), p. 275. Almqvist & Wiksell, Stockholm, 1966.

30. McMASTERS, R. E., WEISS, A. H. and CARPENTER, M. B. Vestibular projections to the nuclei of the extraocular muscles. Degeneration resulting from discrete partial lesions of the vestibular nuclei in the monkey. *Am. J. Anat.* **118**, 163, 1966.

31. PETRAS, J. M. Cortical, tectal and tegmental fiver connections in the spinal cord of the cat. *Brain Res.* **6**, 275, 1967.

32. NYBERG–HANSEN, R. Origin and termination of fibers from the vestibular nuclei descending in the medial longitudinal fasciculus. An experimental study with silver impregnation methods in the cat. *J. comp. Neurol.* **122**, 355, 1964.

33. PRECHT, W., GRIPPO, J. and WAGNER, A. Contribution of different types of central vestibular neurons to the vestibulospinal system. *Brain Res.* **4**, 119, 1967.

34. WILSON, V. J., WYLIE, R. M. and MARCO, L. A. Synaptic inputs to cells in the medial vestibular nucleus. *J. Neurophysiol.* **31**, 176, 1968.

35. GERNANDT, BO. E. Functional properties of the descending medial longitudinal fasciculus. *Expl Neurol.* **22**, 326, 1968.

36. WILSON, V. J. and YOSHIDA, M. Monosynaptic inhibition of neck motoneurons by the medial vestibular nucleus. *Expl Brain Res.* **9**, 365, 1969.

37. WILSON, V. J., WYLIE, R. M. and MARCO, L. A. Organization of the medial vestibular nucleus. *J. Neurophysiol.* **31**, 166, 1968.

38. WILSON, V. J. and YOSHIDA, M. Bilateral connections between labyrinths and neck motoneurons. *Brain Res.* **13**, 603, 1969.

39. MANO, N., OSHIMA, T. and SHIMAZU, H. Inhibitory commissural fibers interconnecting the bilateral vestibular nuclei. *Brain Res.* **8**, 378, 1968.

40. BAKER, R. G., MANO, N. and SHIMAZU, H. Postsynaptic potentials in abducens motoneurons induced by vestibular stimulation. *Brain Res.* **15**, 577, 1969.

41. SHERRINGTON, C. S. *The Integrative Action of the Nervous System.* Scribner's, New York, 1906.

J. psychiat. Res., 1971, Vol. 8, pp. 273–287. Pergamon Press. Printed in Great Britain.

IS PAIN A SPECIFIC SENSATION?

EDWARD R. PERL*

Department of Physiology, University of Utah College of Medicine, Salt Lake City, Utah

PAIN became classified as a sensory quality relatively late in the evolution of ideas on sensation and consciousness. Prior to the Nineteenth Century most authorities had followed Aristotle's view in setting pain opposite to pleasure and assigning it to the realm of emotion. Under impetus of the analyses that followed BELL's (1811)[1] and MAGENDIE's (1822)[2] separation of peripheral sensory and motor pathways in the spinal roots, concepts of nervous organization and function clarified. In company with the increasing dominance of experimentally dictated views of the nervous system, pain came to be more commonly thought of in terms of a sensory phenomenon; however, the specificity of neural mechanisms leading to it has been continually doubted.

As a first step in deciding whether or not pain has the characteristics associated with a specific sensation, it is necessary to set down attributes that might be accepted for this category. Some possible semantic problems may be avoided by starting from an un-ambiguous model. Vision begins with the excitation of structures in the eye, a particular and unique sense organ. Under ordinary conditions the receptive tissue of the eye has a responsiveness limited to a clearly definable set of environmental events. The receptive elements of the retina, in turn, excite a chain of nerve cells that transmit signals related to incoming light to regions of the forebrain. Consequently, a neural sequence from the receptive structure to neurons of the thalamus and cortex are dedicated to the relaying and analysis of information contained in the light reaching the eyes of the organism. Generalizing from this example, a specific sensation has a kind of receptive apparatus (receptor) that is particularly responsive to a limited class of events. Activity generated by specialized receptors then engages a series of neurons forming a projecting system (to higher centers) devoted to the signals initiated by the effective stimuli. Current opinion would agree that the 'special senses' (vision, hearing, smell and taste) are associated with mechanisms fitting this generalization. On the other hand, the situation for somatic sensibility, particularly pain, is less clear.

As the Twentieth Century began, the physiologists and their allies in this cause, the clinical neurologists, apparently had won the argument with the philosophically-oriented over the nature of pain, and it was widely accepted as a sensory experience rather than the emotional reaction opposite to pleasure. At that time there were two viewpoints on the

---

* Present address: Department of Physiology, School of Medicine, University of North Carolina, Chapel Hill, North Carolina.

kind of neural activity that led to pain; variations on these two themes form the bases of currently advocated theories. One concept held that pain results when receptive structures and/or central projections mediating other modalities of somatic sensation are subjected to strong or excessive stimulation. A modern version of this thesis suggests that intense stimulation causes unique patterns of activity in certain fractions of the population of somatic sensory elements. The second hypothesis stemmed from observations of late Nineteenth Century psychophysicists studying cutaneous sensibility. They found that the skin is not uniformly sensitive; spots giving rise to sensation following a given kind of stimulation are separated by areas from which equivalent stimuli do not arouse a response. As the result of such work, von Frey,[3] in particular, proposed a specific receptive and transmission system for various modalities of cutaneous sense, including pain. Unfortunately for his fundamental thesis, von Frey was bold enough to designate a morphologically identifiable end organ for each modality. Subsequent investigations have agreed with the lack of uniformity in skin sensibility but have vigorously denied both the suggested correlation of the functional attributes of a spot to the morphology of underlying sensory structures and the stability of a spot over time. [4-6] Von Frey proposed an end organ for the detection of painful stimuli that differed from other cutaneous sensory endings by the absence of encapsulation. His detractors have pointed out that unencapsulated or 'bare' nerve endings are the only kind found in certain skin regions from which sensations other than pain can be evoked. Furthermore, pain may be initiated by a variety of mechanical, thermal and chemical stimuli; some have found this difficult to equate with a specialization of receptive function.

The question of the nature of the stimuli causing pain raises not only conceptual but practical problems as well. The analysis of sensory function, especially in animals, is unrealistic if the stimulus cannot be given parameters that have meaning in terms of the natural history of the organism. Sherrington[7] came to grips with this some years ago in emphasizing that pain usually results from the threat or fact of tissue destruction. He labeled events *threatening* the integrity of tissue 'noxious'. Noxious stimuli, as common experience dictates, are likely to cause pain and in situations occurring in nature, usually do so. This view of pain-producing stimuli does much to delineate the circumstances associated with the phenomena, and in my opinion, represents the critical point of departure for the consideration of specificity in pain mechanisms. If we are correct in believing that the common denominator for painful stimuli in ordinary or 'normal' circumstances is their noxious quality, then man and animal must have means for distinguishing noxious from innocuous environmental events. It also follows that there must be an unambiguous method for signalling the existence of a noxious event to the central nervous system.

An important clue to the peripheral pathways for pain-producing impulses was provided by morphological observations on mammalian dorsal roots. Ranson[8] noted that dorsal root filaments separated close to their junction with the spinal cord into a medial division containing large diameter myelinated fibers and a lateral division composed of thinly myelinated and unmyelinated fibers. Subsequently, Ranson and Billingsley[9] found that vasomotor and respiratory reactions typical of reactions to painful stimuli were dependent upon the integrity of the dorsal root's lateral division but not its medial one. Another indication of a close relation between impulse conduction in fine afferent fibers of peripheral nerve and pain followed discovery of the significance of the various deflections of the compound action potential. HEINBECKER et al.[10] showed that volleys of impulses elicited by electrical stimulation of a cutaneous nerve had to contain activity in the slowly-conducting (hence, small diameter) myelinated fibers to evoke pain in conscious man or reactions typical of pain in animals. The fact that impulses in the rapidly-conducting, large-diameter myelinated fibers did not lead to pain, while those in more slowly-conducting fibers did, was supported by studies in which differential block of conduction in nerves was produced by pressure or local anesthetic agents during tests for dissociation of sensation in man.[11,12] Unmyelinated afferent fibers were established to convey activity of special importance for the production of pain by similar techniques[13,14] as well as by considerations based on the latency of certain responses to noxious stimuli.[15] The varied nature and persistent recurrence of evidence pointing in the same direction seemed to assure some special significance of impulses in slowly-conducting afferent fibers. Those who favored the concept of a specific neural apparatus for pain (and the adversive reactions normally accompanying it) interpreted them as indicating that receptive terminals (receptors) specialized for the detection of strong stimuli were associated with fine diameter fibers. On the other hand, studies of the responses of single primary afferent units have given ambiguous encouragement for this view. In 1939 ZOTTERMAN[16] reported that noxious stimuli such as burning of the skin evoked impulses in certain receptors with slowly-conducting fibers, including some that were judged to be unmyelinated; however, he also described excitation of afferent units with fibers conducting in the same velocity range by the most gentle mechanical stimulation of the skin. Cutaneous receptors with afferent fibers of slow conduction that are responsive to innocuous manipulation have been repeatedly described.[17-21]. In contrast, a period of active study of individual receptive units brought forth few accounts of 'nociceptive' elements. To be sure, single fibers of various conduction velocities were reported to require intense or damaging stimulation of their terminals for excitation,[18,19,22,23] but their number was small compared to those with low thresholds for naturally occurring events, and their characteristics varied widely. These discrepancies impressed a number of commentators and, along with other inconsistencies, led to articulate attacks on theories proposing specificity for pain mechanisms.[5,6,24]

Similar objections were voiced to the notion of central pathways dedicated to a pain 'system'. There were few who doubted that tracts in the ventrolateral spinal cord and an equivalent one for the afferent input from the head were important for the central conduction of impulses leading to pain, but there was little documentation of a special excitation by noxious stimuli of neurons making up such tracts.[25,26] A theory for pain mechanisms advanced by MELZACK and WALL[25] in 1965 has attempted to reconcile the several kinds of evidence by proposing a continuum of characteristics for somatic receptors and an interplay in their central effects to control a gating system within the dorsal horn of the spinal cord; an appropriate balance of activity in small diameter and large diameter afferent fibers was proposed as necessary for the initiation of ascending activity causing pain. Melzack and Wall's hypothesis found favor with those attracted to generalizations proposing flexibility in neural organization, but its details have been subject to critical attack on the basis of recent experimental data.

The crossed extensor reflex is usually considered part of the flexor withdrawal reaction organized at the spinal cord. My entry into this arena of controversy began some years ago with the observation that this reflex effect depended upon slowly-conducting myelinated fibers in afferent volleys from cutaneous nerves, a finding that was a by-product of an attempt to study neural mechanisms specifically dependent upon input from fine afferent fibers.[27] In the course of the experiments on spinal reflexes, it was also noted that pinching the skin facilitated extensor motoneurons of the opposite side, while brushing hairs did not. Since many slowly-conducting afferent fibers were connected to receptors vigorously excited by the gentle displacement of hairs, only a fraction of that fiber category seemed to form the afferent limb of this reflex. Somewhat later, in studies on activation of thalamic neurons by somatic stimuli after interruption of the dorsal columns, certain cells in the ventrobasal complex were noted to respond only to noxious stimulation of a limited region of the contralateral body half.[28] Latencies of the thalamic responses to electrical stimulation of the intact peripheral nerves at different points suggested that impulses in fibers conducting under 30 m/sec were of critical importance for such discharges. More recently, sympathetic reflexes in spinal animals acting to raise the arterial pressure also were shown to be dependent upon afferent activity in slowly-conducting myelinated fibers.[29] These observations from personal work, in addition to the evidence from the older literature, emphasized the necessity for a close scrutiny of the fine-diameter myelinated portion of the afferent spectrum for its role in the transmittal of sensory information of importance for nociception.

NOCICEPTION BY CUTANEOUS RECEPTORS

A first problem was to find a technique that would facilitate recording from slowly-conducting myelinated fibers so as to permit a careful examination of the responses of their terminals to a variety of stimuli. Microelectrodes inserted into a peripheral nerve prove to be an efficient means of recording impulses from single fibers, provided that proper attention is given to mechanical fixation of the nerve, and to the dimensions of the electrode; if this is done, stable unitary potentials can be obtained in a single experiment from many fibers conducting between 5 and 80 m/sec.[30] A survey in which every unit, identified by a response to electrical shocks of the intact nerve, was tested for the most effective natural stimuli agreed with earlier work in showing that the majority of receptors with myelinated fibers conducting under 40 m/sec (from nerves supplying hairy skin) are very responsive to hair movement or other innocuous stimuli. On the other hand, a significant minority of the same conduction velocity group can be activated only by strong mechanical stimulation of the skin. Figure 1 compares the responses of a receptor with a fiber conducting at 25 m/sec to pressure by a calibrated blunt probe and to a noxious pinch. The mechanical thresholds of elements similar to this type varied from some that were excited only by stimuli causing visible damage to others that responded to moderate pressure; however, all elements of this class increase the number and frequency of discharges as stimuli progress from threshold through overtly damaging intensities. These 'high threshold' receptors had uniquely organized receptive fields consisting of 5–20 or more 'spots', from which responses were most readily evoked, scattered over several square centimeters. Inasmuch as little or no response was initiated by intense thermal or chemical stimuli, such primary afferent units appear to be a special kind of mechanoreceptor.

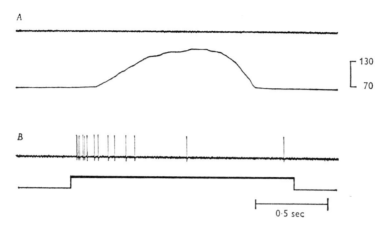

FIG. 1. Responses of a high threshold cutaneous receptor with a myelinated afferent fiber (25 m/sec) to mechanical stimuli. The upper trace of each pair shows the recording from a microelectrode in the posterior femoral cutaneous nerve of cat. *A*—Pinch of a fold of skin containing the receptive terminals with a smooth-surfaced, calibrated tweezers; scale at right indicates grams of force exerted by the tweezer. *B*—Pinch of the same fold of skin with a serrated tissue forceps for duration of the deflection of the lower trace; pressure exerted by the teeth of the tissue forceps was sufficient to penetrate the skin. (From BURGESS and PERL.[30] Figure reproduced by permission of the *J. Physiol. Lond.* **190**, 1967.)

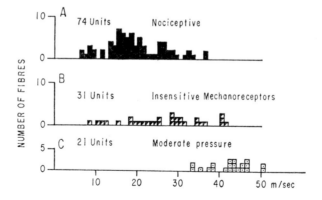

FIG. 2. Conduction velocity of myelinated high threshold mechanoreceptors from the posterior femoral cutaneous nerve of cat. All had a receptive field consisting of points of responsiveness to strong mechanical stimuli separated by areas from which responses could not be evoked by equivalent stimuli. Grouping in arbitrary classes based upon threshold for punctate mechanical stimuli. Sample taken from an analysis of 513 units with afferent fibers conducting under 51 m/sec. (From BURGESS and PERL.[30] Figure reproduced by permission of the *J. Physiol, Lond.* **190**, 1967.)

High threshold mechanoreceptors represented some 30 per cent of 513 units conducting under 50 m/sec from nerves innervating the cat's posterior thigh. A similar survey of cutaneous sensory units in the monkey showed that essentially identical elements are common in the primate, and that their endings appear in both hairy and glabrous areas.[31]. Figure 2 plots the conduction velocity of high threshold mechanoreceptor units from the

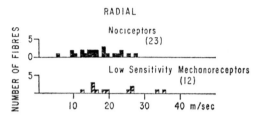

FIG. 3. Conduction velocity of myelinated high threshold mechanoreceptors from the radial nerve of the squirrel monkey. Receptive terminals were located in hairy skin, glabrous skin and bridging both types. Arbitrary division into groups according to threshold for punctate mechanical stimulators. Sample taken from analysis of 209 units with afferent fibers conducting from 4 to over 80 m/sec. (From PERL.[31] Figure reproduced by permission of the *J. Physiol, Lond.* **197**, 1968.)

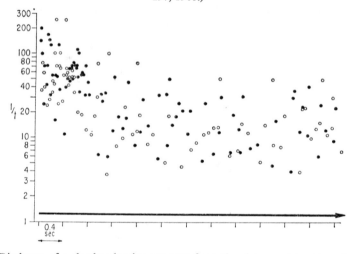

FIG. 4. Discharge of a slowly-adapting receptor from the glabrous skin of a primate with a low threshold for mechanical stimuli. Conduction velocity of the afferent fiber—34 m/sec. Response to moderate pressure across a fold of skin containing the receptive field indicated by filled circles (plotted impulse by impulse as 'instantaneous' frequency); response to noxious pressure across the same fold of skin indicated by open circles. Stimulus was constant throughout the period indicated by the line above the abscissa. (From PERL.[31] Figure reproduced by permission of the *J. Physiol. Lond.* **197**, 1968.)

posterior femoral cutaneous nerve of cat; an arbitrary separation according to mechanical threshold is made in this diagram to illustrate the tendency for threshold to correlate with speed of conduction. Figure 3, taken from the study in the monkey, shows the conduction velocities for units from a nerve supplying both hairy and glabrous skin. The names originally applied to these receptors were conservative. Only those requiring frankly damaging stimuli for threshold excitation were designated as nociceptors, but, in fact, the category as a whole had a singular ability among elements with myelinated fibers to indicate the difference between threatening and innocuous stimuli. This conclusion was drawn from studies of the type exemplified by Fig. 4. The sensory unit of Fig. 4 had an afferent fiber conducting at 34 m/sec and responded to gentle pressure directed at a small area of the glabrous skin of the monkey hand with a slowly adapting discharge; its response to moderate, innocuous pressure is indicated by the filled circles (as the reciprocal of the interval between successive impulses, i.e. 'instantaneous' frequency), while noxious pressure initiated the activity shown by the open circles. No difference in either maximal frequency, adaptation rate, or discharge pattern is apparent. The same results were obtained with all primary sensory units that had low thresholds to some form of natural skin stimulation; noxious stimuli always evoked responses that could be closely mimicked by innocuous stimulation.

There is a clear parallel between the characteristics of the high threshold mechano-receptors and the psychophysics of cutaneous pain, particularly the initial 'pricking' pain elicited by a sharp object. The punctate form of the receptive region for both is one common feature, and the relatively rapid adaptation to a steady stimulus is another. A major difference exists as well: the myelinated high threshold units are not excited by such common pain-producing stimuli as noxious heat or irritant chemicals. Thus, since un-myelinated (C) fibers have also been implicated in the signalling of pain-causing events, exploration of the portion of the peripheral afferent spectrum made up of C fiber elements seemed in order. Previous investigations had reported 'C' high threshold units,[19,20,23] but left important questions unanswered, including the relative numbers of high and low threshold types and the degree to which their characteristics overlap those of receptors associated with myelinated fibers. Gathering an adequate sample of C sensory units was an obstacle inasmuch as previous experience had indicated that adequate isolation of discharges from single C elements could be difficult. Recordings from peripheral nerve using microelectrodes rarely yielded stable recordings from fibers conducting at C velocity, but a modification of the classical technique for dissecting peripheral nerves into fine filaments provided a satisfactory yield of single unit potentials. Quantitative analysis from strands containing more than one active element were then made possible by means of an impulse pattern recognition scheme utilizing a digital computer.[32]

The presence of numerous C sensory units responding vigorously to both the most gentle mechanical stimuli and to moderate cooling was readily confirmed; these elements were not excited by heat and gave responses to noxious mechanical stimuli that were easily duplicated by innocuous manipulation. Figure 5 compares discharge patterns of a low threshold C mechanoreceptor to identical movements (lowermost trace) of a blunt probe (A, B) and a needle (A', B') pressing against the same skin area. The low threshold C mechanoreceptors proved to have interesting properties but they did not appear to be useful for nociception.[33]

Other C sensory units were quite different. Figure 6 shows the discharges of a C receptor evoked by punctate mechanical stimulation of the skin (the bars under each trace indicate the approximate time of stimulation). As indicated, the unit of Fig. 6 differentiated between

H

an innocuous and a noxious mechanical stimulus; moreover, it also responded promptly to intense heat and was excited by irritant chemicals applied to the intact skin. Such elements were labeled 'polymodal nociceptors' and were relatively common forms of C sensory units.

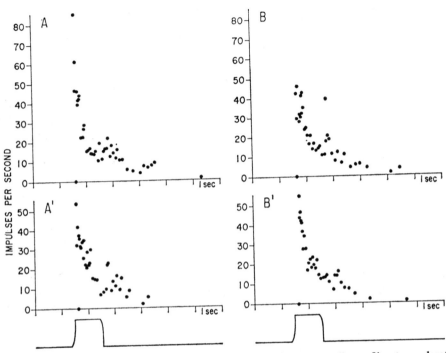

FIG. 5.   Responses from a low threshold mechanoreceptor with a C afferent fiber to moderate and noxious stimuli. Stimuli were 1200 μ indentations of the skin with the time course indicated by the trace below the graphs. *A* and *B* show the responses (as 'instantaneous' frequency) evoked by a blunt (1 mm) tip fitted to the electromechanical stimulating device. *A'* and *B'* show responses evoked by a needle fitted to the stimulator contacting the center of the area stimulated in *A* and *B*. (From BESSOU, *et al.*[33] Figure reproduced by permission of the *J. Neurophysiol.* **34**, 1971. Copyright of the American Physiological Society.)

The polymodal receptors showed a fascinating tendency to increase in responsiveness with successive activations by heat.[32] An illustration of 'sensitization' for a polymodal element is given by Fig. 7: A plots 'instantaneous discharge frequency' against time with a parallel indication of thermode temperature during a cycle of step-wise increases in temperature; B takes the results of A to graph discharge frequency against thermode temperature and C and D do the same with data from subsequent cycles of heating. The display of Fig. 7D shows that after repeated exposure to noxious heat, the discharge activity for the initial activation by heat is nearly duplicated at a stimulus temperature 5°C lower. This kind of enhanced sensitivity to heat sometimes was accompanied by a drop in mechanical threshold. Furthermore, skin damage (by heat or other stimuli) was often associated with a low frequency tonic discharge. It does not stretch the imagination to fit these observations on receptor behavior to the common experience of altered cutaneous sensibility following burns or other insults to the skin.

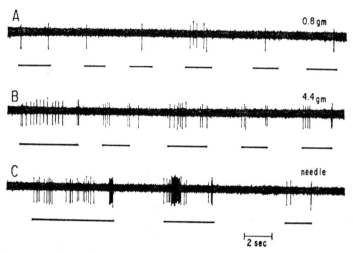

FIG. 6. Responses of a polymodal nociceptor with a C afferent to punctate mechanical stimuli. Bars under each trace mark the approximate time of stimuli, all to one point of the receptive field. The force exerted by the stimulator is indicated to the right of each trace. In C the needle pressure was sufficient to penetrate the skin. (From BESSOU and PERL.[32] Figure reproduced by permission of the *J. Neurophysiol.* **32**, 1969. Copyright of the American Physiological Society.)

Several other types of C fiber receptors from the skin were encountered and in a series of 147 units from hairy skin of cat at least five distinct groups could be recognized with remarkably little overlap in their thresholds for thermal or mechanical stimuli.[32] Approximately 50 per cent of the cutaneous C fiber receptors from hairy regions had elevated thresholds to all forms of stimulation and responded weakly if at all to innocuous stimulation. Approximately the same division between low and high threshold C fiber receptors of hairy skin was also seen during a subsequent series of microelectrode recordings from dorsal root ganglion cells.[33] On the other hand, while polymodal nociceptors with receptive fields in glabrous skin have been identified, other C fiber sensory units of glabrous regions differ from those in hairy skin in their functional characteristics or frequency of occurrence. Such differences emphasize variations associated with the tissue innervated, and suggest that it is unwise to generalize about the types of primary afferent units in a peripheral nerve from a restricted sample.

Thus, with appropriate sampling techniques, it is possible to demonstrate a significant number of 'nociceptors' from the skin. Nociceptors are characterized by an elevated threshold to all forms of stimulation compared to other sensory elements in the same nerve. They do not have a uniform set of characteristics, seeming to show some specialization for the most effective form of stimulation; however, all varieties increase the frequency and/or number of discharges unequivocally as stimuli (most effective for their excitation) progress in intensity from innocuous, though threatening to tissue-damaging.

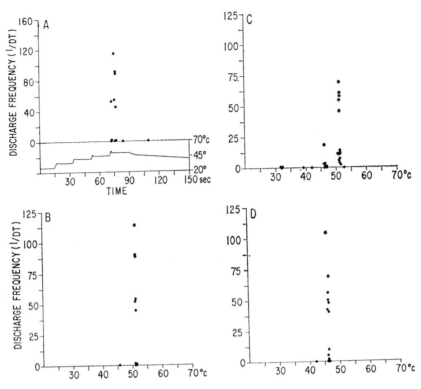

FIG. 7. The response of a polymodal nociceptor with a C afferent fiber during sequential cycles of skin heating by a thermode fixed in contact to one area of skin. *A*—Discharge frequency is indicated on the vertical axis above the dashed line and the thermode temperature below it. The first in a series of three sequential cycles of heating in which similar 5° steps in temperatures were used. *B, C* and *D* are graphs of discharge vs. thermode temperature for the three heating cycles. *B* was taken from the data in *A*. The terminal temperature reached in *D* was approximately 5° lower than for *B* and *C*. (From BESSOU and PERL.[32] Figure reproduced by permission of the *J. Neurophysiol* **32,** 1969.   Copyright of the American Physiological Society.)

SPINAL PROJECTION OF NOCICEPTORS

Our recent emphasis in studies of cutaneous nociceptive mechanisms has been concerned with a spinal cord relay activated by nociceptive and thermoreceptive peripheral sensory units. In this work, no attempt was made to survey spinal cells for their responses to various stimuli. Instead, the initial experiments concentrated on possible projections from high threshold mechanoreceptors with myelinated afferent fibers. Fig. 8 outlines the experimental arrangement for the cat. A cutaneous nerve or dorsal root was exposed, fitted with ordinary electrical stimulating and recording electrodes while its peripheral and central terminations were left intact. The spinal canal was opened and pipette microelectrodes filled with a dye for marking location of the tip were used to record from elements of the dorsal horn.

When a recording of particular interest was made, dye was electrophoretically ejected from the recording electrode; study of histologically-prepared sections after the experiment allowed identification of the recording sites.[34] In a subsequent series, the upper cervical spinal cord could be excited by electrical stimuli to test for antidromic activation of

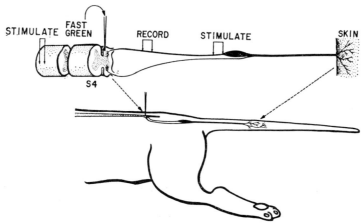

FIG. 8. Schematic diagram of the experimental conditions used to study spinal projections of cutaneous receptors with slowly conducting afferent fibers. A dorsal root of the caudal (coccygeal) level was placed on stimulating and recording electrodes while being left connected to the skin and to the spinal cord. A microelectrode filled with a solution of Fast Green dye in saline was used to penetrate the spinal cord at the dorsal root entrance zone. Stimulating electrodes were placed upon the contralateral spinal cord at the upper cervical level.

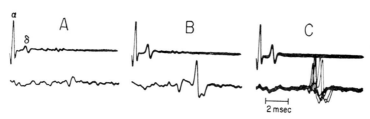

FIG. 9. Responses from the spinal dorsal marginal zone to afferent volleys of graded size. Upper trace of each pair—compound action potential evoked by single electrical shocks to a dorsal root; lower trace—simultaneously recorded activity from a microelectrode in the dorsal horn. The dorsal root component $A\alpha$, fibers conducting over 40 m/sec, is essentially maximal in A; the component $A\delta$, fibers conducting under 25 m/sec, increased progressively from A to C, becoming maximal in the latter. The large unitary responses appeared only with volleys of B size or greater. (From CHRISTENSEN and PERL.[34] Figure reproduced by permission of the *J. Neurophysiol.* **33**, 1970. Copyright of the American Physiological Society.)

elements under study from rostral levels. In these experiments, the recording microelectrode has advanced into the spinal cord while single volleys were initiated in the afferent nerve by two strengths of shocks. Alternately, a weak and a strong shock was delivered; the weaker was sufficient to excite only the rapidly conducting myelinated fibers ($A\alpha$) while the stronger also activated the more slowly conducting myelinated fibers ($A\delta$). Those postsynaptic responses dependent upon the presence of slowly-conducting fibers in the volley were examined further. Recordings obtained from a spinal unit meeting these conditions is shown in the lower traces of Fig. 9; the neuron responded only when the afferent volley (upper traces) included part of the $A\delta$ component (Fig. 9B). With shocks supramaximal for all of the myelinated fibers, the unit responded regularly, but still showed latency variations typical for postsynaptic elements (Fig. 9C). Units of this type were usually recorded close to the point of penetration of the dorsal surface of the spinal cord and, while relatively scarce, were encountered in every preparation near the rostral limit of the segment.[34] They could not be excited by gentle mechanical stimulation of the skin and thus, a significant excitatory input from the $A\delta$ fiber hair receptors was ruled out.

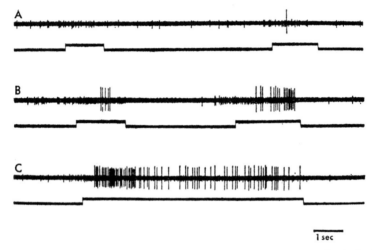

FIG. 10.   Response of a neuron in the spinal dorsal marginal zone to mechanical stimulation of the skin. The lower trace marks the time of stimulation: *A*—firm stroke with smooth rod; *B*—pinch of skin fold with smooth forceps; *C*—pinch of skin fold with tissue (serrated) forceps. (From CHRISTENSEN and PERL.[34] Figure reproduced by permission of the *J. Neurophysiol.* **33**, 1970. Copyright of the American Physiological Society.)

Intense mechanical stimuli did evoke responses. Fig. 10 compares activity generated by firm strokes across the unit's receptive field with a smooth object (A), pinches of a skin fold with a smooth-surfaced forceps (B), and a firm pinch of the same fold by a forceps with teeth (C). The latter (Fig. 10C) was damaging to the cutaneous surface, and the neuron's discharge was much greater than that evoked by the lesser stimuli (Fig. 10A and B). Certain elements located in the same regions of the spinal cord received excitatory inputs from myelinated and from C afferent fibers; these types were activated both by strong mechanical and by intense thermal stimuli. A third class which were excited only when afferent volleys included a C fiber component, responded to innocuous thermal stimuli. Dye marks identifying the recording sites for unitary potentials with specific responses to noxious and thermal stimuli were clustered about the border between the gray and white matter in the spinal dorsal horn (Fig. 11D). Each dot in the schematic drawings of the dorsal horn shown in Fig. 11 indicates a site from which a particular recording was obtained: A gives the relative positions of units responding only to intense mechanical stimuli, B locates units excited by noxious heat and intense mechanical stimuli, while C shows the relative locations of three different kinds of units observed in one experiment (1—responsive to cooling, noxious heat and intense mechanical stimuli; 2—responsive to noxious heat and intense mechanical stimuli; 3—responsive to intense mechanical stimuli only). In some instances, the dye was confined within the outlines of a large (pericornual) cell of the marginal zone, suggesting these cells as the probable source of the unitary potentials. An identical projection to the marginal zone of monkey has been found; the relative ease of locating such elements in the primate implies that they are more common in this species than in cat.

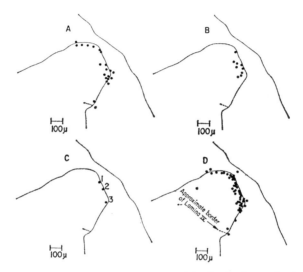

FIG. 11.   Locations of spinal neurons excited by activity in slowly conducting afferent fibers. A—units responding to only strong mechanical stimuli; B—units responding to noxious heat and strong mechanical stimuli; C—relative position of three units in one experiment (1—innocuous cooling, strong mechanical stimuli, noxious heat; 2—strong mechanical aid, noxious heat; 3—only strong mechanical stimuli) D—all marked recording sites in 52 experiments. (From CHRISTENSEN and PERL.[34] Figure reproduced by permission of the *J. Neurophysiol.* **33,** 1970. Copyright of the American Physiological Society.)

About one-fourth of the marginal-zone units receiving specific projections from nociceptors were found to be antidromically excited by electrical stimulation of the contralateral half of the spinal cord at cervical levels. Therefore, at least some of the marginal-zone cells must have processes extending the length of the spinal cord. Dorsal horn marginal cells were suggested as part of the source for a crossed ventrolateral spinal ('spinothalamic') pathway by FOERSTER and GAGEL[35] and by KURU[36] on the basis of retrograde degeneration studies of human cordotomy cases. In the absence of supporting physiological evidence, their proposals for the origin of the ventrolateral systems concerned with pain and temperature sensations did not receive wide acceptance. Its validity is, however, strongly supported by these results showing that cells with specific input from noci- and thermoreceptors preferentially occupy marginal locations in the apex of the dorsal horn.

CONCLUSIONS

The observations presented indicate that both certain primary afferent units and certain higher order cells to which they project are excited solely or most effectively by stimuli strong enough to threaten the integrity of tissue. They are, therefore, functionally suited for nociception. In addition, there is a significant subspecialization within this nociceptive group of neurons. A reasonable correlation exists between the physiological characteristics of the system formed by these elements, and the psychophysical characteristics of pain produced by noxious stimuli in man. Thus, some of the major features of specialized sensory mechanisms are also applicable to a neural organization that informs the central nervous system of mammals about acute environmentally produced threat or injury and the pain such situations usually evoke in man.

The results discussed herein leave many questions about pain and its neural substrate unanswered. Past critics of specificity have pointed out that tissue damage does not always lead to pain. A case in point is the absence of pain from certain neoplasms. On the other hand, it can be argued that the system for nociception evolved long before major threats to the organism were related to processes of development and aging. Another commonly raised objection to the notion of specificity in the pain process is found in the fact, as stories from the battlefield attest,[25] that severe tissue damage does not always result in pain. A retort to such criticism could be the fact that sound does not always penetrate consciousness in an unattentive child. In the same vein one can demand what sensations are aroused in the anesthetized preparations used to study the admitted specificity of the visual and auditory systems? It must be remembered that there is a critical and still mysterious step between input of sensory origin to the higher central nervous system and conscious perception. Finally, what about the 'pain' that appears in the absence of stimulation, or is evoked by normally innocuous stimulation, in certain diseases of the nervous system? A very similar problem also exists in other sensory systems; for example, certain visual or other hallucinations are often reported as a consequence of drug usage. Thus, despite the many unexplained phenomena, it seems reasonable to propose at this juncture that the signalling system leading to pain has many similarities to those existing for the sensory mechanisms subserving the so-called 'specific' sensations. Thus, while much more needs to be done to settle the question in an unequivocal fashion, tentative classification of pain as a 'specific' or distinct modality of sensation seems reasonable.

Acknowledgements—This article was prepared, in part, during tenure of a Visiting Professorship at Faculté des Sciences à St. Jerome, Université de Marseille. The effort was assisted by funds from grant NS 01576-13 from the U.S.P.H.S. I am grateful for the assistance of Mrs. L. Sedivec in the preparation of the manuscript.

REFERENCES

1. BELL, C. Idea of a new anatomy of the brain submitted for the observation of his friends. London, 1811.
2. MAGENDIE, F. *J. Pysiol. expl. Path.* **2**, 366, 1822. As quoted in KEELE, K. D., *Anatomies of Pain*, p. 130, C. C. Thomas, Springfield, 1957.

3. FREY, M. VON. Untersuchungen über die Sinnesfunctionen der Menschlichen Haut. Erste Abhandlung: Druckempfindung und Schmerz. *Berl. sachs. Gess. Wiss. math. phys.* **Kl. 23,** 175, 1896.

4. NAFE, J. P. The pressure, pain and temperature senses. In: *Handbook of General Experimental Psychology,* C. MURCHISON (Ed.) Clark Univ. Press, Worcester, Mass, 1934.

5. SINCLAIR, D. C. Cutaneous sensation and the doctrine of specific energy. *Brain* **78,** 584, 1955.

6. WEDDELL, G. Somesthesis and the chemical senses. *A. Rev. Psychol.* **6,** 119, 1955.

7. SHERRINGTON, C. S. *The Integrative Action of the Nervous System.* Yale Univ. Press, New Haven, Conn., 1906.

8. RANSON, S. W. The tract of Lissauer and the substantia gelatinosa Rolandi. *Am. J. Anat.* **16,** 97, 1914.

9. RANSON, S. W. and BILLINGSLEY, P. R. The conduction of painful afferent impulses in the spinal nerves. *Am. J. Physiol.* **40,** 571, 1916.

10. HEINBECKER, P., BISHOP, G. H. and O'LEARY, J. Pain and touch fibers in peripheral nerves. *Archs Neurol. Psychiat., Chicago* **29,** 771, 1933.

11. HEINBECKER, P., BISHOP, G. H. and O'LEARY, J. Analysis of sensation in terms of the nerve impulse. *Archs Neurol. Psychiat., Chicago* **31,** 34, 1934.

12. ZOTTERMAN, Y. Studies in the peripheral nervous mechanism of pain. *Acta med. scand.* **80,** 1, 1933.

13. CLARK, D., HUGHES, J. and GASSER, H. S. Afferent function in the group of nerve fibers of slowest conduction velocity. *Am. J. Physiol.* **114,** 69, 1935.

14. COLLINS, W. F., NULSEN, F. E. and RANDT, C. T. Relation of peripheral nerve fiber size and sensation in man. *Archs Neurol. Psychiat., Chicago* **3,** 381, 1960.

15. LEWIS, T. *Pain.* Macmillan, New York, 1942.

16. ZOTTERMAN, Y. Touch, pain and tickling: an electrophysiological investigation on cutaneous sensory nerves. *J. Physiol.* **95,** 1, 1939.

17. DOUGLAS, W. W. and RITCHIE, J. M. Non-medulated fibers in the saphenous nerve which signal touch. *J. Physiol., Lond.* **139,** 385, 1957.

18. HUNT, C. C. and McINTYRE, A. K. An analysis of fibre diameter and receptor characteristics of myelinated cutaneous afferent fibres in cat. *J. Physiol., Lond.* **153,** 99, 1960.

19. IRIUCHIJIMA, J. and ZOTTERMAN, Y. The specificity of afferent cutaneous C fibres in mammals. *Acta physiol. scand.* **49,** 267, 1960.

20. IGGO, A. Cutaneous mechanoreceptors with afferent C fibres. *J. Physiol. Lond.* **152,** 337, 1960.

21. HENSEL, H., IGGO, A. and WITT, I. A quantitative study of sensitive cutaneous thermoreceptors with C afferent fibres. *J. Physiol., Lond.* **153,** 113, 1960.

22. DODT, E. Schmerzimpulse bei Temperaturreizen. *Acta physiol. scand.* **31,** 83, 1954.

23. IGGO, A. Cutaneous heat and cold receptors with slowly conducting (C) afferent fibres. *Q. Jl. exp. Physiol.* **44,** 362, 1959.

24. MELZACK, R. and WALL, P. D. On the nature of cutaneous sensory mechanisms. *Brain* **85,** 331, 1962.

25. MELZACK, R. and WALL, P. D. Pain mechanisms: a new theory. *Science* **150,** 971, 1965.

26. WALL, P. D. Organization of cord cells which transmit sensory cutaneous information. In: *The Skin Senses,* KENSHALO, D. R. (Ed.) C. C. Thomas, Springfield, Ill, 1968.

27. PERL, E. R. Crossed reflexes of cutaneous origin. *Am. J. Physiol.* **188,** 609, 1957.

28. PERL, E. E. and WHITLOCK, D. G. Somatic stimuli exciting spinothalamic projections to thalamic neurons in cat and monkey. *Expl Neurol.* **3,** 256, 1961.

29. FERNANDEZ DE MOLINA, A. and PERL, E. R. Sympathetic activity and the systematic circulation in the spinal cat. *J. Physiol.* **181,** 82, 1965.

30. BURGESS, P. R. and PERL, E. R. Myelinated afferent fibers responding specifically to noxious stimulation of the skin. *J. Physiol.* **190,** 541, 1967.

31. PERL, E. R. Myelinated afferent fibres innervating the primate skin and their response to noxious stimuli. *J. Physiol.* **197,** 593, 1968.

32. BESSOU, P. and PERL, E. R. Response of cutaneous sensory units with unmyelinated fibers to noxious stimuli. *J. Neurophysiol.* **32,** 1025, 1969.

33. BESSOU, P., BURGESS, P. R., PERL, E. R. and TAYLOR, C. B. Dynamic properties of mechanoreceptors with unmyelinated (C) fibers. *J. Neurophysiol.* **34,** in press, 1971.

34. CHRISTENSEN, B. N. and PERL, E. R. Spinal neurons specifically excited by noxious or thermal stimuli: marginal zone of the dorsal horn. *J. Neurophysiol.* **33,** 293, 1970.

35. FOERSTER, O. and GAGEL, O. Die Vorderseitenstrangdurchschneidung beim Menschen. *Z. ges. Neurol. Psychiat.* **138,** 1, 1932.

36. KURU, M. *Sensory Paths in the Spinal Cord and Brain Stem of Man.* Sogensya, Tokyo, 1949.

J. psychiat. Res., 1971, Vol. 8, pp. 289–300. Pergamon Press. Printed in Great Britain.

RESPONSES OF PHOTORECEPTORS

M. G. F. Fuortes

Laboratory of Neurophysiology, National Institute of Neurological Diseases and Stroke
National Institutes of Health, Bethesda, Maryland

SIMPLE PHOTOCHEMICAL PROCESSES

When molecules absorb light, their electronic structure is disturbed with consequent alteration of the chemical bonds between their atoms. Common results of the absorption of light are: the splitting of the molecule in its components; the synthesis of a new molecule; the change of configuration of the molecule, etc. For instance:

$$2\ HI \xrightarrow{h\nu} H_2 + I_2 \tag{1}$$

$$CO + Cl_2 \xrightarrow{h\nu} COCl_2 \tag{2}$$

$$\begin{matrix} COOH\text{–}C\text{–}H \\ |\quad| \\ H\text{–}C\text{–}COOH \end{matrix} \xrightarrow{h\nu} \begin{matrix} COOH\text{–}C\text{–}H \\ |\quad| \\ COOH\text{–}C\text{–}H \end{matrix} \tag{3}$$

These and other similar changes are examples of *primary photochemical process*, often called *light reactions*, in which new molecules are *instantaneously* formed by the action of the impinging radiation.

If these new molecules are inactive, all changes terminate as soon as the light is discontinued. But if the newly formed molecules react with one another, with their precursors or with other molecules present in their vicinity, chemical changes may continue to occur after the return to darkness. These delayed processes are called *secondary photochemical processes* or *dark reactions*. In certain cases, the secondary processes take the form of chain reactions: for instance, a single ultraviolet photon absorbed by chlorine in the presence of hydrogen may lead to the formation of hundreds of thousands of hydrochloric acid molecules. This is explained as follows:

$$Cl \xrightarrow{h\nu} Cl^* + Cl$$
$$Cl + H_2 \rightarrow HCl + H$$
$$H + Cl_2 \rightarrow HCl + Cl$$

A chlorine molecule is split by light producing one excited and one non-excited atom. If hydrogen is present, the chlorine atom combines with the hydrogen molecule giving hydrochloric acid and atomic hydrogen. The hydrogen atom combines with chlorine producing a molecule of hydrochloric acid and an atom of chlorine. This combines with a molecule of hydrogen as before, and the reaction proceeds in darkness, terminating only when the free atoms recombine with each other rather than with the hydrogen or chlorine molecules.

VISUAL PIGMENTS

Photochemical reactions are usually produced by ultraviolet but not by visible light. The reason for this is that visible light has irradiated the earth for perhaps four billion years and, therefore, molecules or systems which are unstable under visible light have had small probability to remain on the earth surface. Molecules which are unstable under ultraviolet radiation could instead survive because the ultraviolet light from the sun is absorbed by the atmosphere and, thus, does not reach the surface of the earth. Important exceptions are offered, however, by biological systems, where substances are found which are unstable under visible light. They are still present because they possess a property peculiar to living matter: the ability to regenerate if they are altered or destroyed.

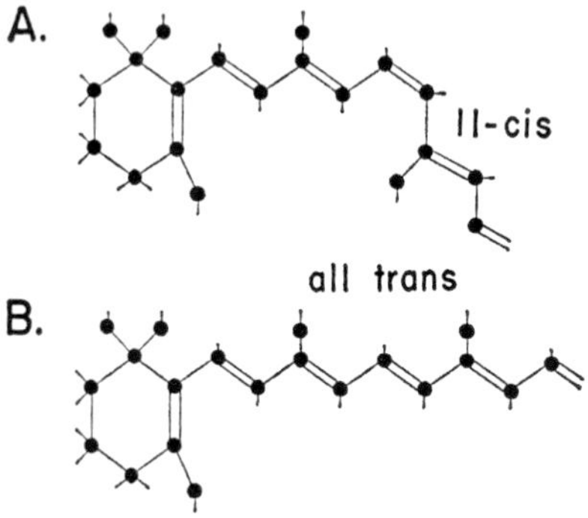

FIG. 1.   Structure of 11-*cis* (A) and all-*trans* (B) retinal.

In animals, the most important photosensitive molecules are the visual pigments. The best known of these is the rhodopsin of vertebrate rods, which consists of two components: a protein called opsin and a carotenoid called retinal.[1] The properties of the protein are largely unknown. Retinal, in contrast, has been thoroughly studied and is known to be a chain of carbon atoms connected by alternating single and double bonds, which in darkness has a so-called 11-*cis* configuration, as illustrated in Fig. 1A. If the molecule absorbs a photon it undergoes isomerization[2] which leads to the all-*trans* configuration of Fig. 1B. It is suggested[3] that the isomerization of retinal alters the forces connecting the chromophore to the protein, with the result that the chromophore detaches and the protein itself changes configuration (Fig. 2). A basic problem in visual physiology is to determine how these light-evoked changes of the visual pigments lead to visual responses. This question is not yet well understood and will be discussed later. It is important to note at this point that the all-*trans* retinal can isomerize back to the 11-*cis* form in two ways: either in darkness, making use of chemical energy which is normally stored in the cell or under the influence of light. In either case, the reformed 11-*cis* retinal attaches spontaneously to the opsin and in this way the original rhodopsin molecule is regenerated.

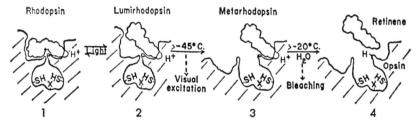

FIG. 2.   Presumed action of light on rhodospin.

In darkness, the chromophore has an 11-*cis* configuration and is firmly attached to the opsin (1). When light is absorbed the chromophore is isomerized and becomes loosely attached to the protein (2). The protein itself changes configuration (3) and finally the chromophore detaches completely (4). (From HUBBARD and KROPF[3]).

PHOTORECEPTOR CELLS

Visual pigments are contained in specialized nerve cells, the photoreceptors, which have the ability to transform light into an electrical signal. In different animals, photoreceptor cells may have very different structure and organization: from the very large and irregularly scattered photoreceptors of the so-called ventral eye of Limulus to the slender and regularly organized receptors in the fovea of primates. They may have an axon several centimeters long (as in the lateral eye of *Limulus*) or their total length may be only a small fraction of a millimeter. In spite of these diversities, all photoreceptors have one morphological feature in common and this is a specialized structure formed by protrusions or infoldings of their membrane. In most invertebrate photoreceptors these take the form of microvilli which typically are 0.1μ in dia. and 1μ–2μ long. In other cases, however, namely in the photoreceptors of ciliary origin,[4] the specialized membrane takes the form of discs (as in the vertebrate rods), folds (as in the cones) or elaborate convolutions of the membrane (as in Pecten). In any case, there are regions in all photoreceptors, in which the area of the membrane is greatly expanded. The purpose of this arrangement is not known but it is reasonable to suppose that the function of the membrane expansions is to support a large number of pigment molecules. This view is derived from the spectrophotometric studies of LANGER and THORELL[5] showing that visual pigments are found in the specialized regions of photoreceptor cells but not elsewhere, and from the experiments of HAGINS and

McGAUGHY,[6] SMITH and BROWN[7] and BLASIE and coworkers[8,9] which indicate that visual pigments are a membrane component.

It seems safe to conclude from all this that light is absorbed by molecules which are contained in the membrane of the specialized regions of photoreceptor cells, and that absorption instantaneously alters the structure of these molecules. It appears possible, therefore, that light might directly alter the electrical properties of the membrane, thereby producing instantaneous visual responses. Studies of the features of the responses of photoreceptors to light, however, do not support this view.*

GENERATOR POTENTIALS

Important insights on the properties of the responses produced by light in photoreceptor cells was obtained when HARTLINE et al.[10] succeeded in recording visual cell responses by means of intracellular microelectrodes. Their work was performed on cells of the

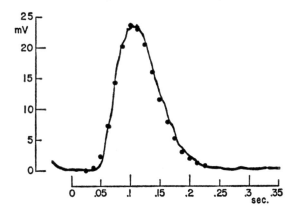

FIG. 3.   Response recorded from a visual cell of *Limulus* following a brief flash.

A flash delivering about $3 \cdot 8 \times 10^6$ absorbable photons was applied at time *O*. The electrical response was recorded by an intracellular microelectrode. The preparation was light adapted and was kept at 25·5°C. It is seen that the electrical response develops with considerable delay, reaching peak about 100 msec after the end of the flash. The filled circles show the output of the model of Fig. 6, with nine stages ($n = 9$). (From BORSELLINO and FUORTES[11]).

lateral eye of *Limulus* and they demonstrated that following illumination these cells become depolarized and may produce nerve impulses. It was also observed in these studies that the depolarization develops slowly following illumination. As a consequence of this, if the light is presented in the form of a brief flash, the electrical response occurs well after

---

* An instantaneous electrical change, the early receptor potential, can, in fact, be recorded from photoreceptors when light is absorbed. It is now established that it arises as a consequence of the charge displacement produced directly by the impinging photons. There is no evidence, however, that the early receptor potential gives rise to a transmitted signal and, therefore, it is not regarded as a visual response.

the flash is over (Fig. 3). Thus, the visual responses of a photoreceptor cell bear analogies
with the dark reaction of photochemistry. It cannot be a direct result of the isomerization
of the visual pigment, which is an instantaneous consequence of light and must arise
instead as a consequence of some secondary process or sequence of processes.

KINETICS OF VISUAL RESPONSES—LINEAR MODELS

Some features of these intermediary events have been studied by means of kinetic studies
of visual responses.

DeLange[12] investigated visual responses in man and observed that the attenuation of
the perception of flicker with increasing frequency is similar to the attenuation of electrical
signals passing through a filter consisting of a sequence of several R–C elements. Later,
DeVoe[13,14] observed that a filter of this type reproduces very satisfactorily the electrical
responses recorded from the eye of the spider Lycosa, including the latency of the responses
evoked by flashes or steps of light. A good agreement was also found to occur between the
output of the filter and the responses recorded from visual cells of *Limulus*.[15] The number
of stages required in order to reproduce the time course of visual responses was found to
be quite large: about ten stages on the average for the visual cells of Limulus. This observation suggests that a correspondingly large number of processes is necessary to bring about
the response of visual cells.

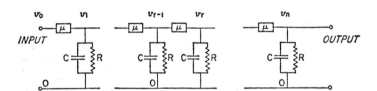

FIG. 4.   Electrical network reproducing the kinetics of visual responses. The network consists

of n identical stages and is characterized by the two parameters: $\lambda_1 = \dfrac{1}{RC}$ and $\lambda_2 = \dfrac{\mu}{C}$.

The components separating the successive stages are amplifiers of infinite input impedance and
of mutual conductance μ. This network, with 10 stages, reproduces the shape of small (linear)
responses evoked by light in visual cells of Limulus. In order to reproduce non-linear responses,

the conductances $\dfrac{1}{R}$ are made linearly dependent upon the voltage of the output or of the

stage just before the output (See Fig. 7). (Modified from FUORTES and HODGKIN[15].)

Since the filter illustrated in Fig. 4 is a linear system, it can simulate visual responses
only over their limited visual range, namely only as long as the response remains
proportional to the stimulus. If this range is exceeded the visual responses deviate sharply
from the output of the model. Further investigations showed, however, that the multi-stage

model has features which are adequate for reproducing the non-linearities of visual responses.

RELATIONS BETWEEN SENSITIVITY AND TIME SCALE

The starting point for this study was the observation that light adaptation decreases sensitivity while it increases temporal resolution. These phenomena are well known in psychophysics, since it can be clearly demonstrated that in the presence of a background light or after a period of intense illumination, a flash becomes less visible but flicker fusion frequency is increased. These results suggest that the response to a flash becomes smaller and faster with light adaptation and in fact these changes can be observed directly by recording the responses of visual cells Fig. 5. It is seen in experiments of this type that the changes of sensitivity and of time course are correlated but the decrease of sensitivity is much greater than the shortening of the time scale. In visual cells of *Limulus*, a decrease of sensitivity by a factor of 500 is associated with an acceleration of the time course by a factor of about 2.

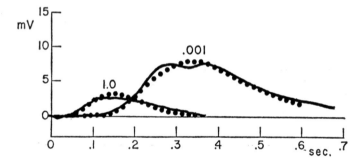

FIG. 5.   Responses evoked in dark and light adaptation.

The larger response was evoked by a flash of intensity 0·001 in a dark-adapted preparation. The other response was elicited by a flash of intensity 1·0 applied a few seconds after a period of strong illumination. It is seen in results of this type that light adaptation decreases sensitivity and shortens the delay of the response. Similar changes of sensitivity and time scale are obtained in the model of Fig. 4 by changing the value of λ_1. The dotted curves in the Figure show the calculated output of the model with $\lambda_1 = 23\cdot5$ sec^{-1} for the dark-adapted response and $\lambda_1 = 53\cdot4$ sec^{-1} for the smaller, light-adapted response. All other parameters were the same in the two cases. (From FUORTES and HODGKIN).[15]

The multi-stage model is quite suitable for reproducing this relation since sensitivity and time course of responses are controlled by the value of the parameter λ_1 representing the rate of decay of the intermediary processes. If λ_1 is increased by two-fold in nine stages, time to peak of the the response to a flash is reduced to one half while sensitivity is decreased by a factor of 512. Thus, the changes of sensitivity and time scale brought about by background illumination can be explained, assuming that the background light increases the rate of decay λ_1 for the majority of the intermediary processes represented by the stages of the system.

NON-LINEAR MODEL

The same general notion can now be utilized for interpreting the well-known non-linearities of visual responses.

It has been known for some time that as light intensity is increased, the response of a photoreceptor cell increases, not in proportion with the stimulus, but approximately as the logarithm of the stimulus.

Experimental observation shows that the non-linearity of visual responses does not develop instantly: at early times, the responses to light are linearly related to light intensity and they start deviating from linearity only when they exceed a certain voltage (Fig. 6). This observation suggests that visual cells are equipped with an automatic gain control which decreases sensitivity as the amplitude of the response increases.

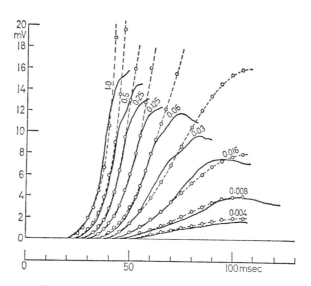

FIG. 6. Early linearity of responses to flashes.

The continuous curves are tracings of responses to flashes of increasing intensity as shown by the figures. The dashed curves show the outputs of the model of Fig. 6 to stimuli of correspondingly increasing strengths. The experimental and theoretical responses are similar for voltages not exceeding 8 mV. (From FUORTES and O'BRYAN[16].)

These non linear features can be reproduced if one adds to it a feedback loop by which the output voltage controls the rate of decay λ_1, and it can be shown that, with this added feature, the responses of the model approximate closely the experimental responses of visual cells over a wide range of light intensities as illustrated in Fig. 7.

J

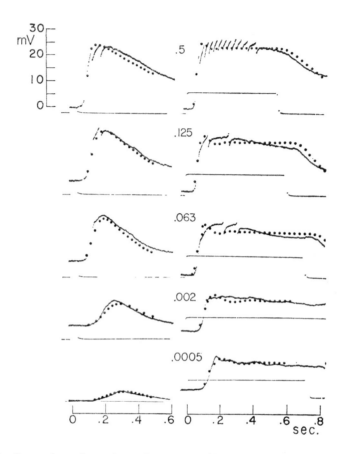

FIG. 7. Comparison of experimental responses with output of the non-linear model.

Solid lines are photographs of responses recorded from a visual cell of *Limulus*. Left-hand column: responses to flashes; right-hand column: responses to steps of light. Light intensity in arbitrary units is indicated near each pair of records. The dotted curves are the outputs of the model of Fig. 4 with a gain control given by the relation

$$\overline{\lambda_1} = \lambda_1 \left\{ 1 + \frac{v_n - 1}{w} \right\}.$$

With this device, the responses of the model fit the experimental responses over a wide range of stimulus intensities.

(Modified from MARIMONT[17].)

It seems, therefore, that a model consisting of a sequence of stages is adequate for reproducing many important features of visual responses.

A CHEMICAL MODEL

It becomes important at this point to ask what processes might correspond to the stages of the model.

One possibility is that the sequence of RC stages in the model represents a succession of chemical reactions. With this view in mind, it is convenient to represent the model as a system of compartments (Fig. 8). The compartments represent different substances and the arrows represent the transitions from one substance to the next. This system is completely analogous to the electrical filter and, therefore, it gives the same input–output relations.

A

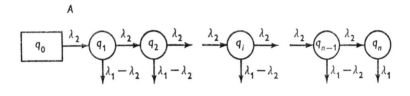

B   C

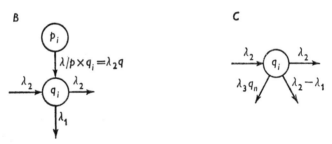

FIG. 8. Compartmental representation of the model of Fig. 6. The parameters of this model correspond to the parameters of the electrical network as follows:

Compartmental model	q_1	λ_1	λ_2	n
Electrical model	v_1	$1/RC$	μ/R	n.

In the electrical model, the elements supply current to the stages $i + 1$ without draining current from the preceding stages. In order to reproduce this feature in the compartmental model, $i + 1$ must receive particles from i, but must not lose particles in the process. Thus, the outflow from i into $i + 1$ ($\lambda_2 q_i$) must be compensated by an equal influx ($-\lambda_2 q_i$). This can be accomplished by subtracting λ_2 from the rate of decay λ_1. One obtains then

$$\frac{dq_i}{dt} = -(\lambda_1 - \lambda_2) q_i - \lambda_2 q_i + \lambda_2 q_i - 1 = -\lambda_1 q_i + \lambda_2 q_i - 1$$

A chemical system satisfying this relation has been described in a previous article and is reproduced in B: a precursor reacts with an enzyme in compartment i to give a new enzyme in compartment $i + 1$ (Borsellino et al.[18]).

The gain control can be incorporated in the compartmental system using the relation

$$\overline{\lambda_1} = \lambda_1 \left(1 + \frac{qn}{w}\right) = \lambda_1 + \lambda_3 qn$$

and a typical compartment of the non-linear system is illustrated in C. (From Borsellino and Fuortes[19].)

The instantaneous effects of a flash of light represented in the compartmental model as the sudden injection of q_1 particles in compartment 1 (where q_1 is proportional to the number of photons in the flash). The following compartments represent successive chemical transformations which lead to the final production of a substance q_n which depolarizes the membrane.

EFFECTS OF TEMPERATURE AND OF DNP ON VISUAL RESPONSES

In this chemical model, the parameters λ_1 and λ_2 represent reaction rates and, therefore, they would be expected to be affected by temperature in accordance with the Arrhenius relation:

$$\lambda = \lambda_o e^{-\frac{E}{kT}}.$$

Study of visual responses at different temperature yields results which are consistent with this expectation. Experiments performed on cells of the lateral eye of *Limulus* show that, as temperature is decreased, the response becomes smaller and slower. These changes can

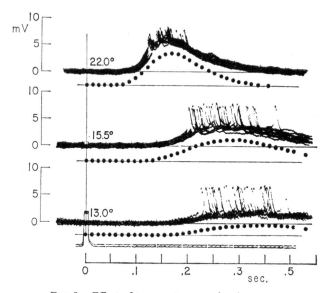

FIG. 9.   Effect of temperature on visual responses.

Responses were evoked by dim flashes at the different temperatures indicated. The temperature was changed slowly and was practically constant during the time required to obtain the several responses superimposed in each record. The response becomes larger and faster when the temperature is increased. Similar changes can be obtained in the model of Fig. 10 by changing the parameters λ_1 and λ_2 in the same proportion, as shown by the dotted curves under each set of records.

be produced in the model, by decreasing the parameters λ_1 and λ_2 approximately in the same ratio (Fig. 9). In the experiments we have performed activation energy was about

1 eV, corresponding to value of Q_{10} of approximately 2. The results of the temperature studies are therefore consistent with the notion that visual responses are brought about by a sequence of chemical reactions.

Since many biological reactions are sustained by metabolism, we investigated the effects of metabolic poisons on visual responses and found that di-nitrophenol rapidly and reversibly abolishes the response to light, without appreciably altering membrane properties, such as membrane potential, membrane resistance or the ability to produce spikes (Fig. 10).

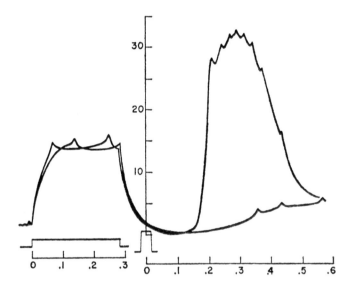

FIG. 10. Action of DNP on the responses of visual cells.

A pulse of depolarizing current and a flash of light were applied to a visual cell. Responses were recorded before and about 7 min after application of DNP in 0·1 mM concentration. The voltage drop was not appreciably altered but the response to light was greatly decreased by the poison. (From BORSELLINO and FUORTES[11]).

Thus, it appears that the view that visual responses are brought about by a sequence of chemical reactions is in general agreement with a number of experimental results.

REFERENCES

1. WALD, G. Distribution and evolution of visual systems. In: *Comparative Biochemistry*, Vol. 1, Chap. 8, FLORKIN, M. and MASON, H. S. (Eds.) Academic Press, New York, 1960.
2. HUBBARD, R. and WALD, G. *Cis–Trans* isomers of vitamin A and retinene in the rhodopsin system. *J. gen. Physiol.* **36**, 269, 1952.
3. HUBBARD, R. and KROPF, A. Molecular aspects of visual excitation. *Ann. N.Y. Acad. Sci.* **81**, 388, 1959.
4. EAKIN, R. M. Evolution of photoreceptors. *Cold Spring Harb. Symp. quant. Biol.* **30**, 363, 1965.
5. LANGER, H., and THORELL, B. Microspectrophotometric assay of visual pigments in single rhabdomeres of the insect eye. In: *The Functional Organization of the Compound Eye*, BERNHARD, C. G. (Ed.) Pergamon, London, 1966.

6. HAGINS, W. A. and McGAUGHY, R. E. Membrane origin of the fast photovoltage of squid retina. *Science*. **159**, 213. 1968.
7. SMITH, T. G. and BROWN, J. E. A photoelectric potential in invertebrate cells. *Nature* **212**, 1217, 1966.
8. BLASIE, J. K. and WORTHINGTON, C. R. and DEWEY, M. M. Planar liquid-like arrangement of photopigment molecules in frog retinal receptor disk membranes. *J. molec. Biol.* **39**, 407, 1960.
9. BLASIE, J. K., WORTHINGTON, C. R. and DEWEY, M. M. Molecular localization of frog retinal receptor photopigment by electronmicroscopy and low-angle X-ray diffraction. *J. molec. Biol.* **39**, 417, 1969.
10. HARTLINE, H. K., WAGNER, H. G. and MACNICHOL, E. F. The peripheral origin of nervous activity in the visual system. *Cold Spring Harb. Symp. quant. Biol.* **17**, 125, 1952.
11. BORSELLINO, A. and FUORTES, M. G. F. Interpretation of responses of visual cells of limulus. *Proc. IEEE.* **56**, No. 6. 1024-1032, 1968b.
12. DELANGE, H. Research into the dynamic nature of the human fovea-cortex system with intermittent and modulated light. *J. opt. Soc. Am.* **48**, 777, 1958.
13. DEVOE, R. D. Linear superposition of retinal action potentials to predict electrical flicker responses from the eye of the wolf spider (Keyserling). *J. gen. Physiol.* **46**, 75, 1962.
14. DEVOE, R. D. Linear relations between stimulus amplitudes and amplitudes of retinal action potentials from the eye of the wolf spider. *J. gen. Physiol.* **47**, 13, 1963.
15. FUORTES, M. G. F. and HODGKIN, A. L. Changes in time scale and sensitivity in the ommatidia of Limulus. *J. Physiol., Lond.* **182**, 239, 1964.
16. FUORTES, M. G. F. and O'BRYAN, P. Generator potentials in invertebrate photoreceptors. *Handbook of Sensory Physiology.* Springer-Heidelberg (in press).
17. MARIMONT, R. Numerical studies of the Fuortes–Hodgkin limulus model. *J. Physiol., Lond.* **179**. 489, 1965.
18. BORSELLINO, A., FUORTES, M. G. F. and SMITH, T. G. Visual responses in limulus. *Cold Spring Harb. Symp. quant. Biol.* **30**, 428, 1965.
19. BORSELLINO, A. and FUORTES, M. G. F. Responses to single photons in visual cells of Limulus. *J. Physiol., Lond.* **196**, 507, 1968a.

J. psychiat. Res., 1971, Vol. 8, pp. 301–307. Pergamon Press. Printed in Great Britain.

SPECIFICITY OF RESPONSES OF CELLS IN THE VISUAL CORTEX

DAVID H. HUBEL

Department of Neurobiology, Harvard Medical School, Boston, Massachusetts

LOOKING at the human brain from the outside, the most striking feature, by far, is the cerebral cortex, partly because it is on the outside, and partly because of its sheer size. A student approaching the nervous system for the first time is bound to be struck by the paucity and unevenness of present-day knowledge of this impressive structure. Despite a century of study by neurologists, neuroanatomists and neurophysiologists, only a very small fraction of the cortex is understood in any detail, and much of it is not understood at all. This ignorance is not confined to the cortex, but is common to a large part of the deeper structures of the brain.

Considering how much is known about most organs of the body, such as the pituitary, pancreas, or kidney, our slowness in coming to grips with the nervous system may seem puzzling. The main source of the difficulty is to be found in the very nature of the nervous system. For most other organs it is enough, broadly speaking, to know the functions of a few classes of cells. If you understand the actions of one salivary gland cell, plus the architecture of the gland's circulation and duct system, you have a reasonable grasp of the whole organ. In the nervous system it is not enough to know how a single cell works, though of course that is essential. One must also study the connections and interrelations between enormous numbers of cells, and this is a matter of comprehending an architecture vastly more complicated than the salivary gland duct system.

In the past few decades much progress has been made in working out what might be called the general cellular physiology of the nervous system, including the ionic mechanisms of impulse conduction and synaptic transmission. This has opened the way towards an attack on the functional architecture of the central nervous system. Today we are in the position of someone who has a reasonable understanding of the components of a radio circuit, the resistors, condensers, transistors and so on, but for the most part does not know how they are strung together, or what the electrical signals passing through them signify, or how the signals are being analysed or transformed.

One difficulty here is that the problem requires a study of many single cells in the intact animal. It does not get us very far to study the pooled activity of many cells at a time—for example with large electrodes placed on or in the brain—since neighbouring cells even if morphologically similar may perform entirely different tasks. Studies of populations of cells in general tell us little about the individuals. Until very recently methods for studying single

cells in the intact brain did not exist, and it was not until around 1950 that single
cortical cells were first recorded. Probably the first finding of profound interest was
Mountcastle's discovery that somatosensory cells are aggregated into columnar groups
according to modality. This was the first indication of a parcellation of cells on a scale
smaller, by an order of magnitude, than the cortical filelds which the architectonic anatomists
and localization neurophysiologists had fought so hard to establish in the previous
decades.

In the past 10 or 15 years techniques have advanced rapidly and much progress has been
made, especially in the sensory systems, where one can examine regions not too remote, in
terms of numbers of synapses, from the input to the nervous system. The visual system,
despite its great analytic capabilities and consequent complexity, has turned out to be
especially amenable to study. This is partly because it has a fairly simple anatomic path,
with flow of information directed mainly from periphery centrally over a number of
relatively discrete stages. In the present paper I wish to illustrate one type of work that is
being done by describing two cells in the visual cortex, one situated in area 18 in the cat,
the other in 17 in the Rhesus monkey. These are not special or exceptional cells, but typical
ones both in their specificity and their great individuality. The experiments were done at
Johns Hopkins and later at Harvard by TORSTON WIESEL and myself.[1,2] In a sense they are a
continuation of studies begun by Hartline in frog and Limulus, and by Kuffler in the
cat retina.

Let me begin with a brief word about methods, some of which were originally developed
for awake unrestrained animals while I was at Walter Reed. We now mainly use
anesthetized animals because for this type of experiment it is very much easier and more
efficient. In the past few years, however, most of the results have been shown to hold in
awake unrestrained animals by WURTZ.[3] The animal (cat or monkey) has its head firmly
supported in a head holder, and the eyes are held open facing a screen one and a half meters
away. Visual stimuli of various shapes, colors and rates of movement are projected upon
this screen and hence onto the retinas. Records are made extracellularly from a tungsten
microelectrode introduced through a small hole in the skull. With these methods it is
possible, in a good experiment, to record over a hundred cells as one penetrates through
2 mm of cortex. A single cell can if necessary be studied for several hours.

Cell I: A 'hypercomplex' cell of area 18 (visual II) in the cat

This cell was recorded from area 18, a region which, in the cat, is situated just lateral to
area 17, and which receives a topographically ordered set of connections both from 17 and
from the lateral geniculate body. The cell, like the great majority of cells in the visual
cortex, gave no detectable response to changes in diffuse light; even shining a bright flash-
light into the eyes of the animal produced no obvious change in spontaneous firing. There
were, however, strong and predictable responses to a specific stimulus within an area of
visual field about 2° by 4° in size, located about 15° below and to the contralateral side of
the center of gaze. (The moon subtends $\frac{1}{2}$° to an observer on earth, and 1° of visual angle
corresponds to about 250μ on the cat retina.) After much trial and error we found that the
most effective stimulus was an edge, oriented in a 2 o'clock—8 o'clock direction, with dark
below and light above, swept slowly up across the rectangular region outlined by dotted

lines in Fig. 1. As the edge's position was varied to include more and more of the left half of the rectangle, the responses became increasingly vigorous, in terms of impulses per second and total number of impulses (Fig. 1, A–C). On extending the edge still further to the right, however, the response began to get weaker, and when it covered the entire dotted region there was no response at all (D–E). It was as if stimulating the right hand area with an edge

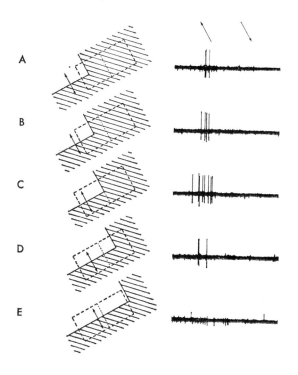

FIG. 1.   Records from a hypercomplex cell in cat visual II. Stimulation of right (ipsilateral) eye. Receptive field, $2° \times 4°$, indicated by interrupted rectangle. Stimulus consisted of an edge oriented at 2:00, with dark below, terminated on the right by a second edge intersecting the first at 90°. A–C: up-and-down movement across varying amounts of the activating portion of the field: D–E: movement across all of the activating portion and varying amounts of the antagonistic portion. Rate of movement 4°/sec. Each sweep, 2 sec (See Ref. 1, Fig. 8).

was able to block the response that would normally have been produced by stimulating the left area. Both regions were orientation specific. If the optimal orientation for the left region was kept constant at 2:00–8:00, while varying the part of the edge crossing the right hand region, it was possible to show that here too a 2:00–8:00 orientation was specific, this time for a complete blocking of the response (Fig. 2).

This cell was maximally responsive, then, to a specifically oriented moving edge terminated on the right at a specific point. If the edge extended to the right of that point the response failed, whereas it could be extended without penalty any distance to the left.

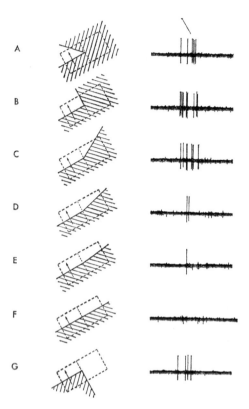

FIG. 2. Same cell as in Fig. 1. Stimulation with two intersecting edges moved up across the receptive field as shown. Inhibition is maximum when the right (antagonistic) half of the receptive field is stimulated with an edge having the same orientation as the optimum edge for the left (activating) half (F). Duration of each sweep, 2 sec. (See Ref. 1, Fig. 9.)

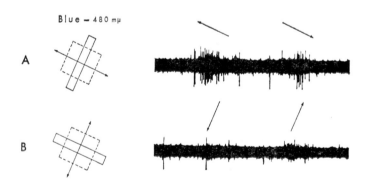

FIG. 3. Complex cell with color coded properties recorded in layer II of monkey striate cortex. Responses to two orthogonal stimulus orientations; wavelength of light, 480 mμ (blue). Size of receptive field, $\frac{1}{2}° \times \frac{1}{2}°$. Time for each record, 5 sec. (See ref. 2, Fig. 6.)

Cell II: A complex color coded cell in monkey cortex

This cell was recorded from monkey striate cortex. Like a typical cell of the type we term 'complex' it gave a brisk, sustained response as a properly oriented line was swept over a restricted region of retina. Here the optimal orientation was 1 o'clock–7 o'clock; a vertical orientation or more oblique ones such as 2 o'clock–8 o'clock, or 4 o'clock–10 o'clock were quite ineffective (Fig. 3). The remarkable feature of this cell was its wavelength specificity. The best responses were obtained with a moving blue line, about 480 mμ in wavelength. Wavelengths of 520 mμ (blue green) or longer were virtually without effect, at any available brightness (Fig. 4). What was especially striking was the ineffectiveness of a *white* line, which could be obtained simply by removing the blue filter from the slide projector, i.e. by adding in the longer wavelengths that the filter had been holding back. It was as if this longer wavelength light was in some way blocking the response the blue light would have produced.

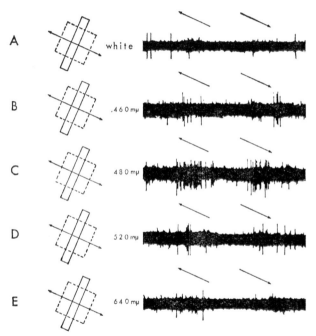

FIG. 4.   Same cell as in Fig. 3. Responses to movement of optimally oriented slits of white light and monochromatic light at various wave-lengths. Monochromatic light made by interposing interference filters in a beam of white light. Stimulus energies are greatest for A, and progressively less for E, D, C and B. None of the responses was improved by lowering the intensity. (See Ref. 2, Fig. 5.)

My main purpose in describing these cells has been to illustrate the characteristic specificity that one finds in cells of the visual path in higher mammals. Frequently this specificity seems to be the result of converging excitatory and inhibitory influences that can cancel each other. In the first example an edge crossing the left area excites, whereas an edge crossing the right area, if presented simultaneously, precisely antagonizes and cancels out this response. A plausible scheme to illustrate the mechanism is given in Fig. 5. It is as if the cell received an excitatory input from a cell with a receptive field in the left area, and an inhibitory input from a second cell with its field in the right hand area. A long line would be expected to fire both these lower order cells, and their influences on the cell we are discussing would cancel, resulting in no response. In the second example a similar antagonism exists between the effects of short and long wavelengths, and we may imagine that a similar convergence of inputs is responsible for the observed behavior. The result of such transformations is that a single cell may possess specificity of response to a large number of variables, such as position on the retina, orientation, speed of movement, wavelength, line length, and so on. All of these may have to be precisely adjusted for the stimulus to work. Our impression is that for each combination of values of these variables there corresponds a cell or set of cells. Of course this calls for a vast number of cells, but that is exactly what a structure like the visual cortex possesses, given many square centimeters of cortex, and some 10^5 cells beneath each square millimeter of surface.

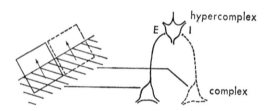

FIG. 5.   Wiring diagram that might account for the properties of a hypercomplex cell. Cell responding to single stopped edge (as in Figs. 1 and 2) receives projections from two complex cells, one excitatory to the hypercomplex cell (*E*), the other inhibitory (*I*). The excitatory complex cell has its receptive field in the region indicated by the left (continuous) rectangle; the inhibitory cell has its field in the area indicated by the right (interrupted) rectangle. The hypercomplex field thus includes both areas, one being the activating region, the other the antagonistic. Stimulating the left region alone results in excitation of the cell, whereas stimulating both regions together is without effect.

By using methods such as those illustrated here to analyse a large number of cells in the visual cortex it has been possible to obtain further insight into the functions of this structure. Little by little one learns what attributes of a visual image are important in producing responses from cortical cells, and one begins to form an idea of how images are analysed. By comparing the properties of neighbouring groups of cells it is also possible to learn something of the functional architecture of the cortex, and to correlate this with morphology. At present we can thus list a number of specific functions of this part of the brain, and give definite and testable suggestions as to how these functions are carried out.

Fortunately for our livelihoods, the work is just beginning. The detailed ultrastructure of the cortex seems vastly more complex than any of the circuits we can propose, and it is likely that the gold in the mine greatly exceeds any that has already been removed. The encouraging thing is that known methods seem to be equal to the task. Moreover, to understand the cortex, despite its complexity, seems well within man's capabilities.

Getting the information is often difficult and sometimes exasperating, but the results are usually simple and elegant. The monkey's solution to the problem of analysing the visual environment is more ingenious than anything a neurophysiologist could possibly dream up.

REFERENCES

1. Hubel, D. H. and Wiesel, T. N. Receptive fields and functional architecture in two non-striate visual areas (18 and 19) of the cat. *J. Neurophysiol.* **28**, 229, 1965.
2. Hubel, D. H. and Wiesel, T. N. Receptive fields and functional architecture of monkey striate cortex. *J. Physiol., Lond.* **195**, 215, 1967.
3. Wurtz, R. H. Visual receptive fields of striate cortex neurons in awake monkeys. *J. Neurophysiol.* **32**, 727, 1969.

J. psychiat. Res., 1971, Vol. 8, pp. 309–322. Pergamon Press. Printed in Great Britain.

ELECTROPHYSIOLOGY OF VISUAL AND PERCEPTUAL ACTIVITY

JOHN C. ARMINGTON

Department of Psychology, Northeastern University, Boston, Massachusetts

THE STUDY of vision is an ongoing process in which knowledge accumulated through experimentation serves both as a basis and as a stimulus for further investigations. The purposes of this article are to review some of the visual research conducted in the Division of Neuropsychiatry at the Walter Reed Army Institute of Research under the leadership of Dr. David Rioch and to describe some of the results of current projects* which have been a direct outcome of the earlier work. In review, the research appears to follow a regular, logical order with one experiment leading sensibly to the next. At the time the experiments were conducted, however, this trend was less evident. It was not always clear what step to take next; some experiments did not lead to a successful outcome; and in fact, the general direction being taken by a series of experiments was often forgotten because of the pressure of immediate technical problems. The data selected for presentation here were chosen not just because they are representative of visual research but because they seem to fit together with common purpose.

Early research in vision at Walter Reed was characterized by several goals. The primary one was to investigate transfer of visual information through the nervous system taking into account as many factors as possible from stimulus to ultimate response. In addition, however, there was an interest in retinal function in its own right, an interest in developing improved and more sensitive recording systems, and an interest in discovering the neural correlates of visual perception. As an attack upon these goals, steady efforts were directed towards developing a means of monitoring the action of the intact human visual system at several of its levels. Furthermore, an attempt was made to use quantitative procedures whenever possible in order to obtain results which could be compared with the psychophysics of vision and perception. At first, electrophysiological observations could only be made conveniently at the retina. Later, as more advanced techniques became available, activity could also be studied successfully at the cortex.

Progress was not merely a matter of designing new experiments, of investigating new stimulus parameters nor of investigating old parameters more thoroughly. Progress was

---

* Current research is supported by PHS Research Grant No. EY 0058903 from the National Institutes of Health.

strongly dependent upon advances in instrumentation. Improvements were made in the manner of presenting stimuli, in the methods of recording and in the ways of evaluating data. In recent years the on-the-line digital computer has been important in advancing all phases of experimentation.

The electroretinogram, a slow wave response to photic stimulation, has provided the indication of retinal activity. Although the electroretinogram is obtained with a single active recording electrode, it is capable of providing several kinds of information as may be seen by considering its complicated waveform. GRANIT,[1,2] more than 30 years ago did experiments which separated the electroretinogram into several components. The results of his analysis are shown in the upper part of Fig. 1. The analysis indicated that the A-wave, a corneal negative potential appearing soon after the stimulus, takes its origin in the receptor layer of the retina and that the positive B-wave which follows immediately after arises within the bipolar layer. His experiments, truly of a pioneering nature, have received strong confirmation in the microelectrode studies of the monkey electroretinogram conducted by BROWN[3] and his associates. Recent work of MILLER and DOWLING[4] indicates that the B-wave is generated by glial cells extending through the retina. The response may be governed chiefly by activity in the bipolar layer, however.

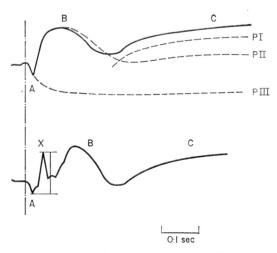

FIG. 1. Wave form of the electroretinogram. The upper half of the figure illustrates the principal features of this response as recognized by Granit. The solid line is the electroretinogram while the dashed lines indicate his analysis of the wave form into three components. The lower half of the figure illustrates some of the additional waves which appear under particular recording conditions.

There is more to the electroretinogram than this, however. Under special recording conditions it breaks up into a number of subcomponents as shown in the lower half of Fig. 1. This particular recording was obtained by presenting red flashes to the partially dark-adapted eye, but the same elements can be seen with varying degrees of prominence under many other conditions. Careful examination of the A-wave shown in the lower tracing reveals that it is composed of two subcomponents. These can be related to the activity initiated by the two main types of receptors found in the retina, the rods and the cones.[5] It will be recalled that the retina has a duality of function. Under high levels of illumination, vision is said to be photopic. Acuity is high, sensitivity is low, and there is good color vision. Vision at photopic levels is mediated by the cones. When the eye has been adapted to darkness, vision is scotopic. Light sensitivity is high, but weak stimuli appear colorless, and their shapes are not easily resolved. Vision at scotopic levels of illumination is chiefly mediated by the rods. One subcomponent of the A-wave accompanies photopic cone activity, and the other accompanies scotopic rod activity. The two early positive components also reflect this duality of visual function. The first, labelled X, appears to reflect photopic activity of the retina while the second, B-wave, is essentially scotopic.[6] Thus, the electroretinogram seems to provide an indication of the separate activities of the scotopic and photopic systems and it may also provide an indication of these activities at both the receptor and bipolar retinal layers.

The human electroretinogram is usually recorded with an electrode supported by a contact lens worn on the subject's eye, and is elicited by a flash of light produced by a visual stimulator. Although recording is not unusually difficult from a technical point of view, interpretation of the results may be. The problem is not so much one of recording as it is of delivering a stimulus of known character to the retina. Electroretinograms obtained by conventional procedures are elicited with intense flashes of light. Stimulation is clearly above normal physiological levels. A stimulator constructed to deliver specified amounts of light to the eye may still produce a distribution of light at the retina which is impossible to describe because of what has been called 'the stray light problem',[7] a term used to call attention to uncontrolled light which is absorbed by the receptors outside of the intended image area. Some of the rays entering the eye are scattered to one side by the optical media before reaching the image area. That portion of the light which does reach the image area is only partially absorbed, some of it being reflected to other retinal regions. Such stray light falling on parts of the retina beyond the image area can be extremely effective as a stimulus because the remote electrodes used for electroretinography respond to the activity of all parts of the retina. Under typical recording conditions a much larger portion of the total illuminated retina area lies outside the image area than within. The large area responding to stray light often contributes more to the actual recording than does the image area. The stray light problem rendered the study of color phenomena difficult[8,9] and for many years made it impossible to deal with problems of visual acuity, perimetry, or of stimulus shape and form. At first, it did not seem to matter where the stimulus was imaged upon the retina, only the total light flux passing the pupil was important.[10]

An approach to the stray light problem became apparent, but it could not be completely realized with the facilities available in the mid-1950's. A study dealing with area-luminance relations gave a clue as to the direction to be taken;[11] it was to try to work with less intense stimuli. During the course of the experiment a determination was made of how the sensitivity of the photopic ERG component (X-wave) varies as stimulus flashes are imaged on different retinal locations. The result is shown in Fig. 2. In this figure relative sensitivity, defined as the reciprocal of the light intensity needed to produce a fixed response amplitude, was plotted against the location of the stimulus along the horizontal meridian of the retina.

K

The lower horizontal straight line describes the sensitivity of 50 μV responses obtained by high intensity stimuli. They were of nearly equal sensitivity, and hence, amplitude, no matter where stimuli were directed to the retina. Response in this case was completely governed by stray light because the numbers of cone receptors which are responsible for releasing photopic responses is not constant across the retina. Concentration is much greater at the center of the retina in and near the fovea than towards the periphery. When weaker stimuli were used, however, the position of the stimulus did make a small difference for 25 μV responses. In this case there is a somewhat higher sensitivity for stimuli near the center of the retina. Evidently, evidence for stimulus localization is better because stray light contributes less to the response with lower intensities. It would have been desirable to continue the investigation at yet lower luminances. There was one problem, however; as the stimulus became weaker, the response became smaller. The low intensity activity shown in Fig. 2 was barely measurable against the background of baseline fluctuations even though the stimuli were still fairly bright. In fact, the response was so small that the stimulus was repeated several times in order to be certain of the results. The points shown in Fig. 2 are average ones based upon several repetitions. The figure suggests that more complete freedom from stray light could have been obtained if weaker stimuli were employed, but this was impossible. Responses produced by weak stimuli were of too low an amplitude for detection.

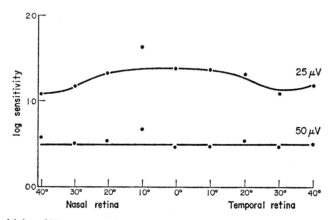

FIG. 2.   Sensitivity of X-waves to stimulation at different points along the horizontal meridian of the retina. This figure shows that the central parts of the retina are slightly more efficient in producing 25 μV responses than the periphery. Sensitivity for 50 μV responses is nearly uniform for all positions.

There was only one way in which electroretinograms of lower amplitude could have been detected: that was to have repeated stimulation many more times and thus to have obtained many more recordings for averaging. Responses are always recorded against a background of irregular baseline activity. If a great many responses are averaged together, a more stable result is obtained because random baseline fluctuations tend to average to zero. The labor and time necessary for such an endeavor at the time of the experiment was prohibitive since all operations had to be performed manually.

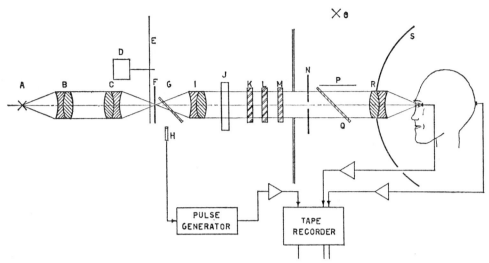

FIG. 3. Diagram of the Maxwellian view stimulator and the initial stages of a recording system used to study average ERG's and VECP's.

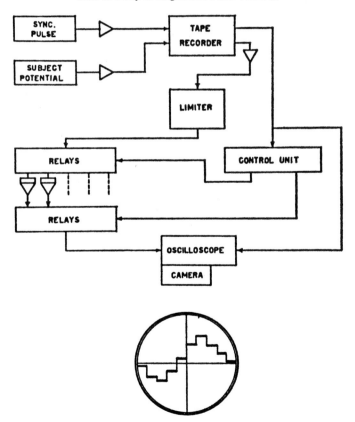

FIG. 4. Block diagram of an early computer system used for averaging electrophysiological signals.

Soon, however, computer technology made averaging procedures practicable. DAWSON[12] in England, had developed a special purpose device for obtaining central nervous system responses to peripheral nerve stimulation. BRAZIER and CASBY[13] developed a system of resonators which made it possible in some instances to detect visual responses of the brain. Following the lead set by these investigators ARMINGTON et al.[14] developed an improved analog device for obtaining average electroretinograms of very low amplitude and could use stimuli of low luminances. It also permitted simultaneous recording of visually evoked cortical potentials. The operation of this device is outlined in Figs. 3 and 4. The method made use of a Maxwellian view stimulator to generate flickering stimuli (Fig. 3). The repeated responses elicited by this flicker could be processed as recorded or stored on magnetic tape for later analysis. Each time the stimulus flashed, it triggered a chain of relays which closed and opened in tandem. They switched consecutive segments of the response recordings to a series of electronic integrators. If the voltages on the integrators were 'read out' after a series of flashes had been presented, an average response waveform could be obtained as shown in the bottom of Fig. 4. Subsequently a digital computer was adapted to accomplish the same result. It produced on-line recordings of average electroretinograms and visually evoked cortical potentials[15-17] even more efficiently.

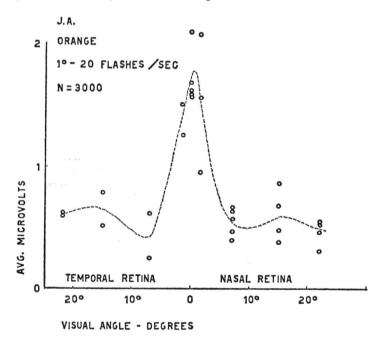

FIG. 5. Average amplitudes of small X-waves produced by flickering 1° stimuli imaged at several positions along the horizontal meridian of the retina.

One of the first tasks attempted, when a computer for determining averaged response wave-form had become available, was that of repeating the retinal mapping experiment of CRAMPTON and ARMINGTON described above.[11] It was now possible to employ stimuli of much smaller diameter and lower luminance. Although the electroretinograms were not nearly as large as those seen before, they were readily detected by average response computation. Their amplitude was found to be strongly dependent upon the position of the stimulus on the retina, the response being much larger when the stimulus was centered on the fovea than when it fell in the periphery, as shown in Fig. 5. Since the responses produced by the flickering light were of a photopic nature, the peaking seen with central stimulation indicated that the effectiveness of stray light had been much reduced. Simultaneous recordings were made of the visually evoked cortical potentials which are picked up from electrodes attached to the occipital scalp. They, too, were largest when the stimulus was centered on the fovea. Further analysis of the data indicated that although stray light stimulation had been greatly reduced with these procedures, it had not been eliminated entirely.[18] Nevertheless, the method was found to be quite useful for studying the development of visual sensitivity in infants[19] and for testing for localized retinal lesions in certain clinical cases.[17]

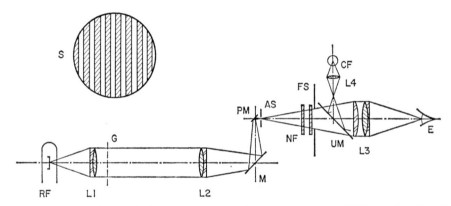

FIG. 6. Diagram of the optical system used to produce alternating stimuli. The symbols identify the following: *RF*, tungsten source light; *L1, L2, L3* and *L4*, lenses: *G*, reticle determining the stimulus pattern; *M*, first surface mirror; *PM*, a pivoted mirror for producing alternation; *AS*, aperture stop; *FS*, field stop; *UM*, an unsilvered mirror used to introduce a fixation point; *CF*, fixation light source; and *E*, the eye of the observer. The insert, *S*, shows how the stimulus appears to the subject.

Computers have also made it possible to use a new form of stimulation which reduces the effectiveness of stray light almost completely.[20,21] The method used for doing this is known as that of stimulus alternation. Apparatus for presenting alternating stimuli is is diagrammed in Fig. 6. The subject is presented with a striped pattern as shown in the insert, *S*. This pattern is imaged on the retina with a Maxwellian view optical system. At regular intervals a pivoted mirror, *PM*, within the optical system is turned with a square wave motion so that the dark and light stripes are interchanged. The retinal receptors which were under the dark stripes now receive more light while those which were under bright stripes receive less. These changes in stimulation elicit retinal and cortical responses. An average response computer, whose sweep is triggered by each stimulus alternation, is used to average the small responses which are produced.

In order to understand why this method is successful, it is important to remember that a change in stimulation is needed to produce visual responses. With stimulus alternation stray light spreads from the image area to other parts of the retina. However, it does not fluctuate as the stripes are exchanged because the total flux entering the eye does not change. Since the stray light is constant, it produces no response. Response comes only from the retinal image area upon which the alternating stripes fall. The method of alternation cannot be used without response averaging because the responses from local retinal areas of a few degrees' diameter are quite small. Substantial proportions of the retina must be activated before responses can be seen without a computer.

The success of the method of stimulus alternation has been demonstrated in a variety of experiments. For example, it may be used to provide an electroretinal indication of the Stiles–Crawford effect,[22] to study photopic spectral sensitivity,[20] and to investigate retinal color mechanisms.[23] The method also offers potential for improved retinal mapping experiments. Under photopic conditions alternating stimuli produce the largest electro-retinograms when they are positioned where cone concentrations are high; under scotopic conditions large electroretinograms are produced with stimuli directed to those retinal regions where rods are most concentrated.[24]

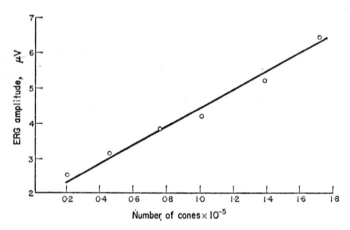

FIG. 7. Amplitude of the local electroretinogram as a function of the number of cone receptors stimulated with fields of increasing diameter.

Perhaps the best demonstration that responses obtained with the method of alternation are nearly independent of stray light is provided by Fig. 7. The data for this figure were obtained through presentation of stimulus fields having different areas but constant luminance.[21] The number of receptors stimulated by each area was computed and plotted along the abscissa. The ordinate shows the amplitude of the electroretinograms produced by each area. Since the response is nearly proportional to the number of cones activated, it appears that stray light is almost without effect.

Although it may be comparatively easy to relate the electroretinograms to simple stimulus and structural factors, visually evoked cortical potentials recorded under the same conditions are not such a simple matter. They seem to depend upon many complicated factors such as the state of the subject's arousal, habituation, task relevancy and other factors.[25] Recent research suggests that stimulus patterning is also a crucial factor in determining evoked potential amplitude.[26-28]

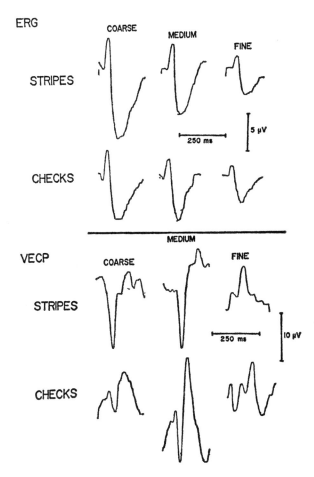

FIG. 8. Electroretinal (upper half) and cortical (lower half) responses produced with striped and checkered patterns of varying texture.

The data now to be shown were obtained by presenting the subject with a series of striped and checkered fields whose elements varied in size. That is, the stimulus field remained of constant diameter but the number of stripes or checks within it was changed. Simultaneous recordings were made of the electroretinogram and the evoked potential. The data show that the texture of the stimulus appearing in the alternating field is important both for the electroretinogram and the evoked potential, but that the responses do not depend upon it in the same way. Some sample responses are shown in Fig. 8. The upper part of the figure shows electroretinograms elicited by checks and stripes having three degrees of fineness. As the structure becomes finer the responses become smaller for both kinds of stimuli. Furthermore, there is no great difference in the amplitude of the electroretinograms produced by checks or stripes whose elements subtend the same visual angle.

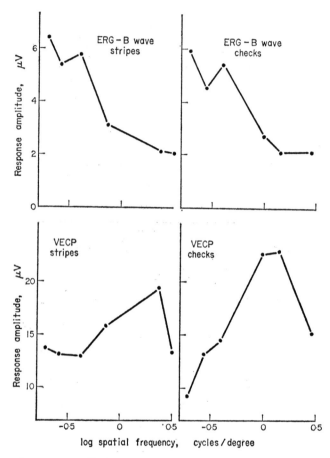

FIG. 9. Plots of response amplitude vs. spatial frequency (stimulus texture) for the ERG and the VECP using stimulus stripes and checks.

Evoked potentials recorded at the same time are shown in the lower part of the figure. Larger evoked potentials are seen towards the middle of the investigated range of textures than at the ends. The evoked potentials for stripes and checks of equal size are not the same. Checkered stimuli in the middle of the range produce larger responses than stripes. Further details are shown in Fig. 9. In this figure, the amplitudes of responses to stimuli of fixed luminance are plotted against spatial frequency, a measure of the closeness of spacing of the stripes and checks. Coarse patterns of stripes or checks have low spatial frequencies and *vice versa*. Data for the electroretinogram are shown in the upper half of the figure. There are two plots, one for checks and one for stripes, and they are quite similar. Coarse stimuli always produced the largest electroretinograms. As spatial frequency was increased to the middle of the range investigated, amplitude decreased only a little, but it dropped off rapidly at the high frequencies. Comparison plots for the evoked potential are presented in the bottom of the figure. For both checks and stripes, small responses are found with low spatial frequencies. Responses became larger within these extremes. It should also be noted that the peak amplitude obtained with checks was considerably higher than that obtained with stripes.

The data shown so far were obtained at maximum available luminance. By examining the recordings produced over a range of luminances it was possible to determine the response sensitivity as a function of stimulus spatial frequency, sensitivity being defined here, as in Fig. 2, as the reciprocal of the adaptation luminance required to produce a constant amplitude of response. Examples for checkered stimuli are shown in Fig. 10. Plots of such determinations result in spatial tuning curves. The visual evoked potential is seen to be sharply tuned to the middle of the range while the electroretinogram is not. If the electroretinogram peaks at any spatial frequency, that frequency lies below the values examined here. Tuning curves were also determined for striped stimuli, but are not shown. That for the electroretinogram was virtually the same as seen with checks; that for the visually evoked cortical potential peaked at the same frequency but less sharply than the one for the checks.

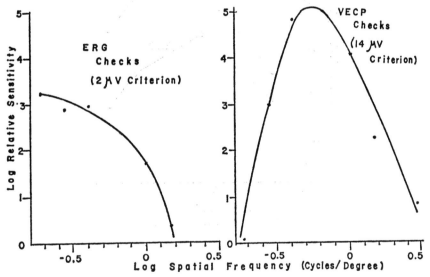

FIG. 10.   Sensitivity of the ERG and the VECP to checkered stimuli of varying interface density.

There are different ways in which data of this sort may be interpreted. The high sensitivity of the evoked potentials to checkered stimuli has been attributed to their large number of edges.[27] Checks of any given spatial frequency have twice as many edges as stripes.

A complete explanation must involve more than this, however. The finest checks produced a stimulus which had more edges than did those in the middle range, yet the latter produced a larger response. Another type of explanation has been advanced by KELLY[29] to account for psychophysical data showing a similar spatial tuning effect. It is based on the notion that the visual system is composed of many overlapping receptive fields. When the size of the checks matches that of the receptive fields, the largest responses are seen. Lateral inhibition between the central part of a field and its surrounding areas reduces the size of the responses unless such a match exists. Stripes can only match the receptor field in one dimension. Hence, the tuning effect is less marked. The fact that no maximum is achieved with the electroretinogram indicates that it has much larger receptive fields than the evoked potential or that its amplitude is not influenced by inhibitory factors.

Earlier experiments have demonstrated a tuning effect in a different but related context. Eye movements, which are generally present in normal viewing, produce a natural displacement of the retinal image and hence, a change in retinal stimulation. Because each eye movement produces a change in the light falling upon individual receptors, it initiates a visual response at the retina and at the cortex. By combining eye movement recording and average response techniques one can observe the visual potentials produced by spontaneous

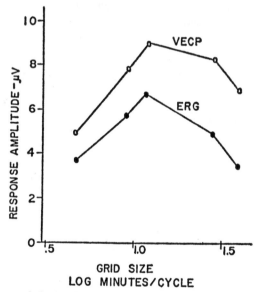

FIG. 11. Dependance of the VECP and the ERG elicited by spontaneous eye movements upon the spatial frequency of striped stimulus patterns.

displacement of the retinal image.[30,31] The eye views a steady striped pattern which neither flashes nor alternates. Its spontaneous movements are recorded with an infrared device which triggers an average response computer whenever there is a saccadic eye movement. The computer averages the electroretinograms and evoked potentials which follow a series of such movements. The amplitude of responses recorded in this way also varies with the stimulus textures both at the retina and at the cortex. As shown in Fig. 11, very fine or very coarse gratings have been found to be less effective than those of moderate spatial frequency. The data shown in the figure when first collected were interpreted in terms of the eye movement amplitudes rather than in terms of inhibitory receptive fields. The size of an eye movement relative to the fineness of the stimulus pattern determines the effective change of retinal stimulation. If the stripe width of a grating pattern viewed by the subject is equal to the excursion produced by a typical eye movement, the positions on the retina which were occupied by bright bars before the eye movement will be exactly filled by black bars afterwards and *vice versa*. Patterns which closely correspond to the size of the average eye movement will produce a maximal change of retinal stimulation and, hence, the largest responses. Patterns of other sizes will not. Taken together data shown in Figs. 8–11, show that both stimulus texture and eye movement can produce spatial tuning effects. In other words, it now appears that sensitivity to patterned stimuli in normal viewing depends both upon neural mechanisms sensitive to the actual texture of the stimulus and upon the relation of the spontaneous shifts of the retinal image to stimulus structure. Present research is directed towards disentangling these two factors.

REFERENCES

1. GRANIT, R. The components of the retinal action potential and their relation to the discharge in the Optic Nerve. *J. Physiol.* **77**, 207, 1933.
2. GRANIT, R. *Sensory Mechanisms of the Retina*. Hafner, New York, 1963.
3. BROWN, K. T. The electroretinogram: its components and their origins. *Vision Res.* **8**, 633, 1968.
4. MILLER, R. F. and DOWLING, J. E. Intracellular responses of the Müller (glial) cells of mudpuppy retina: their relation to *b*-wave of the electroretinogram. *J. Neurophysiol.* **33**, 323, 1970.
5. ARMINGTON, J. C., JOHNSON, E. P. and RIGGS, L. A. The Scotopic *A*-wave in the electrical response of the human retina. *J. Physiol., Lond.* **118**, 289, 1952.
6. ADRIAN, E. D. The electrical response of the human eye. *J. Physiol., Lond.* **104**, 84, 1945.
7. BOYNTON, R. M. Stray light and the electroretinogram. *J. opt. Soc. Am.* **43**, 442, 1953.
8. ARMINGTON, J. C. and BIERSDORF, W. R. Flicker and color adaptation in the human electroretinogram. *J, opt. Soc. Am.* **46**, 394, 1956.
9. BIERSDORF, W. R. and ARMINGTON, J. C. Response of the human eye to sudden changes in the wavelength of stimulation. *J. opt. Soc. Am.* **47**, 208, 1957.
10. ARMINGTON, J. C. and THIEDE, F. C. Effect of stimulus area and intensity upon the light-adapted electroretinogram. *J. exp. Psychol.* **47**, 329, 1954.
11. CRAMPTON, G. H. and ARMINGTON, J. C. Area-intensity relation and retinal location in the human electroretinogram. *Am. J. Physiol.* **181**, 47, 1955.
12. DAWSON, G. D. A summation technique for the detection of small evoked potentials. *Electroenceph. clin. Neurophysiol.* **6,** 65, 1954.
13. BRAZIER, M. A. B. and CASBY, J. U. Crosscorrelation and autocorrelation studies of electroencephalographic potentials. *Electroenceph. clin. Neurophysiol.* **4**, 201, 1952.
14. ARMINGTON, J. C., TEPAS, D. I., KROPFL, W. J. and HENGST, W. H. Summation of retinal potentials. *J. opt. Soc. Am.* **51**, 877, 1961.
15. ROSENBLITH, W. A. Emploi des calculateurs electroniques en neurophysiologie. *Actual. neurophysiol.* **2**, 155, 1960.
16. ARMINGTON, J. C. Relations between electroretinograms and occipital potentials elicited by flickering stimuli. *Documenta ophth.* **18**, 194, 1964.
17. GOURAS, P., ARMINGTON, J. C., KROPFL, W. J. and GUNKEL, R. D. Electronic computation of human retinal and brain responses to light stimulation. *Ann. N.Y. Acad. Sci.* **115**, 763, 1964.
18. ARMINGTON, J. C. Spectral sensitivity of simultaneous electroretinograms and occipital responses. *Clinical Electroretinography* BURIAN, H. M. and JACOBSON, J. H. (Eds.), p. 225. Pergamon, New York, 1966.

19. LODGE, A. ARMINGTON, J. C., BARNET, A. B., SHANKS, B. L. and NEWCOMB, C. N. Newborn infants' electroretinograms and evoked electroencephalographic responses to orange and white light. *Child Dev.* **40**, 267, 1969.

20. JOHNSON, E. P., RIGGS, L. A. and SCHICK, A. M. L. Photopic retinal potentials evoked by phase alternation of a barred pattern. *Clinical Electroretinography*, BURIAN, H. M. and JACOBSON, J. H. (Eds.), p. 75, Pergamon, New York, 1966.

21. ARMINGTON, J. C. The electroretinogram, the visual evoked potential and the area-luminance relation. *Vision Res.* **8**, 263, 1968.

22. ARMINGTON, J. C. Pupil entry and the human electroretinogram. *J. opt. Soc. Am.* **57**, 838, 1967.

23. RIGGS, L. A., JOHNSON, E. P. and SCHICK, A. M. L. Electrical responses of the human eye to changes in wavelength of the stimulating light. *J. opt. Soc. Am.* **56**, 1621, 1966.

24. ARMINGTON, J. C., MARSETTA, R. and SCHICK, A. M. L. Stimulus alternation and low level response. *Vision Res.* **10**, 227, 1970.

25. CHAPMAN, R. M. and BRAGDON, H. R. Evoked responses to numerical and non-numerical visual stimuli while problem solving. *Nature, Lond.* **203**, 1155, 1964.

26. WHITE, C. T. Evoked cortical responses and patterned stimuli. *Am. Psychol.* **24**, 211, 1969.

27. SPEHLMANN, R. The averaged electrical responses to diffuse and to patterned light in the human. *Electroenceph. clin. Neurophysiol.* **19**, 560, 1965.

28. SPEKREIJSE, H. Analysis of EEG responses in man evoked by sine wave modulated light. Junk, The Hague, 1966.

29. KELLY, D. H. Flickering patterns and lateral inhibition. *J. opt. Soc. Am.* **59**, 1361, 1969.

30. GAARDER, K., KRAUSKOPF, J., GRAF, V., KROPFL, W. and ARMINGTON, J. C. Averaged brain activity following saccadic eye movement. *Science* **146**, 1481, 1964.

31. ARMINGTON, J. C., GAARDER, K. and SCHICK, A. M. L. Variation of spontaneous ocular and occipital responses with stimulus patterns. *J. opt. Soc. Am.* **57**, 1534, 1967.

J. psychiat. Res., 1971, Vol. 8, pp. 323–333. Pergamon Press. Printed in Great Britain.

A RE-EVALUATION OF THE CONCEPT OF 'NON-SPECIFICITY' IN STRESS THEORY

JOHN W. MASON

Department of Neuroendocrinology, Walter Reed Army Institute of Research
Walter Reed Army Medical Center, Washington, D.C.

AT THE time of the organization of the Neuropsychiatry Division at Walter Reed in the early 50's, research in Neuroendocrinology was very much dominated by the provocative 'stress' concepts formulated by Hans Selye. Although SELYE first reported the findings which led to his initial formulation of 'stress' theory in 1936,[1] the publication of his monumental volume entitled *Stress* in 1950, followed by the five subsequent *Annual Report on Stress* volumes, made an extraordinary impact on biology and medicine in the early 50's.[2-7] There was an aura of academic excitement and controversy in that period as a result of these publications which was responsible for attracting many young investigators to the study of endocrine regulation and for stimulating a considerable amount of new research in this field. There were perhaps two principal general concepts in 'stress' theory upon which most attention was focussed. The first was the concept of a 'general adaptation syndrome' and the second, that of 'diseases of adaptation'. The general reaction to these concepts was mixed and a number of critical objections were raised from time to time by other scientists.

Yet, as one now looks back over the past 20 years, it is a curious fact that, while there were both strong opponents and proponents of Selye's concepts, the main body of 'stress' theory still stands largely in the position of having been neither conclusively confirmed and generally accepted nor conclusively refuted and rejected on the basis of definitive experimental evaluation. Much of the controversy over 'stress' theory in the 50's was waged by argument rather than by experiment. Individual workers simply tended to assume personal stands more or less intuitively concerning 'stress' theory and there were apparently relatively few sustained and systematic attempts to put specific points in 'stress' theory to rigorous experimental tests, particularly as new methods became available.

Historically, it is perhaps especially noteworthy that 1950 marked an approximate dividing point between two eras in research on endocrine regulation from a methodological standpoint. Prior to 1950, the study of endocrine regulation was based largely on relatively indirect and non-specific methods, such as glandular weight, glandular histology, bioassays, or the metabolic effects of hormones. The period following 1950 was a truly revolutionary one in which such analytical principles as chromatography, isotope techniques, immuno-assay, microspectrophotometry and fluorimetric techniques made possible remarkably precise, sensitive, and specific methods for the measurement of individual hormones in plasma and urine. As it happened, most of Selye's own research leading to the 'stress' concept, as well as a great deal of 'stress' research by others up to the middle 50's, was based upon the use of the older, less direct methods of evaluating pituitary-adrenal cortical function.

As more refined methods for biochemical measurement of the adrenal cortical hormones became available, the need to re-evaluate some of Selye's earlier work based on indirect methods was generally recognized. In particular, a crucial notion which really forms the foundation of 'stress' theory is the concept of the 'non-specificity' of the pituitary-adrenal cortical and certain other bodily responses to a variety of stimuli. This concept was derived by Selye from the observation that increased adrenal cortical activity could be elicited by a remarkably wide variety of different 'nocuous' agents including trauma, hemorrhage, burns, cold, heat, X-rays, nervous stimuli, muscular exercise, anoxia, infections, fasting and various drugs. In his 1950 'stress' volume, Selye described the 'general adaptation syndrome' based largely on the 'non-specificity' concept as follows:

"The general-adaptation-syndrome (G-A-S) is the sum of all non-specific systemic reactions of the body which ensue upon long-continued exposure to systemic stress. One of the most fundamental observations in connection with the G-A-S was the finding that many of the morphologic, functional and biochemical changes elicited by various systemic stressor agents are essentially the same irrespective of the specific nature of the eliciting stimulus." . . . [2]

Selye attached great theoretical importance to this concept of non-specificity in bodily reactions and contrasted it with the concept of specificity in medicine which was introduced by Pasteur, Koch and their contemporaries. "Stress" was defined, then, as the "sum of all non-specific changes caused by function or damage" and the wide variety of stimuli capable of producing the non-specific changes were defined as "stressors".[2]

Many endocrinologists evaluated the effects of the diverse 'stressors' described by Selye upon plasma and urinary corticosteroid levels, using the biochemical methods developed in the 50's. In general, their results appeared to confirm the conclusion that the pituitary-adrenal cortical system responds to a wide variety of apparently different stimuli. Consequently, the notion of the 'non-specific' character of pituitary-adrenal cortical response gained rather wide acceptance among endocrinologists, and interest seemed to wane gradually in the further testing of 'stress' concepts. It is curious, for example, that few if any attempts were made to re-evaluate the concept of the three temporal phases in the general adaptation syndrome (the alarm reaction, the stage of resistance, and the stage of exhaustion) in terms of the associated levels of biochemically measured pituitary-adrenal cortical activity.

In any event, while interest in the re-evaluation of 'stress' concepts has steadily diminished, within the past decade some findings have emerged from the study of endocrine regulation which have important implications concerning the validity of 'stress' theory in general, and the concept of 'non-specificity' in particular. The primary purpose of this paper is to review these recent research developments and to discuss the ways in which they appear to call for revision of 'stress' theory.

The point of departure in our own research in the 'stress' field was the more or less incidental observation reported by Selye that "... Even mere emotional stress, for instance that caused by immobilizing an animal on a board (taking great care to avoid any physical injury), proved to be a suitable routine procedure for the production of a severe alarm reaction".[2] This observation was of considerable interest to many behavioral scientists, for whom it raised the possibility that psychoendocrine mechanisms might exist of a broader scope than was previously realized. Walter Cannon's work had demonstrated earlier that the sympathetic-adrenal medullary system was clearly influenced by psychological factors, but at the time of Selye's reports there were few experimental data to indicate that other endocrine systems were subject to psychological influences. A particularly noteworthy aspect of Selye's observation was that the anterior pituitary, receiving virtually no significant neural input, appeared nonetheless to be influenced by the central nervous system.

In the past 20 years, over 200 research publications have confirmed beyond any question the validity of Selye's observation that psychological stimuli can elicit a substantial pituitary-adrenal cortical response.[8] What has emerged, in fact, is the conclusion that psychological stimuli are among the most potent of all stimuli affecting the pituitary-adrenal cortical system. Not only stimuli strong enough to elicit severe pain or discomfort or emotional reactions, but also the much more subtle psychological stimuli of everyday life can be sensitively reflected in adrenocortical activity. There seems to be little doubt that the potency of psychological influences in the regulation of corticosteroid levels was almost universally underestimated by early workers in the 'stress' research field. In general, as perhaps indicated by Dr. Selye's use of the phrase, "mere emotional stimuli . . . ", physiologists tended to regard psychological variables as negligible factors in their experiments by comparison with such obviously drastic physical variables as trauma, exercise, heat, fasting, and so on. Selye did recognize the possible role of pain in the augmentation of adrenal cortical responses to such stimuli as trauma and infections, but had little reason at that time to suspect the true degree of sensitivity of the pituitary-adrenal cortical response to more ubiquitous and much less drastic psychological influences.

Although the sensitivity of the pituitary-adrenal cortical system to psychological factors was widely acknowledged shortly after 1960, the important implications of psychoendocrine research for the field of endocrine regulation as a whole still seemed not to be generally appreciated. It is likely that the slowness with which psychoendocrine data were incorporated into physiological thinking stems largely from the traditional separation of the behavioral sciences from the rest of biology and medicine. Research on physical stimuli in endocrine regulation is generally confined to endocrinological and physiological laboratories quite far removed from the scene of psychoendocrine studies proceeding in Departments of Psychiatry and Psychology. The territorial separation of the two research areas is almost complete, even to the point of extremely limited communication of published findings between the fields.

Not until our own long-term stress program led us into the study of certain 'physical stressors' did we begin to become more fully aware of the unfortunate consequences of this separation of effort between far-removed disciplines within the field of endocrine regulation. In our initial attempts to study the endocrine responses to such stimuli as exercise, fasting, heat, and cold, we were struck by the fact that it is extremely difficult in the laboratory situation to isolate these stimuli from their natural psychological concomitants. Unless one is extremely mindful of the exquisite sensitivity of the pituitary-adrenal cortical system to psychological influences, one is likely to subject animals or humans to stimuli such as exercise, fasting, cold, heat, etc., under conditions in which either considerable pain, discomfort, or emotional reaction is simultaneously elicited.

For example, in our first effort to study fasting, we simply stopped feeding 2 monkeys out of a group of 8 housed within the same room. The fasting monkeys were, thus, suddenly deprived of their daily food for 3 days while their 6 neighbors were eating as usual. The familiar animal caretaker was coming into the room at the usual times and the sounds, sights, and odors associated with normal feeding were present as usual, but these 2 monkeys found themselves unaccountably being ignored in the passing out of food. As might be expected, under these conditions the deprived animals often vocalized in apparent protest. In addition, after fasting is underway there is the factor of the discomfort of an empty gastro-intestinal tract as another possible basis for psychological reaction. It is not surprising, then, that 'fasting' under these conditions was associated with a marked increase in urinary 17-hydroxycorticosteroid (17-OHCS) levels in the first monkeys so studied.

We next made an effort to minimize these possible psychological variables in two ways. First, we placed the fasting monkeys in a small, private cubicle where they were protected from non-involved monkeys and from other extraneous influences. Second, they were given fruit-flavoured but non-nutritive pellets which were similar in appearance and taste to their normal diet. Although the monkeys ate fewer of these non-nutritive cellulose pellets than they did of their normal diet pellets, they did eat enough to provide some bulk within the gastrointestinal tract. Under these conditions designed to minimize psychological reaction, we found no significant 17-OHCS response to fasting, although other hormonal changes (epinephrine, norepinephrine, insulin, growth hormone) were observed.[9] Fasting *per se*, then, appears to elicit little, if any, adrenal cortical response, but the fasting *situation* as a whole may indeed evoke a marked 17-OHCS response if it includes factors which elicit psychological reaction or arousal of the subject.

This experience proved to be only one of a steadily lengthening series of observations emphasizing the need for painstaking efforts to isolate physical from psychological stimuli in laboratory experiments. Muscular exercise proved to be another case in point. We found it virtually impossible to force monkeys to perform strenuous muscular exercise, such as walking a treadmill or lifting weights for food, without eliciting signs of displeasure or other emotional reactions that could well, quite by themselves, have explained the marked 17-OHCS responses recorded in these experiments. Perhaps the closest we came to minimizing emotional reaction was in the case of a climbing task in which little, if any, urinary 17-OHCS change was observed in some experiments although a considerable amount of work was performed.[10] More recently we have found that in human subjects exercising under relatively pleasant non-competitive conditions, there is little if any change in either plasma or urinary 17-OHCS levels, even at relatively substantial workloads. Plasma 17-OHCS responses occur only at extremely high workload levels, and again it becomes difficult to rule out attendant psychological reactions under such conditions.[11] Before the current data on exercise are accepted as conclusive, however, it would seem particularly advisable to await future results with isotopic secretion rate studies as a check on the validity of present conclusions based upon plasma and urinary hormone measurements.

Perhaps the most compelling data we have obtained thus far along these lines have come from studies of heat as a physical stimulus. In our initial heat experiments, we suddenly elevated the temperature in a chamber housing a chair-restrained monkey from 70° to 85°F within a matter of a few minutes. In this experiment a urinary 17-OHCS elevation was observed, very similar to the response recorded in earlier experiments in which monkeys were abruptly exposed to a cold environment. By this time we had become very alert to the problem of interfering psychological variables and were careful to avoid any unusual handling or change of location or strange activities in the laboratory. The only variable which we might have overlooked as a possible source of spurious psychological reaction appeared to be the rapidity of the temperature change, the sudden 'thrusting', as it were, of an animal into a hotter environment. The experiment was then repeated with a more gradual, but equally large temperature change, at the rate of a 1°F elevation per hr. Under these conditions, there was not only no 17-OHCS elevation in response to heat, but an actual *suppression* of 17-OHCS levels was observed. Furthermore, this suppression of 17-OHCS levels persisted over a period of several weeks during which the temperature was maintained at 85°F, and was terminated only when the temperature was again lowered to 70°F. We have since observed the suppressing effect of heat on 17-OHCS levels in a number of additional experiments.[12]

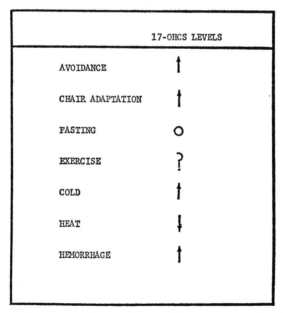

Fig. 1.   Direction of 17-hydroxycorticosteroid responses to various 'stressors'.

In at least two other 'physical stress situations' so far, namely, cold-exposure and hemorrhage, we believe we have been able to minimize factors which might provoke psychological reactions in the monkey. In both of these situations, however, there does appear to be a bona fide elevation in 17-OHCS levels which we presume to be specifically related to the designated physical stimuli and not to be predominantly psychoendocrine responses.

Figure 1 presents a simplified summary of the findings described above, listing seven 'stressors' which have been conventionally included among the variety of 'nocuous' stimuli capable of eliciting a 'non-specific' response of the pituitary-adrenal cortical system. Our initial experiments with all seven stress situations appeared to confirm the prevailing impression that these 'stressors' elicit a pituitary-adrenal cortical response. When, however, a more rigorous experimental approach was taken, mindful of the ubiquitous presence of psychological stimuli in the laboratory situation and in accordance with present knowledge of the sensitivity of 17-OHCS levels to psychological influences, then a different picture was observed. Along with psychological stimuli such as conditioned avoidance and adaptation to the restraining chair, physical stimuli such as cold and hemorrhage also do indeed appear to elicit an elevation in 17-OHCS levels. On the other hand, exercise appears to produce little, or at least questionable changes, fasting even less change, and heat actually elicits a suppression of 17-OHCS levels. While these findings must be regarded as tentative, particularly until they are evaluated in human subjects, in whom psychological reactions can be assessed more reliably, and until secretion-rate measurements of adrenal activity are included, they seem clearly to call attention to the need for some re-evaluation of both earlier stress research and stress theory.

First of all, it appears highly advisable that we view with skepticism the conclusions drawn from all those past and future studies of the role of 'physiological' or 'physical' stimuli in endocrine regulation in which no rigorous efforts were made to minimize or assess the possible role of associated psychological reactions. In some instances, it may prove virtually impossible to isolate certain physical stimuli in 'pure' form. It is very difficult, for example, to conceive of ways of producing trauma without attendant pain and emotional reaction. The malaise, discomfort or apprehension associated with acute infections also seems almost inescapable. Even with other so-called 'physical stresses' such as hypoxia or certain drug injections, such variables as nausea, malaise and related psychological reactions are experimental parameters which deserve attention no less close than that paid to age, sex, body weight, nutrition, room temperature, absence of infection, and other independent variables in our experiments. It is rather ironic that the early stages of psychoendocrine research were marked by a great concern to control for all possible contamination of experiments by attendant physical stimuli. It proved to be feasible and reasonably easy to do this with modern developments in behavioral methodology. Now, more than a decade later, we are faced with the converse problem of eliminating or controlling for psychological stimuli in research on physical stimuli, and it appears that this problem may prove to require a considerably greater amount of painstaking effort if it is to be overcome.

The whole field of 'physical stress' research is really almost completely thrown open to re-evaluation in the light of the developments discussed above. While much more new research is needed before we know the full extent to which psychological factors have entered into 'physical stress' research, even those findings presented in Fig. 1 on fasting, heat, and perhaps exercise, are sufficient to cast serious doubt at present upon the concept of physiological 'non-specificity', which is the very foundation upon which much of stress theory rests. Selye's conclusion that the morphological, functional, and biochemical changes elicited by various systemic stressor agents are essentially the same irrespective of the specific nature of the eliciting stimulus was formulated so as to suggest that these 'non-specific' responses were mediated by physiological mechanisms. All these diverse 'nocuous' stimuli were apparently thought to be conveyed, presumably via humoral or neural pathways, to the anterior pituitary, which responded in a remarkably non-specific way with ACTH release, no matter what the quality of the incoming stimulus. It is perhaps on this point of interpretation that a major fallacy in stress theory exists. There is a great deal of difference, from a biological standpoint, in the conception of many diverse stimuli eliciting a 'non-specific' *endocrine* response as contrasted to eliciting a 'non-specific' *behavioral* response and the recent data I have discussed suggests that this may really be the issue at stake.

In retrospect, it seems possible that the concepts of 'nocuous stimuli' and 'non-specific' bodily changes and the 'stress' concept itself may have served somehow to lull us into a rather uncritical attitude about the mediating body pathways or modes of signal transmission involved in endocrine regulation. For whatever reasons, it does appear that we have failed to really come to grips with the crucial question of what might be called the *afferent* limb of the 'stress' response from a physiological and anatomical standpoint. We have devoted relatively little thought or effort generally in 'stress' research to some basic questions concerning the peripheral receptors, the afferent pathways whereby the messages of received stimuli or 'stressors' are conveyed to neuroendocrine centers, and even the final common neuroendocrine pathways themselves. In the final *Annual Report on Stress* volume in 1956, Selye himself indicated briefly his awareness of this issue, referring to the problem of identifying the "first mediator of Stress–Responses" and summarizing the current state of knowledge as follows:

"We still know virtually nothing about the nature of the 'first mediator(s)' which transmit(s) the impulse for ACTH secretion from the area directly affected by stressors to the hypothalamo-hypophyseal system. Progress has been made mainly in eliminating certain suspected mediators by showing that they could not be *the* first mediator." He cites research indicating that adrenalin, noradrenalin, acetylcholine or histamine are not the 'first-mediator'.[7] Thus, it is clear that, while this issue was largely being by-passed in stress research, the afferent limb of the 'stress' arc was conceived of as involving one or more unknown humoral or physiological 'first mediators'.

What I am suggesting, in other words, is that the 'primary mediator' underlying the pituitary-adrenal cortical response to the diverse 'stressors' of earlier 'stress' research may simply be the psychological apparatus involved in emotional or arousal reactions to threatening or unpleasant factors in the life situation as a whole. The 'primary mediator' may simply be a common body mechanism brought into operation by an experimental variable which was essentially overlooked or underestimated in 'stress' research, namely, the great sensitivity of the endocrine systems to psychological influences which have contaminated many experiments on 'physical stressors'. Perhaps one of the principal points of historical importance concerning 'stress' theory will eventually prove to be in the early calling attention to the sensitivity and ubiquity of psychoendocrine mechanisms.

Be this as it may, we are still left with the basic question of the primary mediating or input mechanisms involved in the elicitation of integrative responses to the various physical stimuli themselves. What is the complete body machinery whereby the messages of cold, heat, fasting, exercise, tissue damage, etc., reach the cells of the anterior pituitary? If we had pursued the question of the organic substratum underlying the 'stress' response along such more mechanistic lines, it seems likely that we might well have foreseen earlier that the concept of 'non-specificity' as developed in stress theory presupposes afferent and central mechanisms which are difficult to visualize in the light of present knowledge. What body mechanisms are known to exist which might convey a quality like 'nocuousness' to neuroendocrine centers? Logically, one must assume the existence of either body receptors which can respond 'non-specifically' to the 'nocuous' quality common to many diverse stimuli, or central neuronal aggregates which can respond 'non-specifically' to a wide variety of humoral and neural inputs representing these diverse 'nocuous' stimuli. While either of these possibilities would be conceivable, such physiological mechanisms have not yet been demonstrated to exist. Of the existing known bodily mechanisms which might be capable of such a 'non-specific' response to 'nocuous' stimuli, the psychological mechanisms of emotional arousal to threat seem to be ideally suited to the task.

I was interested to read recently some autobiographical notes written by Selye concerning the reaction of Walter Cannon to his 'stress' concepts:

"Cannon was my first critic . . . I felt quite frustrated at not being able to convince the Great Old Man of the important role played by the pituitary and the adrenal cortex in my stress syndrome. He gave me excellent reasons why he did not think these glands could help resistance and adaptation in general and even why it would seem unlikely that a general adaptation syndrome could exist. But there was no trace of aggressiveness in his criticisms, no sting that could have blurred my vision to the point of refusing to listen."[13]

This anecdote was of particular interest to me since I had long been troubled by the apparent incompatibility of the 'general adaptation syndrome' with the concept of homeostasis. How could the same hormonal response have adaptive utility in response to diverse stimuli which place such diametrically opposite metabolic needs on the body as do, for example, heat and cold? Ingle's concept of the 'permissive' nature of adrenal cortical hormonal action provided one possible explanation, but still it seems most appealing to think of homeostatic regulatory mechanisms as generally more selectively organized to deal appropriately with metabolic needs or changes in a relatively specific fashion. In a cold environment, for example, there is a bodily need to increase heat production and decrease heat loss, while in a hot environment, decreased heat production and increased heat loss would be expected to have special survival value to the organism. Can the same hormone exert thermogenic effects on one occasion and thermolytic effects on another occasion? Perhaps the only bodily response which might conceivably be equally appropriate, in a homeostatic sense, under conditions of both heat and cold would be a *behavioral* response of emotional arousal or hyperalerting preparatory to flight, struggle or other strenuous exertion which might serve to eliminate the source of heat or cold or to remove the subject from its presence. If the organism perceives the 'physical stress' situation as threatening enough, then perhaps psychoendocrine responses do occur rather universally and are superimposed upon the endocrine and other bodily responses to the pure 'physical' stimulus. If this interpretation is correct, then *the 'stress' concept should not be regarded primarily as a physiological concept but rather as a behavioral concept*. The more correct basic conclusion really appears to be, then, that adrenal cortical responses occur in many different laboratory situations involving a wide variety of stimuli, because emotional reactions (which elicit adrenal cortical responses) occur commonly in a wide variety of laboratory situations in which animals or humans are subjected to 'physical stress'. In this sense, in the sense of the ubiquity of emotional reaction to threat, one is dealing with a 'non-specific' response of a primarily behavioral nature. The above distinction between a 'behavioral' versus a 'physiological' concept is not intended to imply, of course, any fundamental biological difference between psychological and other physiological functions, but simply to call attention to the important question of the *level* within the central nervous system at which neuroendocrine responses to 'stressors' are integrated. It is to emphasize the point that the 'afferent limb' and the integrative processes underlying the 'non-specific' bodily responses to stressors probably involve a *higher level* of central nervous system function than was previously realized.

It will almost certainly yet prove to be true that the pituitary-adrenal cortical system is responsive to more than one stimulus, i.e. to certain 'physical' stimuli as well as psychological stimuli. If adrenal cortical responses to cold, anoxia, and several other stimuli are proven to occur even in the absence of psychological disturbances, this does imply a relative degree of 'non-specifiicity' of response in this system as Selye concluded, but not nearly to the degree that it was originally thought in the development of 'stress' theory. It also seems likely, incidentally, that a number of other endocrine systems will be shown to have an equally broad range of response to multiple stimuli, as current work with insulin, growth hormone, epinephrine, and other hormones suggests.

The future usefulness of the concept of 'non-specificity' in relation to the pituitary-adrenal cortical system is therefore open to question. Certainly, we should be very cautious not to make the same assumptions regarding any additional endocrine systems that prove responsive to a wide variety of 'nocuous' stimuli until possible psychoendocrine factors have been carefully evaluated. It seems advisable in future studies to devote greater attention to the isolation of 'pure' stimuli, physical and psychological, in the study of endocrine regulation. Not only is there an important problem in the identification of psychological factors and their elimination from the stimulus situation, but a number of natural 'physical stress' situations actually involve a variable mixture of several 'pure' stimuli in a physiological sense. Hemorrhage, for example, is a composite mixture of hypoxia, fluid loss, hypoproteinemia, hypotension, etc., so that, in the study of hormonal responses to hemorrhage, one is at a loss to establish precise stimulus–response relationships unless these component stimuli are studied separately under highly controlled conditions. 'Altitude stress' is a mixture of 'pure' stimuli, including hypoxia, barometric pressure changes, and possibly psychological reaction to adverse bodily symptoms or situational factors, and so on. We must first seek to identify the basic 'pure' or 'elemental' stimuli to which body receptors linked to neuroendocrine mechanisms can respond. After the responses evoked by these 'elemental' stimuli are known, then the stimuli can more interpretably be studied in various combinations as they occur under natural conditions.

It also seems advisable in the future that we give greater thought to the identification of the receptors and the afferent pathways whereby the final common pathways leading to altered endocrine activity are affected. We presume now that there are final common pathway neurones in the hypothalamus which, once stimulated, secrete corticotrophin-releasing factor (CRF) which, in turn, through the hypothalamo-hypophyseal portal system stimulates anterior pituitary cells to secrete ACTH. We must answer questions such as: "How many different, discrete, primary stimuli reaching these CRF-secreting cells are capable of altering CRF secretion? What nerve fibers from what sources project to the CRF-secreting cells? Can changes in the chemical composition or temperature of the blood, for example, stimulate such cells?" We now know that these cells are stimulated under conditions of emotional arousal of the organism. Nerve fibers projecting from the amygdaloid complex and the reticular formation are known to influence ACTH release, so that we have a beginning at least in identifying the central processing mechanisms involved in psychoendocrine responses. We need now to think more intensively along the same lines in identifying the *input pathways* in the case of cold, hypoxia and other stimuli which may also truly elicit ACTH release. Can we interrupt neural pathways which prevent ACTH response to cold but not to emotional stimuli, or vice versa? How does the message of hypoxia reach the CRF-secreting cells?

If we think along these lines, it seems likely that we shall find increasingly little need or use for 'stress' concepts or terminology, particularly the 'non-specificity' concept, except perhaps in connection with situations or events that provoke psychoendocrine or psycho-physiological reactions. Our thinking should revert to dealing with discrete stimuli in as irreducible or 'pure' a form as possible, with receptors, with the afferent or mediating linkages between receptor and neuroendocrine systems and with the final common neuroendocrine pathways. If this can be successfully accomplished, it seems likely that we will be in a much better position to place 'stress' theory and Selye's contributions in a more accurate historical and scientific perspective and, most important, we can confidently expect the principles underlying the organization of endocrine regulation to emerge more clearly.

REFERENCES

1. SELYE, H. A syndrome produced by diverse nocuous agents. *Nature, Lond.* **138**, 32, 1936.
2. SELYE, H. Stress. The Physiology and Pathology of Exposure ot Stress. Acta Med. Publ., Montreal, 1950.
3. SELYE, H. *First Annual Report on Stress.* Acta Med. Publ., Montreal, 1951.
4. SEYLE, H. and HORAVA, A. *Second Annual Report on Stress—1952.* Acta Med. Publ., Montreal, 1952.
5. SELYE, H. and HORAVA, A. *Third Annual Report on Stress—1953.* Acta Med. Publ., Montreal, 1953.
6. SELYE, H. and HEUSER, G. *Fourth Annual Report on Stress—1954.* Acta Med. Publ., Montreal, 1954.
7. SELYE, H. and HEUSER, G. *Fifth Annual Report on Stress—1955–56.* MD Publications, New York, 1956.
8. MASON, J. W. A review of psychoendocrine research on the pituitary-adrenal cortical system. *Psychosom. Med.* **30**, 576, 1968.

9. Mason, J. W., Wool, M. S., Mougey, E. H., Wherry, F. E., Collins, D. R. and Taylor, E. D. Psychological vs. nutritional factors in the effects of 'fasting' on hormonal balance. *Psychosom Med.* **30**, 554, 1968.
10. Miller, R. E. and Mason, J. W. Changes in 17-hydroxycorticosteroid excretion related to increased muscular work. *Symposium on Medical Aspects of Stress in the Military Climate.* GPO, Washington, D.C., 1965.
11. Jones, L. G., Hartley, L. H., Mason, J. W., Hogan, R. P., Gerben, M. J. and Kreuz, L. E. The effects of muscular leg exercise on neuroendocrine blood levels. Army Science Conference, 1970.
12. Mason, J. W., Poe, R. O. and Ehle, A. L. Unpublished observations.
13. Selye, H. *Stress and Disease.* McGraw-Hill, New York, 1956.

J. psychiat. Res., 1971, Vol. 8, pp. 335–344. Pergamon Press. Printed in Great Britain.

CHANNELING OF RESPONSES ELICITED BY HYPOTHALAMIC STIMULATION*

ELLIOT S. VALENSTEIN†

Department of Psychology and Neurosciences Laboratory, University of Michigan, Ann Arbor

Michigan

SCIENTIFIC discovery, like mining, often progresses on a discontinuous course. Progress in one direction continues until a point of diminishing returns is reached. A new strike may produce a scurry of activity in another direction. The development of different techniques may prompt the reopening of a closed shaft. Only after a period of such exploration may a more complete picture of the field emerge. The history of the hypothalamus seems to be following such a course.

Prior to the turn of this century, little attention was given to the hypothalamus. The fact that the obesity observed as part of the Fröhlich syndrome was attributed to pituitary difficulties and not related to hypothalamic involvement clearly reflected the prevailing scientific bias. ANDERSON[1] traced the history of this period and quoted the following portion of Fröhlich's remarks in 1940 at a symposium on the hypothalamus: "The discussions that I have attended the past two days have established the fact that we were wrong in 1901, that it was not the pituitary body but the hypothalamus, but then I must remind you that all we knew at that time was that the hypothalamus was an anatomical region lying beneath the thalamus. That is all we knew."

Following the classic work by KARPLUS and KREIDL,[2] RANSON[3,4] and his colleagues, and HESS,[5,6] the hypothalamus became increasingly stressed as a significant area for the expression of emotion and motivated behavior. The fact that electrical stimulation in this region elicited a number of autonomic responses constituted a major portion of the evidence. Earlier reports emphasized the elicitation of isolated responses such as pupillary dilation and constriction, but there was a gradual awareness that stimulation was capable of activating integrated bodily changes characteristic of such states as rage, temperature regulation, eating and somnolence. For a brief period it was claimed that stimulation activated only the motor aspects of these states and not the motivational or affective components;[7] however, later work demonstrated that the behavior elicited by hypothalamic stimulation had many properties in common with behavior motivated by more

*Supported by National Institute of Mental Health Grant M-4529 and Research Scientist Award MH-4947.

†The Author is indebted to Mary Cooper, Sylvia Vaughn, Peter Beal and Dr. Verne C. Cox for their very able aid during various stages of this project.

natural conditions. Animals could be trained to perform learned behaviors either to turn stimulation on[8] or off[9] as well as to obtain access to a goal object necessary to perform the elicited behavior.[10] These observations, supplemented by additional stimulation studies, have led to the conclusion that there are discrete hypothalamic regions which play a primary role in directing such specific behavior as feeding, drinking, attack, maternal responses, hoarding and sex as well as other responses. Although they are not mutually exclusive, various investigators have given different emphasis to explanations of elicited behavior based on the activation of biological 'drives' such as hunger, the sensitization of the neural substrate of specific motor patterns, or the selective filtering of impinging stimuli.

There is some indication that we may be entering a period of retreat from what may have been an overemphasis on the specificity of hypothalamic control. Evidence from several sources suggest that this may be the case. For example, although FLYNN[11] has described the elicitation of attack behavior by hypothalamic stimulation, in conjunction with ELLISON[12] he has pointed out that cats are capable of integrated attack responses following surgical isolation of the hypothalamus. Also, several reports now exist that indicate that extrahypothalamic stimulation at diverse sites is capable of eliciting responses such as eating and drinking which have been traditionally linked with the hypothalamus.[13] It is very likely to be the case that just as the prevailing bias at the turn of the century led to a neglect of the hypothalamus, the prevailing bias during the past two decades has led to a relative neglect of the rest of the nervous system by investigators interested in motivated behavior. Furthermore, hypothalamic areas believed to be primarily responsible for one behavior category have been implicated in processes that have broader application. In this vein, GROSSMAN[14] has questioned the validity of restricting the function of the ventromedial hypothalamic nucleus to a food 'satiety' center and has suggested that the behavioral changes observed following destruction of this nucleus " . . . may be due to an interference affective rather than appetitive mechanisms."

More recently, other evidence[15,16] has been presented which supports the view that it may be necessary to re-examine some of the conclusions based on electrical stimulation studies. Briefly, this evidence has supported the following conclusions: (1) Elicited behavior differs significantly from behavior evoked by motivational states such as hunger and thirst; (2) If sufficient opportunity is provided, the majority of hypothalamic electrodes elicit several different behaviors. These different behaviors do not necessarily share the same motor elements nor do they appear to be linked by any specific motivational state; and (3) Anatomical locus of electrodes does not provide an adequate basis for predicting the elicited behavior.

The present study was designed to elaborate on some factors responsible for the reliable elicitation of a given behavior pattern by hypothalamic stimulation and some determinants of the ease or difficulty in eliciting other responses from the same electrode.

SUBJECTS AND METHODS

Male and female Sprague–Dawley rats (250–350 g) purchased from the Holtzman Company were implanted with electrodes in the lateral hypothalamus and following recovery from surgery, animals were tested to determine if electrical stimulation elicited eating or drinking (stimulus-bound behavior). Stimulation consisted of 60 c/s sine wave with currents ranging during the initial screening between 3 and 25 μA (R.M.S.). Animals displaying stimulus-bound eating or drinking were used in one of two experiments. *It is important to note that once an intensity was found which elicited either eating or drinking, this same intensity was always used on all future tests.* All testing and screening was done when animals were satiated for food and water and displayed no tendency to eat or drink unless stimulated.

EXPERIMENT 1

The purpose of this experiment was to determine if the amount of opportunity provided to display a particular elicited behavior would influence the difficulty of acquiring a new behavior in response to the same stimulation. Eighteen animals were used in this experiment and they were assigned at random to either the *Control Group* (N = 6) or the *Extra-Elicitation Group* (N = 12). After it was determined that an animal displayed either eating or drinking in response to stimulation, all animals received two *Standard Tests*. A *Standard Test* consisted of twenty 30-sec stimulation periods separated by a 60-sec interstimulus interval. In some of these tests (Two Goal Object) both food and water were available, and in others (One Goal Object) only one of these was offered to the animal. The food used was Purina Lab Chow pellets scattered on the floor; water was presented in a single bottle mounted so that the drinking tube extended about two inches into the Plexiglas test chamber. The behavior was scored by an observer, who recorded the occurrence of eating only when it was evident that the rat was biting off and ingesting pieces of the food pellets and drinking when the tube was lapped and water ingested.

All 18 animals were given two Standard Tests with both food and water presented and were selected from a larger group on the basis that only one behavior (either eating or drinking) was elicited by the stimulation. All animals displayed either eating or drinking during at least 75 per cent of the stimulation presentations and did not eat or drink during any of the interstimulus intervals.

The *Extra-Elicitation Group* was then given 30 Standard Tests with only the goal object to which they oriented present in the chamber. Thus, in these One Goal Object Tests if an animal had previously displayed only eating in response to stimulation, food was the only goal object present. The converse was true for animals that had only displayed elicited drinking. The number of tests per day varied, but never exceeded three and they were always spaced at least 1 hr apart.

Animals in the *Control Group* were placed in the test chamber a comparable period of time, with the cable connected to their electrode, but no stimulation was presented. Following these tests (or pseudo tests) all animals were tested with the opposite goal object so that animals which had displayed only eating in response to stimulation were offered only the water bottle. Animals received a 30-sec stimulation train every 90 sec and an observer recorded the occurrence of any behavior. After each hour of stimulation the animals were given a 15 min rest from stimulation with both food and water available. Animals were also given 3–4 hr to rest after 12 hr on the above schedule. This sequence continued until the animal had displayed the new behavior (either eating or drinking) in response to stimulation on at least 3 out of 5 consecutive stimulus trains. The number of stimulations necessary to reach this criterion was recorded. If a new behavior was not in evidence after 1500 stimulations, the testing was discontinued and it was considered that the animal had not exhibited a new stimulus-bound behavior pattern.

Following the emergence of the new elicited behavior, the animals were given a *Standard Test* with only the goal object relevant to the new behavior present. The purpose of this test was to assure that the new behavior was elicited reliably. In every instance stimulation elicited the new behavior on at least 75 per cent (Av. 90 per cent; Range 75–100 per cent) of the presentations. All animals were then given a competitive Two Goal Object Standard Test to determine the relative strengths of the initial and new elicited behaviors.

TABLE 1.   DIFFICULTY OF ESTABLISHING A NEW STIMULUS-BOUND BEHAVIOR PATTERN AS A FUNCTION OF FREQUENCY OF ELICITATION OF ORIGINAL BEHAVIOR

	Av. No. stimulations prior to new behavior	Per cent animals exhibiting new behavior*	Behavior elicited in competition test	
			Per cent original behav.	Per cent new behav.
Extra-elicitation group (N = 12)	500	67	90	10
Control group (N = 6)	167	100	42	58

* If a new behavior was not elicited after 1500 stimulations, the animal was scored as not exhibiting new behavior.

Results

The major findings are summarized in Table 1. It can be seen that the animals which received the extra-elicitation of the original behavior were more resistant to the development and display of a new behavior in response to stimulation. It was only necessary to provide an average of 167 stimulations in order to obtain the reliable elicitation of a new behavior in all the control animals. In contrast, only 67 per cent of the animals in the extra-elicitation group exhibited a new behavior within the limits of our testing and in these instances it was necessary to provide an average of 500 stimulations. Furthermore, when the new and initial behaviors were tested in a competitive stimulation with both food and water available, the control animals exhibited the new behavior in the majority of the instances while the new behavior displayed by the animals in the extra-elicitation group constituted only 10 per cent of the total elicited behavior (Table 1).

EXPERIMENT 2

It was observed that in the majority of instances in which a behavior was elicited by stimulation there seemed to be an initial period during which the elicitation of the behavior became increasingly more reliable. It was the purpose of this experiment to study this process more systematically.

Except where otherwise noted, the experimental methodology was the same as described in the first experiment. Specifically, surgical procedures, stimulation parameters, Standard Tests and subject population were identical to those used in Experiment 1. Two groups of naive animals were compared. The *Minimal Stimulation Group* (N = 5) consisted of animals which had received less than 40 stimulation trains before receiving a 2 week 'rest period' without stimulation. Prior to the rest period these animals were stimulated only until three instances of either eating or drinking were elicited, but they were not used if this criterion was not met prior to the presentation of 40 stimulations. During this initial screening, the stimulus intensity was gradually raised until, judging by the animal's behavior, the probability of eliciting eating or drinking was maximal. Animals in the *Control Group* (N = 8) were given a series of standard tests until they had succeeded in exhibiting elicited behavior on at least 50 per cent (10 out of 20) of the stimulations on 2 consecutive tests. For 1 animal in this group this criterion was reached in 2 Standard Tests, but most required more and 3 subjects received 11 tests. Following the achievement of this criterion the control animals were also given a 2 week respite from stimulation.

After the 2 week rest period, animals in both groups were given standard tests until they exhibited an elicited behavior during 50 per cent of the stimulation periods on two consecutive tests. At the completion of this sequence the animals received slightly different treatment depending upon their performance. In the case of animals that were exhibiting both eating and drinking, the behavior that was exhibited less frequently was selected for additional testing with only one goal object present. Thirty standard tests were given with tests separated by at least 1 hr and no more than three of these one goal object tests given on a single day. Thus, an animal which exhibited less eating than drinking in the two goal object tests following the 2 week rest period was given 30 tests with only food available. Animals that exhibited only one behavior in the two goal object test were stimulated until a new behavior appeared and then they were also given 30 tests with only the goal object of the weaker behavior present. After the 30 tests the animals were given a series of standard tests with both goal objects present until it was clear which behavior was exhibited more frequently.

Results

Figure 1 compares the effect of the 2-week rest period without stimulation following different amounts of initial stimulus-bound behavior experience. It can be seen that animals in the Minimal Stimulation Group, which received only a brief initial screening, exhibit very little stimulus-bound behavior immediately after the rest period. With each successive test after the rest period, the animals in this group exhibit a greater amount of elicited behavior. In contrast, animals in the Control Group displayed a relatively high amount of stimulus-bound behavior immediately after the rest period. These animals received a greater amount of opportunity to display stimulus-bound behavior prior to the rest period, and their performance after 2 weeks was almost exactly what it had been on the last test. The Control Group animals also tended to increase the amount of stimulus-bound behavior displayed on the second test after the rest period, but they were not tested further, as all had achieved criterion level.

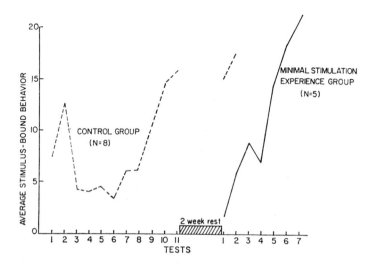

FIG. 1. Comparison of the effect of a 2-week rest period without stimulation, following different amounts of experience. Prior to the rest period, animals in the Minimal Stimulation Group received only a brief initial screening consisting of less than 40 stimulations (eating and/or drinking were elicited only 3 times). Animals in the Control Group received a series of standard tests until they achieved criterion (cf. text). The variability in the curve of the control group prior to the rest period was caused by a reduction in the number of animals as criterion was achieved. All individual records were consistent with the trend depicted by the group averages (cf. Fig. 2). Twenty stimulations were administered on each test. Animals displaying stimulus-bound eating and drinking could achieve a score above 20 if both behaviors were displayed during stimulus periods.

Figure 2 illustrates the performance of an individual animal from the Minimal Stimulation Group and an individual animal from the Control Group. The performance of animal 14JJ is consistent with the group average illustrated in Fig. 1. This animal received only the minimal stimulation involved in the initial screening, and after the 2-week rest period stimulus-bound eating was not evident at all on the first test. Gradually over successive tests, eating was elicited by stimulation more and more reliably. No stimulus-bound drinking was observed even though the water bottle was available. Following these tests, stimulation in the presence of the water bottle, but with no food available, was continued until some evidence of stimulus-bound drinking was observed. Thirty tests with only the water bottle available were then administered, and it can be seen from Fig. 2 that drinking was elicited more and more reliably over this testing sequence. In the competitive tests with food and water both available, which followed the 30 single goal object test, stimulus-bound drinking tended to be displayed more frequently. Thus a behavior that was not seen at all during the initial competitive tests became the more dominant pattern.

The tendency for repeated testing of one stimulus-bound behavior pattern to produce a dominance was not always evident, as can be noted from the performance of animal 71JJ (Fig. 2). This animal was in the Control Group and it can be seen that prior to the 2-week rest period stimulus-bound drinking was elicited more reliably over successive tests.

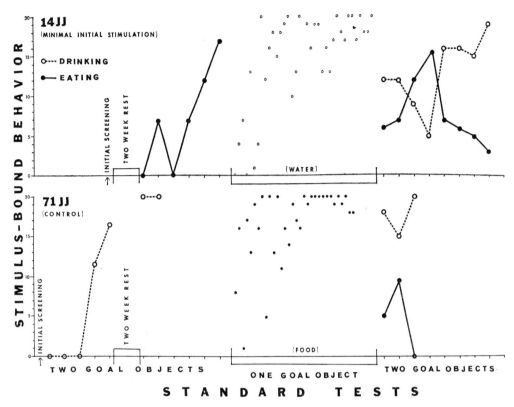

FIG. 2.   Individual animal records illustrating effect of a 2-week rest period following different amounts of experience. Also shown are two different results of attempts to strengthen weaker behavior by providing 30 additional standard tests with only one goal object prior to competitive tests with both goal objects (cf. text).

At the end of the rest period a high level of stimulus-bound drinking was exhibited immediately. As described for 14JJ, a new stimulus-bound behavior (eating) gradually emerged and then was observed to be elicited more reliably over the successive 30 single goal object tests. In this instance, however, the new behavior was elicited less frequently in the final competitive tests. No pattern could be described that permitted a prediction of the behavior that dominated in the final competitive tests. In some cases the new and in others the initial pattern dominated and this seemed to be independent of the testing history of the animal.

DISCUSSION

Several important points emerge from the results of the two experiments described in the present report. It is evident from the data obtained in Experiment 1 that the likelihood of observing a second or new behavior pattern elicited by hypothalamic stimulation is influenced by the amount of opportunity an animal has had to display only the initially elicited behavior. Animals that have had a great amount of experience displaying a given stimulus-bound behavior pattern are more resistant to adopting a second pattern, as they seem to persist in ignoring other alternatives. These results have both methodological and theoretical implications. With respect to the former, it would seem that there is a definite possibility that the amount of specificity of function attributed to a given hypothalamic area can easily be exaggerated with some testing procedures. This would be particularly true, for example, when interest is restricted to one behavior and only at a later time is it thought important to test for the possibility that additional behaviors might be elicited from activation of the same site. As can be seen from Table 1, if animals are tested for only one behavior it may take more than 500 stimulations before a second behavior starts to be elicited reliably. This is likely to involve considerably more effort than is usually expended in testing for the presence of other stimulus-bound behaviors.

ROBERTS[17] has argued that the testing of animals with several goal objects simultaneously available may be misleading, as a weaker response to the same stimulation may not have an opportunity to be expressed. He recommends that animals be tested with each object separately before concluding that the stimulation did not have the capacity to elicit a second behavior initially. This is probably good advice, but it should be clear that in the cases we have described there was no evidence that the stimulation had the capacity to elicit the second behavior from the outset. Even when tested with only one goal object available, it characteristically took a large number of stimulations before the second behavior was first displayed and usually it was elicited only during a small percentage of the stimulations. This trend is particularly evident in Experiment 2, where it was noted that the elicitation of stimulus-bound behavior normally went through a process of 'strengthening' (cf. Figs. 1 and 2). After the animal had sufficient opportunity to display the new behavior in response to stimulation it was likely to be exhibited in the competitive situation, often predominantly, in spite of the fact that it had not been displayed at all in the initial competitive tests. It is unlikely that this strengthening process is simply reflecting the animals' increasing familiarity with the testing cage, goal objects or even the location of the goal objects. Animals were always provided with sufficient opportunity to explore the test chamber and the location of the food and water should have posed no problem as the familiar Purina Lab Chow pellets were scattered all over the floor and the water was in the same type of bottle that was attached to the home cage. Animals were also observed eating and drinking on occasion during habituation and rest periods in the chamber without stimulation. The animals in brief seem to know the relevant spatial information prior to stimulation. To obtain the food and water, no unfamiliar instrumental responses were required that could explain the necessity for several hundred (considerably above 500 in many instances) stimulations to be presented before the new stimulus-bound behavior appeared.

Nor is there any reason to believe that the postulation of a developing 'incentive motivation' would be helpful. In the present context, the term 'incentive motivation' implies that the capacity of the goal objects (food and water) and the testing situation to elicit eating or drinking has been enhanced. There does not seem to be any evidence to support the view that this is a major factor in the emergence of stimulus-bound behavior. VALENSTEIN and COX[18] have shown, for example, that placing animals on a regimen where they received all their food and/or water in a distinctive test chamber and at a particular time during the day did not increase the probability of obtaining stimulus-bound behavior by local brain stimulation.

Another conclusion that may be drawn from Experiment 2 is, that once a stimulus-bound behavior pattern becomes well established, it tends to retain a significant position in an animal's response hierarchy even though not exercised repeatedly. It was seen in Fig. 1 that animals in the Control Group which were tested until the percentage of stimulus-bound behavior had reached criterion level, exhibited the same amount of elicited behavior after a 2-week rest period. The same conclusion can be drawn from the fact that when animals have not had an opportunity to display the initial stimulus-bound behavior for an extended period during the establishment and 'strengthening' of a second behavior, the initial pattern is generally still displayed in later competitive tests (Fig. 2).

It is difficult to prove conclusively that all the stimulus-bound patterns that eventually emerge are not reflecting pre-existing connections between the hypothalamic area stimulated and the neural substrate underlying the elicitation of the responses. Our own experience with this phenomenon has led us to conclude that it is unnecessary to make such an assumption. The many instances we have observed where a stimulus-bound behavior emerges only after a very long period of testing, and then gradually becomes elicited with greater frequency suggests that in some ways an association is being developed. It seems to us that the assumption that there always exists a fixed association between the hypothalamic area stimulated (or the state induced by such stimulation) and the specific expression of a particular response pattern that finally is elicited, is gratuitous. It is not implied that any arbitrarily selected response can be associated with stimulation at any hypothalamic site, and indeed some limitations have been discussed by the author elsewhere.[19] It is suggested, however, that evidence is accumulating which indicates that it is possible to establish and strengthen the association between the effects of hypothalamic stimulation and a specific mode of expression. The mode of expression has to be consistent with the state induced by stimulation, but it is not predetermined. This is what is implied by the title: 'Channeling of Responses Elicited by Hypothalamic Stimulation.'

It may not be accidental that most stimulus-bound behaviors that have been studied have been observed in conjunction with the stimulation of hypothalamic sites judged to be 'reinforcing' by self-stimulation performance. Once a behavior pattern is elicited with a degree of consistency, this response seems to be highly resistant to extinction. Perhaps the association of certain response patterns with the activation of a neural system involved in a basic reinforcement process creates the underlying condition for the maintenance of the behavior when the animal is in the same state. This is what may be involved in stereotyped, compulsive behaviors.

REFERENCES

1. ANDERSON, E. Earlier ideas of hypothalamic function, including irrelevant concepts. In: *The Hypothalamus*. HAYMAKER, W., ANDERSON, E., NAUTA, W. (Eds.) Charles Thomas, Springfield, Ill., 1969.
2. KARPLUS, J. P. and KREIDL, A. Gehirn und Sympathicus. I. Mitteilung: Zwischenhirnbasis und Halssympathicus. *Pflügers Arch. ges. Physiol.* **129**, 138, 1909.

M

3. RANSOM, S. W. Some functions of the hypothalamus. *The Harvey Lectures*, 1936–1937, p. 241 Williams & Wilkins, Baltimore, 1937.

4. RANSON, S. W. and MAGOUN, H. W. The hypothalamus. *Ergebn. Physiol.* **41,** 56, 1939.

5. HESS, W. R. *Diencephalon. Autonomic and Extrapyramidal Function.* Grune & Stratton, New York, 1954.

6. GLOOR, P. Autonomic functions of the diencephalon. A summary of the experimental work of Prof. W. R. Hess. *A.M.A. Archs Neurol. Psychiatry* **71,** 773, 1954.

7. MASSERMAN, J. H. Is the hypothalamus a center for emotion? *Psychosom. Med.* **3,** 1, 1941.

8. OLDS, J. and MILNER, P. Positive reinforcement produced by electrical stimulation of septal area and other regions of rat brain. *J. comp. physiol. Psychol.* **47,** 419, 1954.

9. DELGADO, J. M. R., ROBERTS, W. W. and MILLER, N. E. Learning motivated by electrical stimulation of the brain. *Am. J. Physiol.* **179,** 587, 1954.

10. COONS, E. E., LEVAK, M. and MILLER, N. E. Lateral hypothalamus: Learning of food-seeking response motivated by electrical stimulation. *Science* **159,** 1117, 1968.

11. FLYNN, J. P. The neural basis of aggression in cats. In: *Neurophysiology and Emotion,* GLASS, D. C. (Ed.) Rockefeller Univ. Press, New York, 1957.

12. ELLISON, G. D. and FLYNN, J. P. Organized aggressive behavior in cats after surgical isolation of the hypothalamus. *Archs ital. Biol.* **106,** 1, 1968.

13. ROBINSON, B. W. and MISHKIN, M. Alimentary responses to forebrain stimulation in monkey. *Expl. Brain Res.* **4,** 330, 1968.

14. GROSSMAN, S. P. The VMH: A center for affective reactions, satiety, or both? *Physiol. Behav.* **1,** 1, 1966.

15. VALENSTEIN, E. S. Behavior elicited by hypothalamic stimulation: A prepotency hypothesis. *Brain Behav. Evol.* **2,** 295, 1969.

16. VALENSTEIN, E. S., COX, V. C. and KAKOLEWSKI, J. W. Reexamination of the role of the hypothalamus in motivation. *Psychol. Rev.* **77,** 16, 1970.

17. ROBERTS, W. W. Are hypothalamic motivational mechanisms functionally and anatomically specific? *Brain Behav. Evol.* **2,** 317, 1969.

18. VALENSTEIN, E. S. and COX, V. C. Influence of hunger, thirst and previous experience in the test chamber on stimulus-bound eating and drinking. *J. comp. physiol. Psychol.* **70,** 189, 1970.

19. VALENSTEIN, E. S. Behavior elicited by hypothalamic stimulation: A prepotency hypothesis. *Brain Behav. Evol.* **2,** 295, 1969.

J. psychiat. Res., 1971, Vol. 8, pp. 345–361. Pergamon Press. Printed in Great Britain.

NEUROCHEMISTRY OF REWARD AND PUNISHMENT: SOME IMPLICATIONS FOR THE ETIOLOGY OF SCHIZOPHRENIA*

Larry Stein

Wyeth Laboratories, Philadelphia, Pennsylvania

Over the past two decades, physiological,[1,2] anatomical,[3,4] and psychopharmacological[5-8] research findings have resulted in the identification of systems in the brain tentatively associated with reward and punishment. While the reward system has been characterized

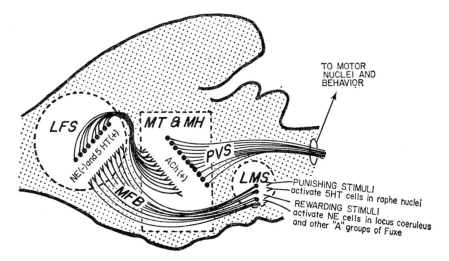

Fig. 1. Diagram representing hypothetical relationships between reward and punishment mechanisms and behavior. Signals of positive reinforcement release behavior from periventricular system (PVS) suppression by the following sequence of events: (1) Activation of norepinephrine-containing cells in lower brain stem (LMS) by stimuli previously associated with reward (or the avoidance of punishment) causes release of norepinephrine (NE) into amygdala and other forebrain suppressor areas (LFS) via the medial forebrain bundle (MFB). (2) Inhibitory (−) action of norepinephrine suppresses activity of the LFS, thus reducing its cholinergically-mediated excitation (+) of medial thalamus and hypothalamus (MT and MH). (3) Decreased cholinergic (ACH) transmission at synapses in MT and MH lessens the activity of the periventricular system, thereby reducing its inhibitory influence over motor nuclei of the brain stem. Signals of failure or punishment increase behavioral suppression by the release of serotonin (5-HT), which either excites suppressor cells in the LFS or disinhibits them by antagonizing the inhibitory action of norepinephrine.

---

* The work which provided the basis for this paper was done in collaboration with Dr. C. David Wise, who generously assisted in the preparation of this presentation.

as mainly noradrenergic,[9,10] the punishment system appears to be cholinergic,[10] and, if preliminary indications are correct, partially serotonergic as well.[11] The cells of origin of the reward system are located in the locus coeruleus and reticular formation of the lower brain stem, and the axons ascend via the medial forebrain bundle to form nora-drenergic synapses in the hypothalamus, limbic system, and frontal cortex. The cells of the serotonergic punishment system originate in the raphe nuclei, but the fibers ascend in the medial forebrain bundle and distribute in the forebrain in parallel fashion to those of the noradrenergic system. This parallel innervation may permit reciprocal control of behavior by norepinephrine and serotonin neurons along lines generally suggested by BRODIE and SHORE,[12] and illustrated diagramatically in Fig. 1.

FACILITATION OF SELF-STIMULATION BY INTRAVENTRICULAR NE

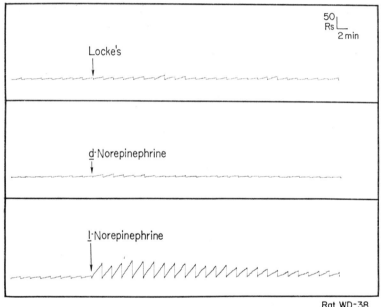

Rat WD-38

FIG. 2.   Facilitation of self-stimulation of the lateral hypothalamus (at the level of the ventro-medial nucleus) by an intraventricular injection of *l*-norepinephrine HCl (10 μg). Control injections of Ringer–Locke solution (10 μl) or *d*-norepinephrine HCl (10 μg) had negligible effects. Pen cumulates self-stimulation responses and resets automatically every 2 min (see key).

Evidence in support of these conclusions has been reviewed elsewhere.[10,11,13,14] Briefly, electrical stimulation of the medial forebrain bundle serves as a powerful reward, and also elicits species-typical consummatory responses, such as feeding and copulation, which produce pleasure and permit the satisfaction of basic needs. Similar effects are produced pharmacologically[15] by potentiation of the noradrenergic activity of the medial forebrain bundle system, as illustrated in Figs. 2 and 3. On the other hand, electrolytic lesions of the medial forebrain bundle cause severe deficits in goal-directed behavior and the loss

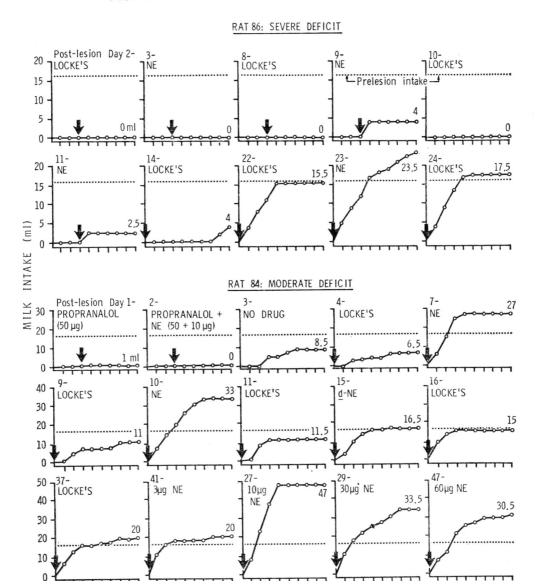

FIG. 3. Recovery of feeding by intraventricular administration of norepinephrine (NE) after lateral hypothalamic lesions. Curves are cumulative plots of milk intake during 45-min tests in successive 5-min periods. Numbers over curves indicate 45-min intakes. Arrows indicate time of intraventricular injections. All doses are 10 μg unless noted otherwise. (Rat 86) Reversal of aphagia by l-norepinephrine (NE) in a rat with severe hypothalamic damage. Postoperative feeding occurs for the first time on Day 9 as a result of the norepinephrine injection, although a similar injection on Day 3 failed to induce feeding. (Rat 84) Reversal of anorexia and extensive overeating induced by l-norepinephrine in a case of moderate damage. On Day 15, d-norepinephrine had no effect. The bottom row of plots indicates that norepinephrine is effective over a wide range of doses, with optimal effect at 10 μg (From BERGER et al.[15])

of consummatory reactions;[16] again, similar effects are produced by pharmacological blockade of noradrenergic function or potentiation of serotonergic function, as shown in Fig. 4. There is some evidence that these findings in animals may be extrapolated to man.[17,18]

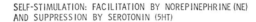

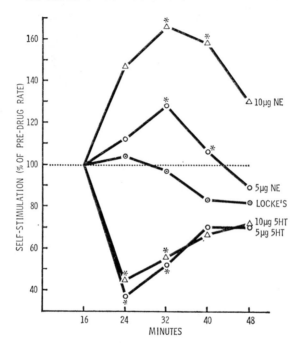

FIG. 4.   Facilitation of lateral hypothalamic self-stimulation by l-norepinephrine HCl (NE) and suppression by serotonin HCl (5-HT). Intraventricular injections were made 16 min after the start of the test. Data are expressed as a percent of the self-stimulation rate in the second 8-min test period (8–16 min after start of test); the curves were obtained by averaging per cent scores for the group of 11 rats. Starred points differ significantly from Locke's control at 0·05 level or beyond.

How may these systems influence behavior? Briefly, we assume that they provide feedback to ongoing behavior based on the consequences of the behavior in the past.[19,20] The feedback is positive in the case of reward or negative in the case of punishment—'go' or 'stop'. That is, one may think of the noradrenergic medial forebrain bundle fibers as part of a behavior-facilitating or 'go' mechanism. The mechanism is activated or engaged by ongoing behavior if that behavior previously produced pleasure or avoided pain. Activation of the 'go' mechanism initiates facilitatory feedback, which increases the probability that the behavior will run off to completion. On the other hand, behavior associated with failure or punishment engages the serotonergic 'stop' mechanism. This generates negative feedback that tends to cut the unsuccessful behavior short. The adaptive nature of these regulatory mechanisms is obvious. It is equally obvious that malfunction of these mechanisms could have serious consequences for normal behavior. We will argue that schizophrenia is one such extreme consequence, and that it is caused by selective chemical damage to the noradrenergic reward mechanism.

ROLE OF HEREDITY IN SCHIZOPHRENIA

Genetic studies provide indirect support for the idea that an impairment of noradrenergic function may be involved in schizophrenia. The early impression that schizophrenia is inherited has been verified by systematic family studies[21,22] and studies of adopted children,[23,24] which establish ". . . the importance of genetic factors in the development of schizophrenia . . . beyond reasonable dispute."[23] Several modes of inheritance have been proposed, but some authorities currently favor the idea that a main gene of large effect, modified either by a second gene,[25] or by multiple factors,[23] is responsible for schizophrenia and borderline schizoid disorders. In any case, the conclusion that schizophrenia is hereditary necessarily implies a biochemical aberration, since no other mechanism is known for the expression of genetic traits.

A CHEMICAL THEORY OF SCHIZOPHRENIA

Recently, Dr. David Wise and I have proposed a novel physiological and chemical etiology for schizophrenia.[26] Our work is based on THUDICHUM's[27] concept that "many forms of insanity" are caused chemically by "poisons fermented within the body." The essential properties of the offending chemical have been outlined by HOLLISTER:[28] "In short, what is required is an endogenous toxin, highly active and highly specific in its action at minute doses, continuously produced, for which tolerance does not develop."

Current biochemical theories, which use mescaline or LSD as a model, generally attribute hallucinogenic or psychotomimetic properties to the toxic metabolite,[29-32] a formulation which has been critically reviewed by KETY.[33] Two grounds appear to provide a basis for criticism. First, in view of the chronic and even life-long duration of schizophrenia, it seems unlikely that a mescaline-like substance would be produced in adequate quantities continuously over many decades without the development of tolerance. Secondly, many authorities now question the assumption that hallucinogenic drugs induce a 'model psychosis'. These agents do not reproduce the fundamental symptoms of schizophrenia, and the differences between the drug states and schizophrenic reactions are easily distinguished.[34] The wide variety of mental changes caused by the drugs, such as hallucinations and delusions, tend rather to resemble the accessory symptoms of schizophrenia.

According to BLEULER,[35] ". . . the fundamental symptoms consist of disturbances of association and affectivity." Specifically, this author suggests that schizophrenic associations lose their continuity because the thoughts "are not related and directed by any unifying concept of purpose or goal." At the same time, emotional responsivity is diminished and eventually reduced to indifference, so that ". . . many schizophrenics in the later stages cease to show any affect for years and even decades." In RADO'S[36] view, the disturbance of affect stems from the fact that the "pleasure resources are inherently deficient." Finally, Bleuler and others emphasize that the course of the disease "is at times chronic, at times marked by intermittent attacks which can stop or retrograde at any stage, but do not permit a full *restitutio ad integrum*."

As noted previously, damage to noradrenergic reward mechanism causes deficits in goal-directed behavior and rewarding consummatory reactions in animals. By analogy, chemical damage of the reward mechanism in the schizophrenic could produce deficits in goal-directed thinking and behavior, and in the capacity to experience pleasure. Furthermore, if the chemical toxin were continuously or episodically produced, and if the damage to the reward mechanism were at least partially irreversible, the disorder would be progressive and chronic.

POSSIBLE CHEMICAL CAUSE OF SCHIZOPHRENIA

Several lines of biochemical evidence suggest that 6-hydroxydopamine (2, 4, 5-trihydroxy-phenethylamine) is the aberrant metabolite that causes schizophrenia.* This compound is an autoxidation product and metabolite of dopamine, and "its formation can occur to a significant extent in the intact animal."[37] 6-Hydroxydopamine induces a specific degeneration of peripheral sympathetic nerve terminals with a marked and long-lasting depletion of norepinephrine.[38] When injected intraventricularly into the rat brain, 6-hydroxydopamine similarly causes a prolonged or permanent depletion of brain catecholamines. Only catecholamine-containing neurons are affected, and brain norepinephrine is more severely depleted than dopamine.[39] Electron microscopic evidence reveals that norepinephrine (but not dopamine) nerve terminals in the brain degenerate and eventually disappear after repeated doses of 6-hydroxydopamine.[40] Single doses of 6-hydroxydopamine of 200 μg or less, however, may decrease brain norepinephrine without apparent ultrastructural damage.[41]

Surprisingly, despite the profound damage to central noradrenergic neurons, rats treated with 6-hydroxydopamine are reported to be 'grossly indistinguishable' from controls 'except for a slight decrease in body weight and a lack of self-grooming'.[40,42,43] If sensitive behavioral tests are used, however, marked deficits are obtained after single or repeated doses of 6-hydroxydopamine.[44,45] Behavioral tests in the unanesthetized rat also may be made more sensitive by use of permanently-indwelling cannulas, which permit injection of solutions into the lateral ventricle with minimum disturbance.

In our experiments, 6-hydroxydopamine as a hydrochloride salt is dissolved in 10 μl of Ringer–Locke solution containing 0·1 per cent ascorbic acid (pH 4·5). Control animals

---

* Closely related compounds, such as 6-hydroxynorepinephrine and 2-hydroxydopamine, cannot yet be ruled out with certainty. 6-Hydroxynorepinephrine is extremely reactive and difficult to prepare. The biochemistry and pharmacology of 2-hydroxydopamine and other analogs of 6-hydroxydopamine are currently under investigation in collaborative studies with Drs. C. D. Wise, H. Smith and R. P. Stein of Wyeth Laboratories.

are injected intraventricularly with 10 μl of the vehicle solution. Under these conditions, large deficits in behavior are readily observed after 6-hydroxydopamine, either in acute experiments with small doses, as shown in Table 1, or in chronic experiments with larger or repeated doses as illustrated in Fig. 5.

TABLE 1. ACUTE SUPPRESSANT ACTION OF 6-HYDROXYDOPAMINE ON FEEDING*

Rat No.	Dose (μg)	Milk intake (ml)				
		No drug (2 tests)		Ascorbic acid Vehicle	6-Hydroxydopamine 1st Test	2nd Test
W–31	6·3	13	14·5	16	6	17
W–36	12·5	24	21·5	23	18·5	22·5
W–35	25	17	13·5	13·5	12	17·5
W–34	50	17·5	19·5	19	6	20†
W–32	100	26	22·5	30	12	13·5

* Rats were trained to drink milk from a graduated tube in a 45-min test until intakes stabilized. Tests were made 3 hr after injections of 6-hydroxydopamine or the vehicle solution. First and second tests were separated by 1 week. The suppressant effects of lower doses showed evidence of tolerance in the second test.

† Received 6·3 μg rather than 50 μg.

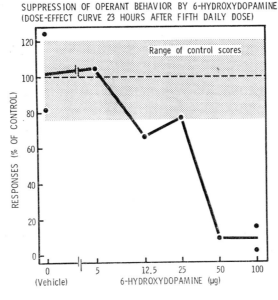

FIG. 5. Suppression of food-rewarded operant behavior by repeated doses of 6-hydroxydopamine. After stabilization of response rates on a 2-min variable-interval schedule, the animals were injected intraventricularly with the dose indicated 1 hr after the daily 72-min test. Plot gives dose–effect curve obtained 23 hr after the fifth dose. Each point represents one rat.

Most directly relevant to the present argument are studies of the chronic effects of 6-hydroxydopamine on 'self-stimulation'[2] behavior maintained by rewarding electrical stimulation of the medial forebrain bundle. A single 200 μg dose of 6-hydroxydopamine reduced the rate of self-stimulation by 58·9 per cent on the first day after the injection, and recovery of the pre-drug rate was only gradual and incomplete over the next 5 days, as shown in Table 2. In a related experiment, 7 daily doses of 25 μg caused progressive suppression of the self-stimulation rate to 67 per cent of control. The suppression persisted for at least 5 days after dosing was discontinued, as illustrated in Fig. 6. In a third study, an

TABLE 2. SUPPRESSANT EFFECT OF 6-HYDROXYDOPAMINE ON SELF-STIMULATION. A SINGLE DOSE OF 200 μG WAS INJECTED INTRAVENTRICULARLY 23 HR BEFORE THE FIRST POSTDRUG TEST

Treatment	Rats (No.)	Postdrug Test day	Mean self-stimulation rate (per cent of predrug)					
			1	2	3	4	5	6
6-hydroxydopamine (200 μg)	5		41·1* ±12·7	71·2* ± 8·8	69·2 ±14·3	71·0 ±18·3	65·6 ±21·1	65·7 ±10·9
Ascorbic acid vehicle (10 μl)	3		96·5 ±25·3	98·6 ±11·5	99·4 ± 8·9	—	—	—

* Differs from vehicle mean at 0·05 level (t-test, single-tailed).

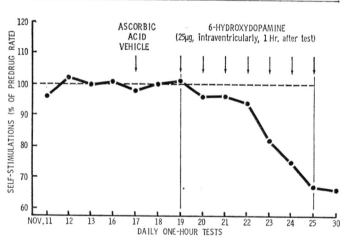

FIG. 6. Suppression of self-stimulation by repeated doses of 6-hydroxydopamine (averaged data of 3 rats). (From STEIN and WISE.[26])

intraperitoneal injection of the monoamine oxidase inhibitor pargyline potentiated for several days the suppressive action of a series of 400 μg doses, as shown in Fig. 7; during most of this time, the rat displayed a catatonic syndrome of 'waxy flexibility', illustrated in Fig. 8. It is evident from these results that 6-hydroxydopamine markedly impairs self-stimulation and other rewarded behaviors. Furthermore, because the drug-induced impairment is long-lasting, it probably is caused at least in part by a selective destruction of the noradrenergic binding sites and eventually the terminals of the medial forebrain bundle. It thus seems reasonable to assume that if 6-hydroxydopamine were formed endogenously in sufficient amounts in the immediate vicinity of noradrenergic nerve endings, it would cause progressive and at least partially irreversible damage to the reward mechanism. As noted, such damage could produce the primary symptoms of schizophrenia.

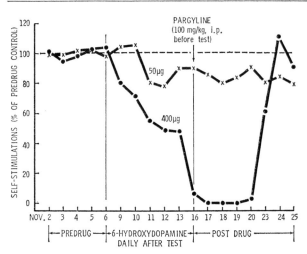

FIG. 7. Suppression of self-stimulation by repeated doses of 6-hydroxydopamine and potentiation of suppression by the monoamine oxidase inhibitor pargyline. The rat that received 400 μg exhibited a catatonic syndrome of 'waxy flexibility' (See Fig. 8) for several days after the injection of pargyline. In these tests, injection of 6-hydroxydopamine immediately after self-stimulation appeared to reduce its toxic action (compared with Fig. 2). (From STEIN and WISE.[26])

The isolation and identification of a specific odorous substance (*trans*-3-methyl-2-hexenoic acid) in the sweat of schizophrenics[46] provides a second thread of evidence that links 6-hydroxydopamine to schizophrenia. Dr. Herchel Smith has suggested hypothetical pathways for the formation of this substance by known biochemical reactions from 6-hydroxydopamine or 2-hydroxydopamine, as illustrated in Fig. 9.

A third line of evidence is suggested by recent studies of Shulgin and his associates[32] on mescaline-like psychotomimetics. This work reveals that phenethylamine derivatives with the same 2,4,5-substitution pattern as 6-hydroxydopamine have consistently high hallucinogenic activity in man. Indeed, SHULGIN, *et al.*, postulate that 6-hydroxydopamine may be an intermediate metabolite in the formation of a possible endogenous psychotogen 2-hydroxy-4,5-dimethoxyphenethanolamine. Although it is not inconceivable that metabolites of 6-hydroxydopamine are hallucinogenic and contribute to the accessory symptomatology, our theory emphasizes the role of 6-hydroxydopamine itself as the agent that causes the fundamental symptoms of schizophrenia.*

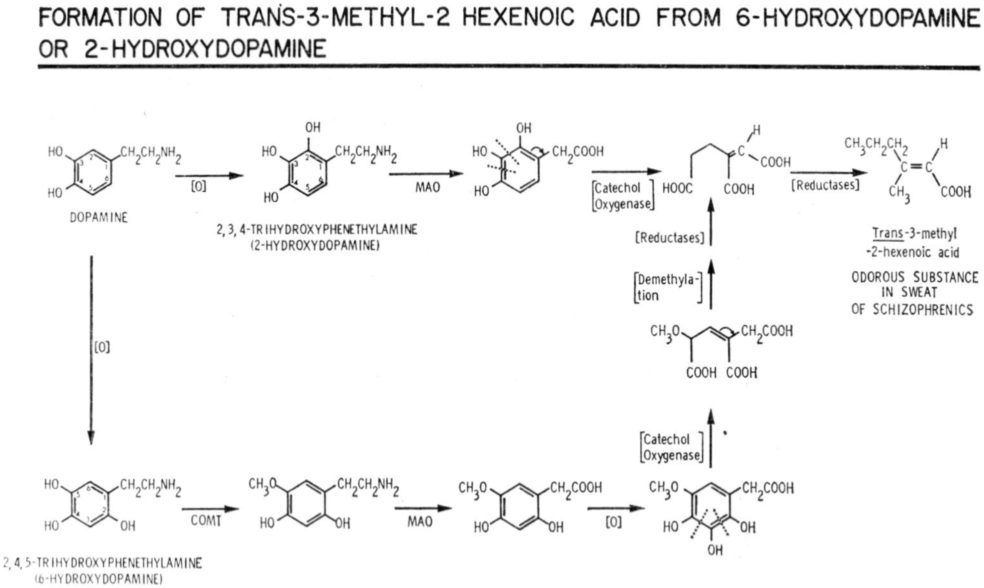

FORMATION OF TRANS-3-METHYL-2 HEXENOIC ACID FROM 6-HYDROXYDOPAMINE OR 2-HYDROXYDOPAMINE

FIG. 9. Hypothetical pathways for the formation of *trans*-3-methyl-2-hexonoic acid from either 6- or 2-hydroxydopamine. The postulated steps involving reductases are unlikely to occur in man, but may be mediated by bacteria in the sebaceous or sweat glands. (From STEIN and WISE.[26])

POSSIBLE MODE OF ACTION OF ANTIPSYCHOTIC PHENOTHIAZINES

The observation[48] that chlorpromazine antagonizes the norepinephrine-depleting action of 6-hydroxydopamine provides a fourth line of biochemical evidence for our theory. Chlorpromazine, the drug of choice in the treatment of schizophrenia,[49] is an inhibitor of the neural norepinephrine uptake process;[50] hence, it has been assumed that chlorpromazine prevents the depletion of peripheral norepinephrine by limiting the access of 6-hydroxydopamine to the noradrenergic nerve terminal.[48] The drug may exert its central antipsychotic effect by the same mechanism. According to this idea, chlorpromazine protects the reward system of the schizophrenic by blocking the uptake of endogenously formed 6-hydroxydopamine into the noradrenergic nerve ending. Hence, although formation of 6-hydroxydopamine may continue in the chlorpromazine-treated schizophrenic, the toxic substance no longer would have entry to the vulnerable site.

---

* Hallucinations, and possibly other accessory symptoms, might be caused by a relative predominance of the serotonin system after impairment of the norepinephrine system by 6-hydroxydopamine. See, for example, work of AGHAJANIAN and SHEARD[47] on the reduction of habituation to auditory stimuli after increases in serotonin activity.

CATATONIC BEHAVIOR INDUCED BY 6-HYDROXYDOPAMINE AND A MONOAMINE OXIDASE INHIBITOR

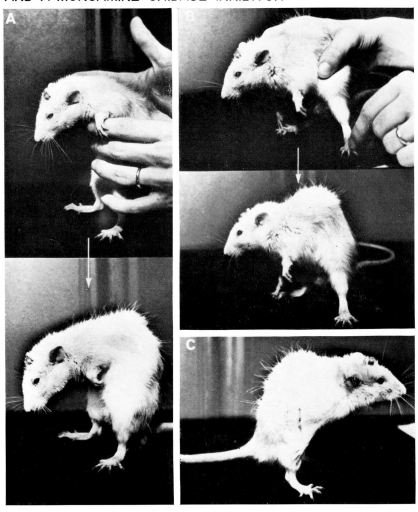

FIG. 8. Induction of catatonic behavior ('Waxy flexibility') after daily intraventricular injections of 6-hydroxydopamine (400 μg) and a single injection of pargyline (100 mg/kg, i.p.). (From STEIN and WISE[26]).

As the first test of this idea, we attempted to protect self-stimulating rats from the toxic action of 6-hydroxydopamine by pretreating them with chlorpromazine. One week before the start of a 6-hydroxydopamine test series, 4 rats received daily injections of chlorpromazine hydrochloride (3 mg/kg, i.p.) immediately after the self-stimulation test. Three controls were given injections of saline. During the next 7 days, 6-hydroxydopamine (25 μg) was administered intraventricularly to all rats 1 hr after injection of chlorpromazine or saline. Injections and self-stimulation tests were discontinued for a 5-day interval, and then reinstated during a second 3-day test period. Self-stimulation rates in the chlorpromazine group were not significantly reduced in either test period, whereas the rates of unprotected control animals declined progressively with successive doses of 6-hydroxydopamine, as shown in Fig. 10. We assume that the behavioral deficit in the unprotected group is due to depletion of brain norepinephrine after 6-hydroxydopamine, and that the absence of a deficit in the chlorpromazine group is evidence that norepinephrine levels were not substantially depleted. These conclusions are supported by biochemical experiments, summarized in Table 3, which demonstrate that chlorpromazine largely prevents the depletion of brain norepinephrine by 6-hydroxydopamine.

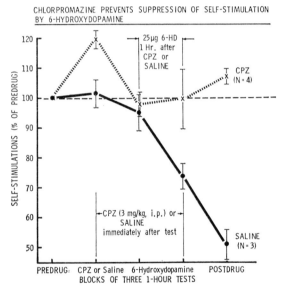

FIG. 10. Prevention of chlorpromazine of 6-hydroxydopamine-induced suppression of self-stimulation. Postdrug means of chlorpromazine and saline groups differ significantly at the 0·005 level. See text for details of experiment. (From STEIN and WISE.[26])

Finally, the present theory of the mode of action of chlorpromazine may explain why the antipsychotic effect of the drug usually takes weeks to develop, and why its abrupt withdrawal usually does not cause immediate deterioration.[51] In animal studies, after electrolytic lesions of the medial forebrain bundle,[15] or after chemical damage by 6-hydroxydopamine (e.g. Fig. 6 and Table 2), recovery of feeding and goal-directed behavior takes place gradually over days or weeks. By analogy, recovery of normal behavior in schizophrenic patients may take weeks to develop after the toxic action of endogenous 6-hydroxydopamine has been blocked by chlorpromazine; in this regard, it is of interest that the half-life of central noradrenergic vesicles in the rat is about 3 days. Furthermore, after chlorpromazine is discontinued, deterioration should become manifest only gradually as the 6-hydroxydopamine regains entry to the noradrenergic storage sites. Finally, the theory explains why the efficacy of chlorpromazine is reduced in 'burnt-out' schizophrenics, if it may be assumed that in these cases the noradrenergic reward terminals have suffered irreversible damage.

TABLE 3. PREVENTION BY CHLORPROMAZINE OF 6-HYDROXYDOPAMINE-INDUCED DEPLETION OF BRAIN NOREPINEPHRINE*

Treatment	Rats (No.)	Mean concentration in diencephalon and forebrain			
		Norepinephrine		Dopamine	
		μg/g	(per cent of control)	μg/g	(per cent of control)
Control (no drug)	3	0·314 ± 0·024	—	0·923 ± 0·066	—
Chlorpromazine + vehicle	3	0·329 ± 0·013	(104)	0·938 ± 0·183	(101)
Chlorpromazine + 6-hydroxydopamine (200 μg)	3	0·251 ± 0·048	(80)	0·812 ± 0·314	(88)
Saline + 6-hydroxydopamine (200 μg)	4	0·093 ± 0·007	(29)	1·550 ± 0·127	(168)
†Saline + 6-hydroxydopamine (100 μg)	4	0·103 ± 0·001	(33)	0·982 ± 0·025	(106)

* Chlorpromazine injected in 2 doses (15 and 30 mg/kg, respectively, i.p.) 24 hr and 1 hr before intraventricular injection of 6-hydroxydopamine (200 μg). Control animals received two injections of saline before the injection of 6-hydroxydopamine. Animals sacrificed 5 days later.

† Animals received 100 μg of 6-hydroxydopamine and were sacrificed 2 days later.

POSSIBLE ENZYME DEFICIT IN SCHIZOPHRENIA

Taken together, the foregoing lines of evidence provide reasonable support for the theory that chemical damage to the noradrenergic reward system by endogenous 6-hydroxydopamine causes schizophrenia. If this hypothesis were correct, it would be logical to ask (i) how 6-hydroxydopamine gains access to the noradrenergic nerve endings of the reward system, and (ii) why toxic quantities of the substance are formed only in the schizophrenic and not in the normal.

Although one can only speculate in the absence of data, the answer to the first question may be relatively straightforward: 6-hydroxydopamine has access to the noradrenergic reward terminal because it is formed from dopamine in the noradrenergic nerve. After its release into the synaptic cleft, dopamine could be converted (by autoxidation or by an enzymatic reaction) to 6-hydroxydopamine, which then could be taken up by the norepinephrine uptake mechanism. In the normal brain, only negligible amounts of 6-hydroxydopamine would be formed in this way. The conversion of dopamine to norepinephrine by dopamine-β-hydroxylase normally is not the rate-limiting step in the synthesis of norepinephrine;[52] hence, only a negligible amount of dopamine would be stored in noradrenergic binding sites under ordinary physiological conditions. In the schizophrenic brain, however, the step from dopamine to norepinephrine could be rate-limiting if dopamine-β-hydroxylase activity, or the capacity to induce the enzyme under stress, were drastically reduced by a pathological gene.*

POSTULATED ETIOLOGY OF SCHIZOPHRENIA

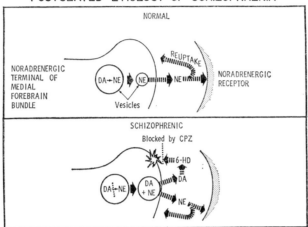

FIG. 11.   Hypothetical diagram of noradrenergic transmission in normal and schizophrenic brain. *Normal:* Virtually all dopamine (DA) is converted to norepinephrine (NE) by dopamine-β hydroxylase. *Schizophrenic:* Pathological gene causes reduced synthesis or aberrant formation of dopamine-β-hydroxylase, resulting in only incomplete conversion of DA to NE. Hence, nerve impulses release both DA and NE into synaptic cleft. Autoxidation or enzymatic conversion of dopamine produces 6-hydroxydopamine, which, when taken up by noradrenergic terminal, destroys it. (From STEIN and WISE.[26])

In such a case, dopamine would be released from noradrenergic nerve endings into the synaptic cleft and converted into 6-hydroxydopamine. Continuous uptake of this substance over a long period of time could damage the binding capacity and, eventually, the structural integrity of the noradrenergic terminal, as suggested diagramatically in Fig. 11.† These concepts are supported by the frequent observation of psychosis in alcoholics after overdoses

---

* The theory as a whole obviously does not rest on the validity of this assumption. All that is required is that the schizophrenic, by some genetic aberration, either produces excessive 6-hydroxydopamine or is hypersensitive to amounts that normally are produced. Direct proof of this assumption would be the demonstration of reduced activity (or reduced induction) of dopamine-β-hydroxylase relative to that of tyrosine hydroxylase or DOPA decarboxylase in samples of schizophrenic blood, spinal fluid, or brain obtained shortly after death.

† Early in the process, reward function may be paradoxically augmented by various mechanisms: 6-Hydroxydopamine may displace norepinephrine from its storage sites, it may potentiate the release of norepinephrine by nerve impulses, or it may promote the development of receptor supersensitivity. In this phase, one might see manic and agitated states, euphoria, paranoid delusions of grandeur, etc. This phase would not necessarily occur in all cases. However, in all cases, the lesioning process would progressively destroy reward capacity—sometimes intermittently, as the formation of 6-hydroxydopamine waxes and wanes depending on stress and other factors. In the end, goal-directed thinking and behavior would become increasingly impaired and the mood would flatten, resulting in apathy or depression.

of the dopamine-β-hydroxylase inhibitor disulfiram. According to ANGST,[53] disulfiram psychosis can be symptomatically indistinguishable from schizophrenia. Furthermore, HEATH and his associates[56] report that disulfiram produces extreme mental and physical changes, including an increase in psychotic symptoms, in schizophrenic patients, but only minimal changes in a prisoner control group.

POSSIBLE ETIOLOGY OF MANIC-DEPRESSIVE PSYCHOSIS AND PARKINSON'S DISEASE

A similar process of neural impairment involving 6-hydroxydopamine also may be operative in manic-depressive psychosis and Parkinson's disease. Manic-depressive psychosis has a close similarity to schizophrenia with many overlapping symptoms.[25] Recent histochemical studies suggest that central noradrenergic neurons form two important ascending systems: a dorsal pathway which mainly innervates the cerebral cortex and the hippocampus, and a ventral pathway which mainly innervates the hypothalamus and the ventral parts of the limbic system.[54] It is possible that primary damage to the dorsal system leads to thought disorders (schizophrenia), whereas primary damage to the ventral system produces affective disorders (manic-depressive psychosis). In any case, the therapeutic use of tricyclic antidepressants in manic-depressive psychosis parallels the use of phenothiazine antipsychotics in schizophrenia, and their mechanism of antidepressant action might similarly depend in part on a capacity to block the uptake of 6-hydroxydopamine into noradrenergic terminals.[48] Moreover, as in the case of phenothiazines, the well-established delay in the onset of the antidepressant action may be explained by the time that would be required to synthesize new vesicles and transport them to active sites.* Finally, in Parkinson's disease, the normal resistance of dopamine neurons to the toxic action of 6-hydroxydopamine may be weakened after viral infection or as a result of a pathological gene.

SUMMARY

A novel biochemical etiology for schizophrenia and manic-depressive psychosis, which permits an explanation of the mode of action of antipsychotic phenothiazines and tricyclic antidepressants, is described. The theory assumes: (i) that, in the psychotic, a pathological gene leads to a marked reduction in the activity of dopamine-β-hydroxylase, or in the

---

* These considerations suggest that antipsychotics and antidepressants could be used interchangeably or in combination in schizophrenia and manic-depressive psychosis. In certain types of depression, such combinations (e.g., perphenazine and amitriptyline) have in fact become the treatment of choice. Tricyclic antidepressant drugs are used in schizoaffective and cyclophrenic psychosis and in the depressive hypochondriacal states of chronic paranoid schizophrenic patients.[55] In general, however, imipramine-like drugs are not regarded as useful in the treatment of schizophrenia, possibly for the following reasons: (i) By a noradrenergic-facilitating action, imipramine may potentiate the manic or agitated early phases of some schizophrenias and (ii) the recommended imipramine dose of 75–300 mg per day for depression is well below the effective antipsychotic dose of chlorpromazine of 400–1000 mg per day,[49] although the ED_{50} for blockade of 6-hydroxydopamine uptake by mouse heart is 2·8 mg/kg for imipramine vs. 1·8 for chlorpromazine.[48] In this regard, it is interesting to note that the norepinephrine uptake inhibitor cocaine fails to antagonize the norepinephrine-depleting action of 6-hydroxydopamine[48].

capacity to induce the enzyme under stress, (ii) that, therefore, a mixture of dopamine and norepinephrine is stored in noradrenergic terminals of the reward system, (iii) that release of dopamine into the synaptic cleft permits the formation (by autoxidation or enzymatic reaction) of toxic quantities of 6-hydroxydopamine, (iv) that continuous or episodic uptake of 6-hydroxydopamine over long periods damages the binding capacity and, eventually, the structural integrity of the noradrenergic terminal, (v) that the resulting progressive damage to the noradrenergic reward mechanism is responsible for the fundamental symptoms and long-term downhill course of schizophrenia and manic-depressive psychosis, and (vi) that phenothiazines and tricyclic antidepressants exert their therapeutic action by blocking the entry of 6-hydroxydopamine into the noradrenergic terminal. A similar destructive process involving 6-hydroxydopamine may be operative in senile psychosis and Parkinson's disease. In the latter disorder, the normal resistance of dopamine neurons to the toxic action of endogenous 6-hydroxydopamine may be weakened after viral infection or as a result of a pathological gene.

Acknowledgements—I thank Dr. HERCHEL SMITH for suggesting a pathway from a catecholamine to *trans*-3-methyl-2-hexenoic acid. His suggestion of a trihydroxydopamine intermediate helped to stimulate the idea that 6-hydroxydopamine may be the chemical cause of schizophrenia. I also thank Dr. R. P. STEIN for useful discussions and the preparation of trihydroxydopamines, Mrs. E. BUCKLEY for editorial assistance, and ALFRED T. SHROPSHIRE, NICHOLAS S. BUONATO, WILLIAM J. CARMINT, HELEN C. GOLDMAN, HERMAN MORRIS, JANET D. NOBLITT and LOIS E. WEHREN for expert technical assistance.

REFERENCES

1. DELGADO, J. M. R., ROBERTS, W. W. and MILLER, N. E. Learning motivated by electrical stimulation of the brain. *Am. J. Physiol.* **179**, 587, 1954.
2. OLDS, J. and MILNER, P. Positive reinforcement produced by electrical stimulation of septal area and other regions. *J. comp. physiol. Psychol.* **47**, 419, 1954.
3. NAUTA, W. J. H. Central nervous organization and the endocrine nervous system. In: *Advances in Neuroendocrinology*, NALBANDOV, A. V. (Ed.), p. 5, University of Illinois Press, Urbana, 1963.
4. HILLARP, N. A., FUXE, K. and DAHLSTRÖM, A. Demonstration and mapping of central neurons containing dopamine, noradrenaline and 5-hydroxytryptamine and their reactions to psychopharmaca. *Pharmac. Rev.* **18**, 727, 1966.
5. POSCHEL, B. P. H. and NINTEMAN, F. W. Norepinephrine: A possible excitatory neurohormone of the reward system. *Life Sci.* **3**, 782, 1963.
6. STEIN, L. Self-stimulation of the brain and the central stimulation action of amphetamine. *Fed. Proc. Fedn. Am. Socs exp. Biol.* **23**, 836, 1964.
7. STEIN, L. and SEIFTER, J. Possible mode of antidepressive action of imipramine. *Science* **134**, 286, 1961.
8. WISE, C. D. and STEIN, L. Amphetamine: Facilitation of behavior by potentiated release of norepinephrine from the medial forebrain bundle. In: *Amphetamine and Related Compounds*, COSTA, E. and GARATTINI, S. (Eds.), p. 463. Raven Press, New York, 1970.
9. STEIN, L. Psychopharmacological substrates of mental depression. In: *Antidepressant Drugs*, GARATTINI, S. and DUKES, N. M. G. (Eds.), p. 130. Excerpta Medica Foundation, Amsterdam, 1967.
10. STEIN, L. Chemistry of reward and punishment. In: *Psychopharmacology: A Review of Progress*, 1957–1967, EFRON, D. H., (Ed.), p. 105. U.S. Government Printing Office, Washington, 1968.
11. WISE, C. D., BERGER, B. D. and STEIN, L. Brain serotonin and conditioned fear. *Proc. 78th Ann. Meeting, Am. Psychol. Ass.* **5**, 821, 1970.
12. BRODIE, B. B. and SHORE, P. A. A concept for a role of serotonin and norepinephrine as chemical mediators in the brain. *Ann. N.Y. Acad. Sci.* **66**, 631, 1957.

N

13. HOEBEL, B. G. Feeding: Neural control of intake. *Ann. Rev. Physiol.* **33**, 533, 1971.

14. OLDS, J. Hypothalamic substrates of reward. *Physiol. Rev.* **42**, 554, 1962.

15. BERGER, B. D., WISE, C. D. and STEIN, L. Norepinephrine: Reversal of anorexia in rats with lateral hypothalamic damage. *Science* **172**, 281, 1971.

16. TEITELBAUM, P. and EPSTEIN, A. N. The lateral hypothalamic syndrome: Recovery of feeding and drinking after lateral hypothalamic lesions. *Psychol. Rev.* **69**, 74, 1962.

17. HEATH, R. G. and MICKLE, W. A. Evaluation of seven years' experience with depth electrodes studies in human patients. In: *Electrical Studies On The Unanesthetized Brain*, RAMEY, E. R. and O'DOHERTY, D. S. (Eds.), p. 214. Hoeber, New York, 1960.

18. SEM-JACOBSEN, C. W. and TORKILDSEN, A. Depth recording and electrical stimulation in the human brain. In: *Electrical Studies On The Unanesthetized Brain*, RAMEY, E. R. and O'DOHERTY, D. S. (Eds.), p. 275. Hoeber, New York, 1960.

19. MOWRER, O. H. *Learning Theory and Behavior.* Wiley, New York, 1960.

20. STEIN, L. Reciprocal action of reward and punishment mechanisms. In: *Role of Pleasure in Behavior*, HEATH, R. G. (Ed.), p. 113. Hoeber, New York, 1964.

21. KALLMANN, F. J. *The Genetics of Schizophrenia.* Augustin, New York, 1938.

22. KALLMAN, F. J. The genetic theory of schizophrenia: An analysis of 691 schizophrenic twin index families. *Am. J. Psychiat.* **103**, 309, 1946.

23. HESTON, L. L. The genetics of schizophrenic and schizoid disease. *Science* **167**, 249, 1970.

24. KETY, S. S., ROSENTHAL, D., WENDER, P. H. and SCHULSINGER, F. The types of prevalence of mental illness in the biological and adoptive families of adopted schizophrenics. In: *The Transmission of Schizophrenia*, ROSENTHAL, D. and KETY, S. S. (Eds.), p. 345. Pergamon Press, New York, 1968.

25. KARLSSON, J. L. *The Biological Basis of Schizophrenia.* Thomas, Springfield, Illinois, 1966.

26. STEIN, L. and WISE, C. D. Possible etiology of schizophrenia: Progressive damage of the noradrenergic reward mechanism by endogenous 6-hydroxydopamine. *Science* **171**, 1032, 1971.

27. THUDICHUM, J. W. L. *A Treatise On The Chemical Constitution of The Brain.* Balliere, Tindall & Cox, London, 1884.

28. HOLLISTER, L. E. *Chemical Psychoses.* Thomas, Springfield, Illinois, 1968.

29. FRIEDHOFF, A. J. and VAN WINKLE, E. Isolation and characterization of a compound from the urine of schizophrenics. *Nature* **194**, 897, 1962.

30. HOFFER, A. and OSMOND, H. The adrenochrome model and schizophrenia. *J. nerv. ment. Dis.* **128**, 18, 1959.

31. OSMOND, H. and SMYTHIES, J. R. Schizophrenia: A new approach. *J. ment. Sci.* **98**, 309, 1952.

32. SHULGIN, A. T., SARGENT, T. and NARANJO, C. Structure-activity relationships of one-ring psychotomimetics. *Nature* **221**, 537, 1969.

33. KETY, S. S. Biochemical theories of schizophrenia. *Science* **129**, 1528, 1590, 1959.

34. HOLLISTER, L. E. Drug-induced psychosis and schizophrenic reactions: A critical comparison. *Ann. N.Y. Acad, Sci.* **96**, 80, 1962.

35. BLEULER, E. *Dementia Praecox, Or The Group of Schizophrenias.* International Universities Press, New York, 1950.

36. RADO, S. Hedonic self-regulation of the organism. In: *The Role Of Pleasure In Behavior*, HEATH, R. D. (Ed.), p. 257. Hoeber, New York, 1964.

37. SENOH, S., CREVELING, C. R., UDENFRIEND, S. and WITKOP, B. Chemical enzymatic and metabolic studies on the mechanism of oxidation of dopamine. *J. Am. Chem. Soc.* **81**, 6236, 1969.

38. PORTER, C. C., TOTARO, J. A. and STONE, C. A. Effect of 6-hydroxydopamine and some other compounds on the concentration of norepinephrine in the hearts of mice. *J. Pharmac. exp. Ther.* **140**, 308, 1963.

39. URETSKY, N. J. and IVERSEN, L. L. Effects of 6-hydroxydopamine on noradrenaline-containing neurons in the rat brain. *Nature, Lond.* **221**, 557, 1969.

40. BLOOM, F. E., ALGERI, S., GROPPETTI, A., REVUELTA, A. and COSTA, E. Lesions of central norepinephrine terminals with 6-OH-dopamine: Biochemistry and fine structure. *Science* **166**, 1284, 1969.

41. BARTHOLINI, G., RICHARDS, J. G. and PLETSCHER, A. Dissociation between biochemical and ultrastructure effects of 6-hydroxydopamine in the rat brain. *Experientia*, **26**, 142, 1970.

42. BREESE, G. and TRAYLOR, T. D. Effect of 6-hydroxydopamine on brain norepinephrine and dopamine: Evidence for selective degeneration of catecholamine neurons. *J. Pharmac. exp. Ther.* **174**, 413, 1970.

43. URETSKY, N. J. and IVERSEN, L. L. Effects of 6-hydroxydopamine and catecholanaine containing neurons in the rat brain. *J. Neurochem.* **17**, 269, 1970.
44. SCHOENFELD, R. I. and ZIGMOND, M. J. Effect of 6-hydroxydopamine (HDA) on fixed ratio (FR) performance. *Pharmacologist* **12**, 227, 1970.
45. TAYLOR, K. M., SNYDER, S. H. and LAVERTY, R. Dissociation of the behavioral and biochemical actions of 6-hydroxydopamine. *Pharmacologist* **12**, 227, 1970.
46. SMITH, K., THOMPSON, G. F. and KOSTER, H. D. Sweat in schizophrenic patients: Identification of the Odorous substance. *Science* **166**, 398, 1969.
47. AGHAJANIAN, G. K. and SHEARD, M. H. Behavioral effects of midbrain raphe stimulation—dependence on serotonic. *Comm. Behav. Biol.* **1**, 37, 1968.
48. STONE, C. A., PORTER, C. C., STAVORSKI, J. M., LUDDEN, C. T. and TOTARO, J. A. Antagonism of certain effects of catecholamine-depleting agents by antidepressant and related drugs. *J. Pharmac. exp. Ther.* **144**, 196, 1964.
49. COLE, J. O. and DAVIS, J. M. Clinical efficacy of the phenothiazines as antipsychotic drugs. In: *Psychopharmacology: A Review of Progress, 1957–1967*, EFRON, D. H. (Ed.), p. 1057. U.S. Government Printing Office, Washington, 1968.
50. GLOWINSKI, J. and BALDESSARINI, R. J. Metabolism of norepinephrine in the central nervous system. *Pharmac. Rev.* **18**, 1201, 1966.
51. DOMINO, E. F. Substituted phenothiazine antipsychotics. In: *Psychopharmacology: A Review Of Progress, 1957–1967*, EFRON, D. H. (Ed.), p. 1045. U.S. Government Printing Office, Washington, 1968.
52. UDENFRIEND, S. Tyrosine hydroxylase. *Pharmac. Rev.* **18**, 43, 1966.
53. ANGST, VON J. Zur frage der psychosen bei behandlung mit disulfiram (antabus). *Schweiz. med. Wschr.* **46**, 1304, 1956.
54. FUXE, K., HÖKFELT, T. and UNGERSTEDT, U. Morphological and functional aspects of central monoamine neurons. *Int. Rev. Neurobiol.* **13**, 93, 1970.
55. BAN, T. A. *Psychopharmacology.* Williams Wilkins, Baltimore, 1969.
56. HEATH, R. G., NESSELHOF, W., BISHOP, M. P. and BYERS, L. W. Behavioral and metabolic changes associated with administration of tetraethylthiuram disulfide (Antabuse). *Dis. Nerv. System* **26**, 99, 1965.

J. psychiat. Res., 1971, Vol. 8, pp. 363–384. Pergamon Press. Printed in Great Britain.

EMOTION REVISITED*

JOSEPH V. BRADY

The Johns Hopkins University School of Medicine, Baltimore, Maryland

THROUGHOUT the long history of psychology and psychiatry, few concepts have enjoyed the central role which has been accorded emotion. The use and abuse of emotion constructs however, has continued to betray a deplorable lack of understanding with regard not only to obvious realities but to many subtleties which have remained elusive for want of a more operational language. Indeed, the ambiguity and confusion which has attended even the quasi-technical usage of such emotion expressions as 'anxiety' for example, can be seen to have produced a jumble of fundamental distinctions and not-so-fundamental metaphors. Few of neuropsychiatry's scholars have been more aware of the need to tease apart the strands of this tangle than David McKenzie Rioch. A symposium honoring this innovator of research endeavors dedicated in large measure to such operational objectives would seem to provide an appropriate occasion for revisiting and reviewing the conceptual status of emotion as it has been affected by the investigative efforts which he made possible.

The experimental observations which provide the basis for this overview emerged from an analysis of interrelated behavioral and physiological processes in laboratory animals exposed to a broad range of emotional conditioning situations. The biological components and psychophysiological dimensions identified in the course of such an operational analysis seemed to require that a distinction be made between at least two basic aspects of the emotion complex which have been a traditional and persistent source of confusion. In keeping with more or less conventional usage, the terms 'feelings' and 'emotional behavior' may be suggested for these two classes of behavioral events following recent conceptual[1] and experimental[2] differentiations. A host of semantic, linguistic, and taxonomic problems have of course been occasioned by the interchangeable use of such terms. And much of the endless polemic exchange which has continued at least since the controversies of JAMES[3] and CANNON[4] would seem to have its origins in the failure to make what now appears to be a useful and experimentally supportable distinction between at least these two categories of emotion interactions based simply on the localization of their primary effects or consequences.

Figure 1 summarizes diagrammatically some of the distinctions and interrelationships suggested by this proposed dichotomy. Although both 'feeling' and 'emotional behavior' involve psychological interactions, their effects would seem to be meaningfully differentiated in terms of the boundary relationship between organism and environment. 'Emotional

* The research described in this report was supported in part by Grant No. HE–06945 from the National Heart and Lung Institute.

behavior' is here represented within a broad class of *effective* interactions, the primary consequences of which can be clearly identified *outside* the skin at the interface with the external environment. Such 'emotional behavior' events may be uniquely defined in terms of changes or perturbations, characteristically abrupt and episodic, in the organism's ongoing relationship to this *external* environment. 'Feelings' or *affective* behaviors, on the other hand, are distinguished as a generic class of interactions, the principal effects of which are localizable *within* the skin. Many different subclasses of 'feelings' may be identified within this broad affective category characteristically associated with a range of interrelated endocrine, proprioceptive, and autonomic-visceral activities. A host of recent

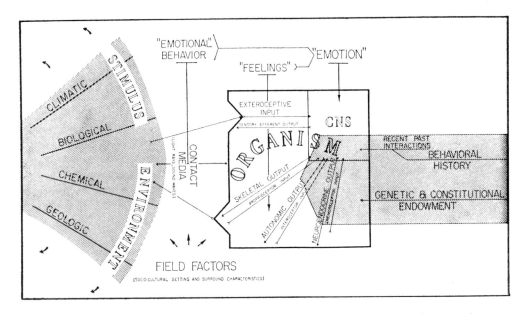

FIG. 1. Diagrammatic representation of a 'behavioral universe' emphasizing organism-environment interactions. 'Emotional behavior' is represented at the interface between organism and environment, while 'feelings' are localized within the reacting organism.

conditioning studies[5-10] have documented the ease with which such interoceptive processes can acquire discriminative control over behavior and the flexibility which characterizes the loose integration of 'feeling' responses with exteroceptive environmental events. Indeed, the persistent confusion between 'feelings' on the one hand, and 'emotional behavior' on the other, can be attributed, in part, at least, to the prominence of such interoceptive participation in a broad range of effective response patterns. But such psychophysiological activity need not constitute a defining property of 'emotional behavior', characterized by the external localization of its primary effects and identified, usually, by abrupt changes in ongoing interactions with the exteroceptive environment. Viewed within this dualistic framework, the wide scope of 'emotion' phenomena becomes susceptible to a functional analysis of their conditions of occurrence in relationship to explicitly-defined interactions between physiological and environmental operations.

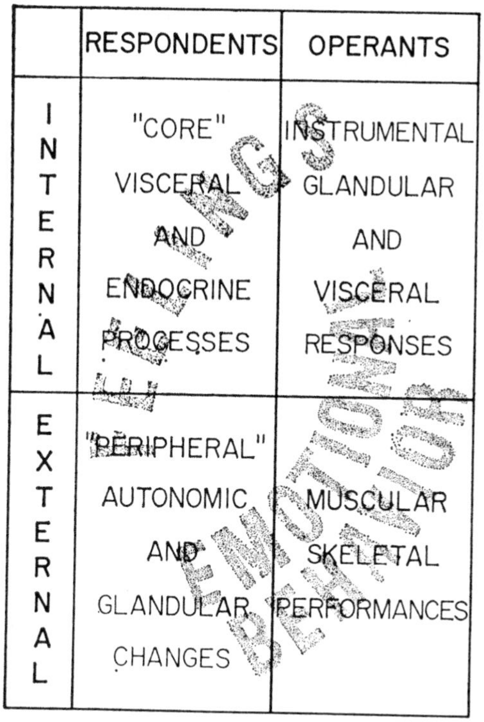

	RESPONDENTS	OPERANTS
I N T E R N A L	"CORE" VISCERAL AND ENDOCRINE PROCESSES	INSTRUMENTAL GLANDULAR AND VISCERAL RESPONSES
E X T E R N A L	"PERIPHERAL" AUTONOMIC AND GLANDULAR CHANGES	MUSCULAR SKELETAL PERFORMANCES

FIG. 2. Categorization of interacting biological 'feelings' and 'emotional behavior' components.

One systematic derivative of this operational basis for identifying biological components of the 'emotion' complex is suggested in Fig. 2 which calls attention to at least four general classes of interrelationships between the indicated 'internal–external' parameter (i.e. 'inside' and 'outside' the skin) and the traditional 'respondent–operant' categorization of behavioral interactions. Classical respondent or Pavlovian conditioning[11] ('involuntary' activity *elicited* by *prior-occurring* stimulus events) has emphasized the flexible organization of visceral and glandular changes. These autonomic-endocrine processes appear to be concerned primarily with regulation of the internal economy and correspond well with the present characterization of 'feelings' components. Operant or instrumental conditioning[12] ('voluntary' performances maintained by environmental changes which occur *following* response *emission*) on the other hand, involves a prominent focus upon the somatic musculature. These striated muscle responses are explicitly organized and closely integrated with exteroceptive stimulus events, thus providing a basis for differentiating the 'emotional behavior' class characterized by external localization of primary effective changes. The four-fold categorization depicted in Fig. 2 however, suggests that the differential characterization of 'feelings' and 'emotional behavior', based principally upon the distinction between 'internal respondents' ('core' visceral and endocrine processes) and 'external operants' (muscular skeletal performances), may be complicated somewhat by the involvement, in part, of at least two other classes of interacting biological events.

'External respondents' ('peripheral' autonomic and glandular changes) have, of course, long occupied the attention of 'emotion theorists,[13-16] and recent studies on instrumental conditioning of visceral and glandular responses[10,17] have generated an ever-expanding interest in the 'internal operant' class. Certainly, a comprehensive account of 'emotion' phenomena could hardly exclude these contributing elements, though an analysis of the major components of the process, as characterized by the present formulation, would seem to require a continuing emphasis upon 'internal respondents' and 'external operants'.

Of course, the obvious differences between affective and effective response patterns cannot occlude the evident operational interrelationships between 'feelings' and 'emotional behavior'. Complex behavioral situations invariably involve close associations and inter-actions between the two, though their respective conditions of occurrence can often be distinguished temporally and localized spacially. Clearly, the internal consequences of prior-occurring *affective* feeling interactions (i.e. 'respondents') may well provide the discriminative occasion for *effective* emotional behaviors (i.e. 'operants') which change the organism's relationship to the external environment. And the abrupt, often chaotic effects of emotional behaviors (i.e. 'operants') certainly produce eliciting stimuli which in turn control the occurrence of feeling responses (i.e. 'respondents'). At least some of the psychophysiological dimensions which define the broad range of interactions between these different classes of events are represented in Fig. 3 which provides an operational framework, suggested by two-factor learning formulations,[9] for laboratory analysis of the problem.

		APPETITIVE OPERANTS	AVERSIVE OPERANTS
APPETITIVE	RESPONDENTS	BEHAVIORAL FACILITATION AND PHYSIOLOGICAL ACTIVATION??	BEHAVIORAL SUPPRESSION AND PHYSIOLOGICAL DEACTIVATION???
AVERSIVE	RESPONDENTS	BEHAVIORAL SUPPRESSION AND PHYSIOLOGICAL ACTIVATION	BEHAVIORAL FACILITATION AND PHYSIOLOGICAL ACTIVATION?

FIG. 3. Categorization of interacting psychophysiological 'appetitive' and 'aversive' dimensions.

The 'appetitive–aversive' dimension of operant–respondent interactions, represented in Fig. 3, is by no means, of course, the only or even possibly the most important 'emotion' parameter to be considered. It has however, played a central role in systematic accounts of emotion,[18-20] and does suggest a range of experimental manipulations which have been productive of an empirical analysis involving behavioral and physiological processes basic to emotional interactions. Significantly, the characterization of psychophysiological interaction effects represented within the 'cells' of Fig. 3, while grossly overgeneralized and in dire need of both behavioral and physiological refinement, does find at least some support in the experimental analysis of such interrelationships.

The extensive experimental literature[9,12,21-23] which has emerged over the past three decades on both the behavioral and physiological analysis of 'contiditioned suppression' models[24-26] for the laboratory study of 'fear' or 'anxiety', based upon the operational interaction between 'appetitive operants' and 'aversive respondents' for example, generally confirms the 'behavioral suppression and physiological activation' characterization represented for this well-worked 'emotion' dimension (lower left 'cell', Fig. 3). In addition, several studies[27-32] have also confirmed the 'behavioral facilitation' (i.e. response rate acceleration) produced by the interaction between 'appetitive respondents' and 'appetitive operants', though the 'physiological activation' aspects of this 'joyful' emotion dimension (upper left 'cell', Fig. 3) have received much less direct experimental attention.[33-36] Topographically similar accelerations (i.e., 'behavioral facilitation') in the rate of an instrumental shock-avoidance performance ('aversive operant') produced by the interacting effects of Pavlovian 'fear' conditioning ('aversive respondent') have also been repeatedly described,[9,37-46] and recent studies of endocrine and autonomic changes in closely related aversive conditioning situations[47,36] provide at least some support for the 'physiological activation' property of this characteristically 'aggressive' emotion dimension (lower right 'cell', Fig. 3). That the 'physiological activation' characterizing these latter two classes of operant-respondent interactions (upper left and lower right 'cells', Fig. 3) may be distinguished psychophysiologically, at least to some extent, is suggested however, by reports of markedly different cardiovascular response patterns ('internal respondents') in experiments comparing appetitively and aversively maintained instrumental performances ('external operants') with virtually identical muscular skeletal properties. WENZEL[34] described directional differences in heart rate changes during behavioral conditioning based on food and shock with cats, and two recent studies[36,48] involving measures of both heart rate and blood pressure changes in dogs and baboons confirm the differential autonomic 'respondent' patterns emerging with strikingly similar 'operant' performances under such appetitive and aversive control conditions.

Only limited experimental attention has been directed to the analysis of interaction effects involving 'appetitive respondents' and 'aversive operants' (upper right 'cell', Fig. 3), though at least two recent reports[49,50] have described effects of a classically-conditioned stimulus, previously paired with food, upon instrumental avoidance responding. Indeed, both these experiments and a study conducted in our own laboratories confirm the hypothesized 'behavioral suppression' effect of superimposing a classically-conditioned 'food reflex' upon a shock-maintained instrumental avoidance performance. In our own study, two Rhesus monkeys, restrained in standard primate chairs, were first trained to press a lever to avoid shocks to the feet which occurred every 50 sec unless the animal pressed the lever within that interval to postpone shock another 50 sec. When this procedure had generated a stable lever pressing performance, presentations of a 30-sec flickering light (terminated contiguously with delivery of 5 1-g food pellets) were intermittently super-imposed upon the on-going avoidance baseline. Figure 4 shows the suppressing effect of the intermittent light-food pairings upon the avoidance lever pressing rate which developed with animal S-7 after such 'respondent conditioning' sessions and which remained stable in both monkeys over several weeks of daily experimental exposures. As yet, no physio-logical data is available on the endocrine or autonomic patterns characterizing this 'appetitive respondent–aversive operant' interaction effect, though the experimental analysis of at least heart rate and blood pressure changes under such conditions is presently receiving attention.

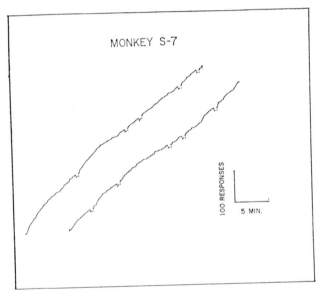

FIG. 4.   Suppressing effect of light-food pairings (displaced segments of cumulative response record) upon shock-avoidance lever-pressing in monkey S-7.

It must of course be recognized that such a laboratory experimental approach necessarily oversimplifies the obviously complex 'emotion' process. Yet the heuristic value of this research effort would appear to lie not only in the generation of interesting operational data but also in the experimental analysis of such fundamental concepts as the proposed distinction between 'feelings' and 'emotional behavior'. Indeed, the experimental findings which have emerged from such an analysis may be seen both to provide support for this basic dichotomy and illucidate somewhat, the defining properties of the participating behavioral and physiological events. For the most part, the relevant evidence has been derived from psychophysiological studies focusing upon interaction models involving 'appetitive operants' and 'aversive respondents' (lower left 'cell', Fig. 3). More recent experiments however, have also emphasized aversively-maintained operant performances in relationship to endocrine and autonomic respondent participation (e.g. lower right 'cell', Fig. 3) in the analysis of such 'emotion' models.

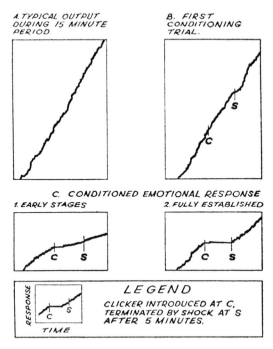

FIG. 5. 'Conditioned anxiety' model showing development of typical behavioral suppression during auditory warning stimulus (clicker) presentations, followed by shock, superimposed upon an ongoing appetitively-maintained lever-pressing performance in a laboratory rat.

Experimental observations related to the 'conditioned anxiety' model illustrated in Fig. 5, for example, have now clearly established the differential effects of a variety of psychophysiological manipulations upon the 'aversive respondent' and 'appetitive operant' components of such 'emotion' segments. Electroconvulsive shock treatments[51-53] limbic system lesions[54-55] electrical stimulation of the brain[56-58] and drug administration[59-61] have all been shown to selectively alter the strength of the 'aversive respondent' component of the 'conditioned anxiety' model while affecting the 'appetitive operant' baseline either not at all or in opposite directions. In addition, the attenuating effect of reserpine upon the conditioned 'anxiety' model (Fig. 5) clearly differentiates this 'aversive respondent' interaction from a topographically similar suppression of the 'appetitive operant' by a stimulus based upon 'discriminated punishment' (i.e. shocks produced only by lever responses during stimulus presentation). Experimental comparisons of such drug effects have shown that the behavioral suppression produced by 'punishment' is essentially unaffected by the same dose of reserpine which virtually eliminates the conditioned 'anxiety' response.[62]

This broad range of experimental findings is consistent with the postulation of selective effects upon those distinguishable aspects of the emotion complex which appear to depend heavily upon 'internal respondent' components and emphasizes the separability of such 'feeling' events from the essentially unaffected 'instrumental behavior' aspects of the emotion complex. Indeed, such an interpretive view finds further support in the results which have emerged from a more direct experimental analysis of the physiological processes presumed to mediate the 'feelings'. This series of recent studies concerned with endocrine and autonomic measurements focused initially upon variants of the 'conditioned anxiety' procedure, illustrated in Fig. 5, with Rhesus monkeys. The development of this conditioned 'anxiety' response was first studied in relationship to changes in plasma 17-hydroxycorti-costeroid (17-OH-CS) levels occurring during a series of acquisition trials consisting of 30-min lever-pressing sessions with auditory stimulus and shock pairing occurring once during each session approximately 15 min after the start. Seven such conditioning trials were accompanied by the withdrawal of blood samples immediately before and immediately after each 30-min session, and 17-OH-CS levels associated with successive stages in the acquisition of the conditioned emotional behavior were determined. The progressive *suppression* of lever pressing in response to presentation of the auditory stimulus during each successive trial (reflecting development of the conditioned 'anxiety' response) was found to be consistently and systematically related to a progressive increase in the 17-OH-CS levels during each of the seven sessions.[63]

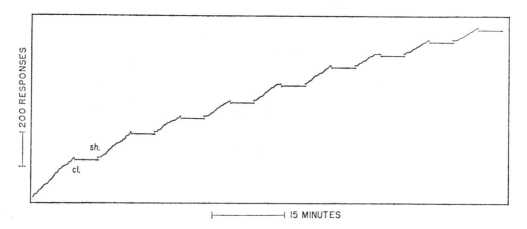

FIG. 6. Cumulative response record showing typical behavioral suppression effect of repeated clicker–shock pairings upon an ongoing appetitively-maintained lever-pressing performance in a Rhesus monkey.

This relationship between emotional behavior segments and the activity of the pituitary–adrenal cortical systems has been further confirmed in a series of experiments[64] with monkeys in which the conditioned suppression of lever pressing had been previously established. Five such animals were studied during 1-hr lever-pressing sessions for food reward involving alternating 5-min periods of auditory-stimulus-presentation and no-auditory-stimulus, as illustrated in Fig. 6. Blood samples taken before and after several such sessions with each animal during which *no* shock followed any of the auditory stimulus presentations, revealed substantial corticosteroid elevations related to the *conditioned* emotional behavior alone. And the rate of rise of this behaviorally-induced steroid elevation was strikingly similar to that observed following administration of large ACTH doses in these same animals. Such behaviorally-induced pituitary–adrenal stimulation was found to cease shortly after termination of the emotional interaction however, with hormonal levels returning to normal within an hour. Significantly, when the conditioned 'anxiety' response was markedly attenuated by repeated doses of reserpine administered 20–22 hr before such experimental sessions, the 17-OH-CS response to the auditory stimulus was also eliminated.[65]

When measurements of plasma epinephrine and norepinephrine levels were added to the corticosteroid determinations in experiments with this conditioned emotional behavior model, the potential contributions of a 'hormone pattern' approach to such psycho-physiological analyses became evident. Observations in the course of a rather rudimentary conditioning experiment[63] involving a loud truck horn and electric foot shock with monkeys suggested the differential participation of adrenal medullary systems in conditioned and unconditioned aspects of such emotional behavior patterns. Exposure to the horn or the shock alone *prior* to the conditioned pairing of the two produced only mild elevations in catecholamine levels. Following a series of conditioning trials, however, during which horn-sounding for 3 min was terminated contiguously with shock, presentation of the horn alone markedly increased norepinephrine levels without eliciting any epinephrine response. This hormone pattern approach has been extended in a series of experiments[66] in which concurrent plasma epinephrine, norepinephrine, and 17-OH-CS levels were determined during monkey performance on the alternating 5-min 'on', 5-min 'off' conditioned 'anxiety' response procedure illustrated in Fig. 6. The results obtained during 30-min control and experimental sessions involving such recurrent emotional behavior segments confirm the differential hormone response pattern characterized by marked elevations in both 17-OH-CS and norepinephrine but little or no change in epinephrine levels.

Observations of autonomic changes related to this same conditioned 'anxiety' model have recently been obtained with a series of monkeys catheterized for cardiovascular measurements.[67-68] Heart rate and both systolic and diastolic blood pressure were recorded continuously during experimental sessions involving both lever pressing alone and exposure to the conditioned 'anxiety' procedure. The stable lever-pressing performances recorded during control sessions before introduction of the emotional conditioning procedure were found to be accompanied by equally stable heart rate and blood pressure values throughout each session. Following a series of only 5–8 emotional conditioning trials involving 3-min presentations of a clicking noise terminated contiguously with foot shock superimposed upon the lever-pressing performance, however, complete suppression of lever pressing during clicker presentations was observed to be accompanied by a dramatic drop in heart rate and a somewhat less vigorous blood pressure decrease. But continued pairings of clicker and shock superimposed upon the lever-pressing performance produced abrupt reversals in the direction of these autonomic changes with cardiac acceleration and blood pressure elevation appearing and persisting in response to the clicker during the later stages of emotional conditioning. Figure 7 shows the sequence of changes in the form of the autonomic responses for one such animal in the course of 50 such emotional conditioning exposures. Blood pressure, heart rate, and lever-pressing rate for successive conditioning trials are shown as changes during the 3-min clicker period as compared to the average value for each measure obtained during the 3-min interval immediately preceding the clicker (the 'O' point on each panel of the graph). The blood pressure and heart rate values are shown as absolute changes in millimetres of mercury and beats per minute, respectively. The lever-pressing values are shown as percent changes in response rate

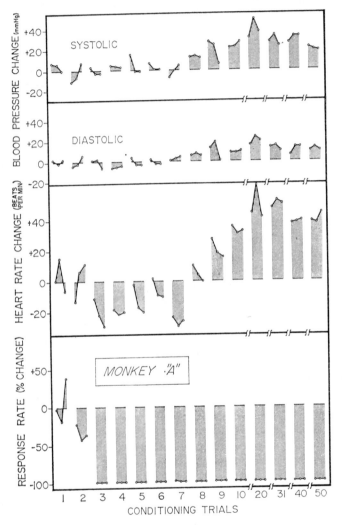

FIG. 7. Minute-by-minute changes in blood pressure, heart rate, and lever-pressing response rate for Monkey A on successive 3-min clicker-shock trials during acquisition and maintainance of the conditioned emotional response.

during the clicker as compared to the pre-clicker baseline. Figure 7 shows complete cessation of lever pressing during the clicker developing by the third conditioning trial for Monkey A and the maintenance of this behavioral suppression response throughout the entire course of 50 clicker-shock pairings. The autonomic changes can be seen to follow a more varied but nonetheless systematic course during this acquisition phase with Monkey A. A marked deceleration in heart rate first appeared during presentation of the clicker on the third conditioning trial corresponding to the initial development of complete behavioral suppression. During the next four trials, a similar decelerative change in heart rate accompanied the behavioral response with little or no change apparent in either diastolic or systolic blood pressure. During the 8th conditioning trial, however, an abrupt change in the direction of the cardiac response to the clicker was reflected in both heart rate and blood pressure measures. Increases in heart rate approximating 40 beats per minute developed in response to the clicker by the 10th conditioning trial and persisted throughout the remainder of the 50 acquisition trials. Both systolic and diastolic blood pressure showed correspondingly consistent and dramatic elevations in response to the clicker developing between the 8th and 10th conditioning trial and persisting through trial fifty.

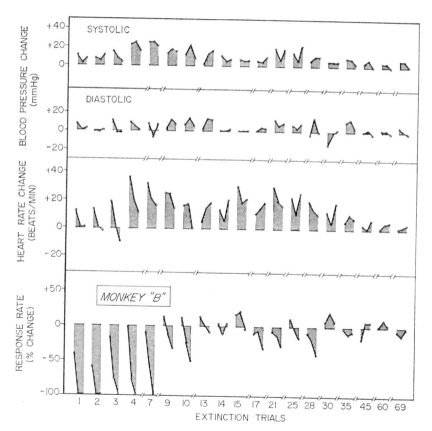

FIG. 8. Minute-by-minute changes in blood pressure, heart rate, and lever-pressing rate for Monkey B on successive 3-min presentations of the clicker alone without shock during extinction of the conditioned emotional response.

When the conditioned 'anxiety' response was extinguished by repeated presentations of clicker alone without shock during daily lever-pressing sessions with such animals following extended exposure to recurrent emotional conditioning of this type, a further divergence between autonomic and behavioral response to emotion was observed. Figure 8 illustrates this characteristic difference in extinction rates for the cardiovascular and instrumental components of the conditioned emotional response with Monkey B. Although virtually complete recovery of the lever-pressing rate in the presence of the clicker can be seen to have occurred within 10 such extinction trials, both heart rate and blood pressure elevations

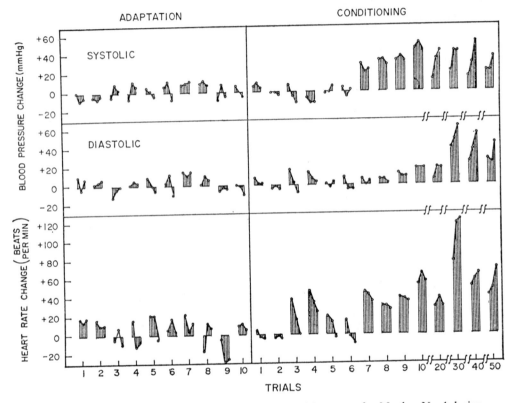

FIG. 9. Minute-by-minute changes in blood pressure and heart rate for Monkey No. 1 during adaptation and on successive 3-min clicker-shock trials *without* lever-pressing performance baseline.

in response to the clicker alone persisted well beyond the 40th extinction trial. Finally, reconditioning of the 'anxiety' response with such animals rapidly produced behavioral suppression accompanied immediately by the tachycardia and pressor responses. Significantly, the initial cardiac decelerative response characteristic of the early trials during original emotional conditioning failed to appear during reconditioning with any of the animals. And when two additional monkeys were exposed to the 'aversive respondent' conditioning procedure alone by repeated presentations of clicker-shock pairings *without*

MONKEY S-300

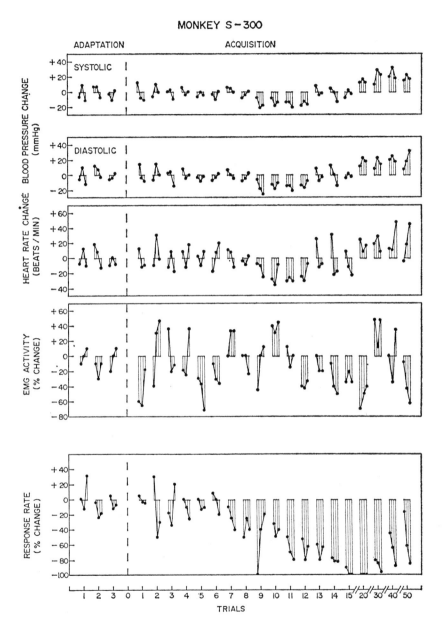

FIG. 10. Minute-by-minute changes in blood pressure, heart rate, electromyographic activity, and lever-pressing response rate for Monkey S-300 on successive 3-min clicker–shock trials during acquisition of the conditioned emotional response.

requiring a concurrently maintained 'appetitive operant' performance (i.e. no lever-pressing baseline interaction), again, only the accelerative cardiovascular pattern was observed. Dramatic increases in heart rate and blood pressure for both monkeys appeared by the 7th or 8th conditioning trial following extensive adaptation (as illustrated in Fig. 9 for one of the animals) without any indication of the initial cardiac deceleration which had developed when clicker–shock pairings were superimposed upon the ongoing instrumental lever-pressing behavior (e.g. Fig. 7). These findings would seem to suggest a possible differentiation between two distinguishable psychophysiological patterns (i.e. internal 'feeling' respondents) related, at least in part, to interacting operant performance processes.

Further evidence for essentially independent control of the autonomic-visceral and somatic-musculature components of such emotional response patterns has recently emerged in the course of an experiment[69] designed specifically to articulate the relationship between the biphasic cardiovascular changes accompanying acquisition of the classical conditioned 'anxiety' model (Fig. 5) and concurrently measured skeletal muscle activity recorded electromyographically. Three monkeys implanted with femoral artery catheters and lumbar paraspinal muscle electrodes received a series of 50 clicker–shock pairings super-imposed upon an ongoing instrumental lever pressing performance. Figure 10 shows the development of the characteristic operant behavioral suppression and biphasic cardio-vascular change accompanying acquisition and maintenance of conditioned 'anxiety' in one of the animals. In addition, changes in electromyographic activity, recorded con-currently during each conditioning trial, are also shown in Fig. 10, emphasizing the striking lack of any systematic relationship to the observed heart rate and blood pressure pattern. Essentially similar findings, characterized by the entire range of possible combinations of cardiac and EMG activity change (e.g. heart rate and blood pressure increases accompanied by EMG decreases, EMG increases accompanied by cardiac suppression, etc.) during emotional conditioning, were obtained with all three monkeys. And the polygraph records shown in Fig. 11 for one of the two remaining animals, comparing the 'early' (i.e. 'trial 10') and 'late' (i.e. 'trial 40') cardiovascular and electromyographic response patterns to emotional conditioning, confirm the absence of any differential EMG changes under the same conditions which can be seen to produce first, systematic blood pressure decreases (accompanying the early development of behavioral suppression during trial 10) and then, systematic blood pressure increases (accompanying later maintenance of behavioral suppression during trial 40). Clearly, the independent variations in these visceral and somatic components is consistent with the current formulation of distinguishable (and separable) components of such emotional response patterns.

The conditioned 'anxiety' model which provided the initial focus for analyzing psycho-physiological dimensions of the emotion complex characteristically emphasizes the behavioral suppression effects of the interaction between 'aversive respondents' and 'appetitive operants'. More recent experimental attention to behavioral facilitation effects produced by interacting 'aversive respondents' and 'aversive operants' has resulted in intensive psychophysiological analyses of conditioned 'avoidance' models which provide additional support for the present conceptual formulation of emotion and illucidate many subtle aspects of participating physiological processes. The free-operant avoidance pro-cedure first described by SIDMAN[70] for example, has been extensively studied in relationship

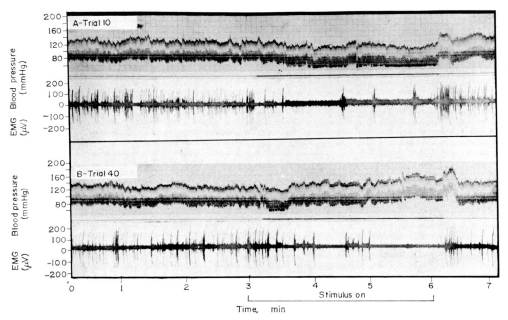

FIG. 11. Polygraph records of blood pressure changes and electromyographic activity for Monkey S-300 during emotional conditioning trials 10 and 40.

to endocrine and autonomic changes of obvious relevance to the 'feelings' components of emotional interactions, as herein formulated. Briefly, the basic 'avoidance' conditioning procedure has involved programming shocks to the feet of a chair-restrained monkey every 20 sec unless the animal pressed a lever within that interval to postpone shock another 20 sec. The stable and durable lever pressing performance generated by this procedure has been shown to be consistently associated with twofold to fourfold rises in 17-OH-CS levels for virtually all animals during 2-hr experimental sessions even in the absence of shock.[23,64] And repeated exposure to extended experimental sessions requiring continuous 6-hr avoidance performances alternating with 6-hr 'rest' periods over several weeks has been found to produce an increase in the concentration of free acid in the gastric juice[71] and a high incidence of pathological gastrointestinal changes in animals subjected to such 'stress' conditions.[72-74]

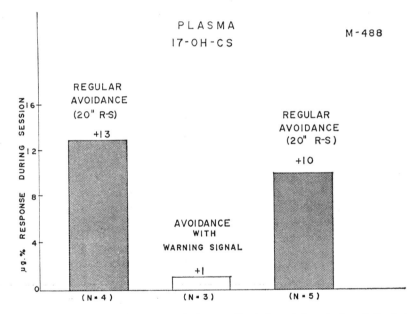

FIG. 12. Plasma 17-OH-CS responses during nondiscriminated ('regular') and discriminated ('warning signal') avoidance sessions.

It has also been possible to demonstrate quantitative relations between the rate of avoidance responding in the monkey and the level of pituitary–adrenal cortical activity independently of the shock frequency.[75] Marked differences in the hormone response have been observed,[63] however, when the avoidance procedure included a discriminable exteroceptive warning signal presented 5 sec prior to administration of the shock whenever 15 sec had elapsed since the previous response. Figure 12 compares the 17-OH-CS levels measured during 'regular' and 'discriminated' avoidance sessions with the monkey and shows the consistently reduced corticosteroid response associated with programming such a warning signal. Conversely, superimposing so-called 'free' or unavoidable shocks upon a well-established avoidance baseline without a warning signal has been observed[63] to amplify markedly the 17-OH-CS elevations. Figure 13, for example, shows that the presentation of such 'free shocks' during 2-hr avoidance sessions more than doubles the corticosteroid response as compared to the regular non-discriminated avoidance procedure. Significantly, these systematic, wide-ranging variations in the internal milieu have been observed to occur under conditions which involve only minimal changes in the behavioral performance, thus providing further experimental support for the basic distinction between separable internal ('feelings') and external ('emotional behavior') components of such interaction segments.

PLASMA 17-OH-CS

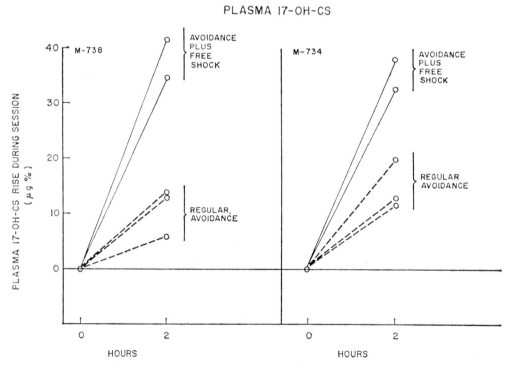

FIG. 13. Plasma 17-OH-CS responses during 'regular' nondiscriminated avoidance and during avoidance with 'free shocks'.

This relative independence of endocrine-autonomic-visceral participants on the one hand, and skeletal-behavioral processes on the other, appears also to be manifest in comparing concurrent biochemical determinations, involving plasma corticosteroid and catecholamine levels, during avoidance performances, with the same biochemical measures made during exposure to the conditioned 'anxiety' procedure. Despite the obvious behavioral differences between these two emotional conditioning situations (i.e. behavioral suppression vs. behavioral facilitation), virtually identical biochemical patterns, characterized by 17-OH-CS and norepinephrine elevations with no change in epinephrine levels, have been observed to occur in response to the two procedures.[66] Variations in these behavioral procedures, however, have been shown to produce significant deviations from this common 'emotion' hormone pattern. When a well-trained monkey was presented with the avoidance signal following removal of the response lever from the restraining chair, for example, making his learned 'coping' response impossible under circumstances which had previously required such a performance, an elevation in epinephrine was observed with no change in nore-pinephrine.[63] This effect occurred within 1 min of the signal presentation and could not be observed after 10 min of exposure to such conditions. Other variations in the pattern of catecholamine levels were observed in a series of experiments which involved the adminis-tration of 'free' or unavoidable shocks to a well-trained monkey, producing dramatic elevations in both epinephrine and norepinephrine even though the animal received no more shock than during previous regular avoidance sessions characterized by high nor-epinephrine and 17-OH-CS levels and no change in epinephrine.[63] More complex emotional behavior situations, involving ambiguity with respect to which of several components in a required performance sequence would follow presentation of a 'ready' signal, have also been observed to produce marked elevations in both epinephrine and norepinephrine, though epinephrine levels invariably fall precipitously once the first unambiguous perform-ance signal is presented.[66] Within the framework of the present 'emotion' formulation, these several variations in hormonal patterns would be consistently viewed as reflecting the internal 'feelings' component of such behavioral interactions.

An even broader spectrum of hormonal and autonomic changes in relationship to emotional behavior situations has been examined in a series of experiments with monkeys involving continuous exposure to extended sessions (72 hr or more in duration) of required shock avoidance performances. The pattern of corticosteroid and pepsinogen changes observed before, during, and after such a continuous 72-hr avoidance experiment for example, has been found to be characterized by the expected elevation in 17-OH-CS throughout the 72-hr session while pepsinogen levels were consistently depressed below baseline levels during this same period. Marked and prolonged elevations in pepsinogen levels (enduring for several days beyond the 48-hr period required for post-avoidance recovery of the preavoidance corticosteroid baseline) were observed however, during the post-avoidance recovery period.[76] Repeated exposure to such continuous 72-hr avoidance requirements over extended periods up to and, in some cases, exceeding 1 yr has also been studied in relationship to the pattern of thyroid, gonadal, and adrenal hormone secretion. One group of animals participated in the 72-hr avoidance experiment on six separate occasions over a 6-month period with an interval of approximately 4 weeks intervening between each exposure. Another group of animals performed on a schedule which repeatedly programmed 72-hr avoidance cycles followed by 96-hr non-avoidance 'rest' cycles (3 days 'on', 4 days 'off') for periods up to and exceeding a year.

The first group of animals exposed to repeated 72-hr avoidance sessions at monthly intervals for 6 months showed a progressively increasing lever-pressing response rate over the 6 successive exposures,[77] though the hormone changes developed as a consistent and replicable pattern.[78] Twofold to threefold elevations in 17-OH-CS levels occurred repeatedly during the 72-hr avoidance and returned to near baseline levels within 4–6 days after termination of the 3-day experimental session. Significant changes were also observed in catecholamine, gonadal, and thyroid hormone levels, though the recovery cycles in some instances (thyroid) extended well beyond 3 weeks following cessation of the 72-hr avoidance performance. The remaining group of monkeys required to perform on the 3-day 'on', 4-day 'off' avoidance schedule showed an initial increase in lever-pressing response rate for approximately the first 10 avoidance sessions similar to that seen in the animals exposed to the repeated monthly sessions. Within 30 weeks however, the lever-pressing response rates for these animals during the 72-hr avoidance periods had decreased to a level well below that observed during the initial sessions and the performance stabilized at this new low level for the ensuing weeks of the experiment.[77] The initial 72-hr avoidance sessions characterized by progressive increases in lever-pressing rates were invariably accompanied by elevations in 17-OH-CS levels, as shown typically in Fig. 14 for monkey M-157. By the 20th weekly 'avoidance-rest' cycle however, steroid levels typically dropped below even the initial basal levels and no elevation occurred during the avoidance performance. By the 30th weekly session, however, 17-OH-CS levels generally returned to their pre-experimental basal values, though continued exposure to the 3-day 'on', 4-day 'off' schedule

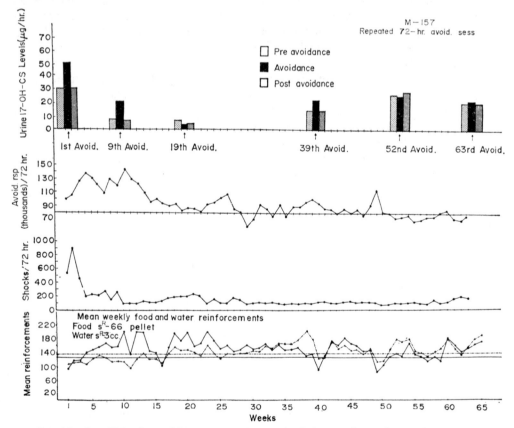

FIG. 14.   Steroid levels, avoidance response rates, shock frequencies, and water intake levels for animal M-157 throughout 65 weekly 72-hr avoidance sessions.

failed to produce any further steroid elevation in response to the 72-hr avoidance requirement even after 65 or more weeks of continuous performance on the program. Significantly,
Fig. 14 also reflects the fact that shock frequencies remained at a stable low level following
some initial adjustments during the early sessions, and normal food and water intake were
maintained essentially unchanged throughout the extended course of the experiment.

Both the results obtained in these more prolonged studies and the observations emerging
from less protracted psychophysiological experiments would seem to provide at least some
general support for the proposed formulation of the emotion process in terms of separable
but interacting physiological and behavioral components. The characterization of identity
relationships between these distinguishable participants on the one hand, and the so-called
'feelings'—'emotional behavior' dichotomy on the other, is of course both oversimplified
and somewhat artificial. It seems clear however, that a comprehensive operational account
of emotion events must proceed by defining the properties of such identifiable constituents
and examining in detail the interrelationships between behavioral interactions with the
external environment and the broader patterning or balance of secretory and visceral
change in the several interdependent endocrine and autonomic systems which in concert
regulate the internal milieu. Indeed, the differentiation of such 'internal' and 'external'
components in relationship to the historical and situational aspects of behavioral interactions[79,80] can, it would seem, provide a meaningful basis for analyzing and integrating
both the 'physiological' and 'cognitive' aspects of emotion.

REFERENCES

1. KANTOR, J. R. Feelings and emotions as scientific events. *Psychol. Rec.* **16**, 377, 1966.
2. BRADY, J. V. Emotion: Some conceptual problems and psychophysiological experiments. In: *Feelings and Emotions*, ARNOLD, M. (Ed.), p. 69. Academic Press, New York, 1970.
3. JAMES, W. The physiological basis of emotion. *Psychol. Rev.* **1**, 516, 1894.
4. CANNON, W. B. The James-Lange theory of emotions: A critical examination and alternate theory. *Am. J. Psychol.* **39**, 106, 1927.
5. RAZRAN, G. The observable unconscious and the inferable conscious in current Soviet psycho-physiology: Interoceptive conditioning, semantic conditioning, and the orienting reflex. *Psychol. Rev.* **68**, 2, 81, 1961.
6. HEFFERLINE, R. F. and PERERA, T. B. Proprioceptive discrimination of a covert operant without its observation by the subject. *Science* **139**, 834, 1963.
7. SCHUSTER, C. R. and BRADY, J. V. The discriminative control of a food reinforced operant by interoceptive stimulation. *Pavlov J. higher nerv. Activ.* **14**, 448, 1964.
8. SLUCKI, H., ADAM, G. and PORTER, R. W. Operant discrimination of an interoceptive stimulus in rhesus monkeys. *J. exp. Analysis Behav.* **8**, 405, 1965.
9. RESCORLA, R. A. and SOLOMON, R. L. Two-process learning theory: Relationship between Pavlovian Conditioning and instrumental learning. *Psychol. Rev.* **74**, 151, 1967.
10. KATKIN, E. S. and MURRAY, E. N. Instrumental conditioning of autonomically-mediated behavior, *Psychol. Bull.* **70**, 52, 1968.
11. PROKASY, W. F. *Classical Conditioning.* Appleton-Century-Crofts, New York, 1965.
12. HONIG, W. *Operant Behavior: Areas of Research and Application.* Appleton-Century-Crofts. New York, 1966.
13. DUNBAR, H. F. *Emotions and Bodily Changes*, 4th Ed., Columbia, New York, 1954.
14. LINDSLEY, D. B. Emotion. In: *Handbook of Experimental Psychology*, STEVENS, S. S. (Ed.), Wiley, New York, 1951.
15. GOLDSTEIN, M. L. Physiological theories of emotion: A critical historical review from the standpoint of behavior theory. *Psychol. Bull.* **69**, 23, 1968.

16. FEHR, F. S. and STERN, J. A. Peripheral physiological variables and emotion: The James-Lange theory revisited. *Psychol. Bull*, **74**, 411, 1970.

17. MILLER, N. E. Learning of visceral and glandular responses. *Science* **163**, 434, 1969.

18. BEEBE-CENTER, J. G. *The Psychology of Pleasantness and Unpleasantness*. Van Nostrand, New York, 1932.

19. YOUNG, P. T. *Emotion in Man and Animal*. Wiley, New York, 1943.

20. ARNOLD, M. B. *Feelings and Emotions*. Academic Press, New York, 1970.

21. DAVIS, H. Conditioned suppression: A survey of the literature. *Psychonomic Monograph Suppl.* **2**, 283 (Whole Number 30), 1968.

22. LYON, D. O. Conditioned suppression: Operant variables and aversive control. *Psychol. Rec.* **18**, 317, 1968.

23. BRADY, J. V. Operant methodology and the production of altered physiological states. In: *Operant Behavior: Areas of Research and Application*, HONIG, W. (Ed.) Appleton-Century-Crofts, New York, 1966.

24. ESTES, W. K. and SKINNER, B. F. Some quantitative properties of anxiety. *J. exp. Psychol.* **29**, 390, 1941.

25. HUNT, H. F. and BRADY, J. V. Some effects of electroconvulsive shock on a conditioned emotional response ('anxiety'). *J. comp. physiol. Psychol.* **44**, 88, 1951.

26. LYON, D. O. CER methodology. *Psychol. Rep.* **20**, 206, 1967.

27. ESTES, W. K. Discriminative conditioning. II. Effects of a Pavlovian conditioned stimulus upon a subsequently established operant response. *J. exp. Psychol.* **38**, 173, 1948.

28. HERRNSTEIN, R. J. and MORSE, W. H. Some effects of response independent positive reinforcement on maintained operant behavior. *J. comp. physiol. Psychol.* **50**, 461, 1957.

29. MORSE, W. E. and SKINNER, B. F. Some factors involved in the stimulus control of operant behavior. *J. exp. Analysis Behav.* **1**, 103, 1958.

30. BRADY, J. V. Motivational-emotional factors and intra-cranial self-stimulation. In: *Electrical Stimulation of the Brain*. SHEER, D. E. (Ed.) Univ. Texas Press, Austin, 1961.

31. MELTZER, D. and BRAHLEK, J. A. Conditioned suppression and conditioned enhancement with the same positive UCS: An effect of CS duration. *J. exp. Analysis Behav.* **13**, 67, 1970.

32. HENTON, W. W. and BRADY, J. V. Operant acceleration during a pre-reward stimulus. *J. exp. Analysis Behav.* **13**, 205, 1970.

33. GANTT, W. H. Cardiovascular component of the conditioned reflex to pain, food, and other stimuli. *Physiol. Rev.* **40**, 266, 1960.

34. WENZEL, B. M. Changes in heart rate associated with responses based on positive and negative reinforcement. *J. comp. physiol. Psychol.* **42**, 638, 1961.

35. SNAPPER, A. G., SCHOENFELD, W. N., FERRARO, D. P. and LOCKE, B. Cardiac rate of the rat under DRL and non-contingent temporal schedule of reinforcement. *Psychol. Rep.* **17**, 543, 1965.

36. ANDERSON, D. E. and BRADY, J. V. Differential preparatory cardiovascular responses to aversive and appetitive behavioral conditioning. *J. Appl. Physiol.* (submitted).

37. SIDMAN, M., HERRNSTEIN, R. J. and CONRAD, D. G. Maintenance of avoidance behavior by unavoidable shocks. *J. comp. physiol. Psychol.* **50**, 553, 1957.

38. SIDMAN, M. Normal sources of pathological behavior. *Science* **132**, 1960.

39. SOLOMON, R. L. and TURNER, L. H. Discriminative classical conditioning in dogs paralyzed by curare can later control discriminative avoidance responses in the normal state. *Psychol. Rev.* **69**, 202, 1962.

40. WALLER, M. B. and WALLER, D. F. The effects of unavoidable shocks on a multiple schedule having an avoidance component. *J. exp. Analysis Behav.* **6**, 29, 1963.

41. BELLEVILLE, R. E., ROHLES, F. H., GRUNZKE, M. B. and CLARK, F. C. Development of a complex variable schedule in the chimpanzee. *J. exp. Analysis Behav.* **63**, 348, 1963.

42. RESCORLA, R. A. and LoLORDO, V. M. Inhibition of avoidance behavior. *J. comp. physiol. Psychol.* **59**, 406, 1965.

43. OVERMIER, J. B. and LEAF, R. C. Effects of discriminative Pavlovian fear conditioning upon previously or subsequently acquired avoidance responding. *J. comp. physiol. Psychol.* **60**, 213, 1965.

44. GROSSEN, N. E. and BOLLES, R. C. Effects of a classical conditioned 'fear signal' and 'safety signal' on non-discriminated avoidance behavior. *Psychonomic Sci.* **11**, 321, 1968.

45. KAMANO, D. K. Effects of an extinguished fear stimulus on avoidance behavior. *Psychonomic Sci.* **13**, 271, 1968.

46. POMERLEAU, O. F. The effects of stimuli followed by response-independent shock on shock-avoidance behavior. *J. exp. Analysis Behav.* **14,** 11, 1970.

47. BRADY, J. V. Endocrine and autonomic correlates of emotional behavior. In: *Physiological Correlates of Emotion.* BLACK, P. (Ed.) Academic Press, New York, 1970.

48. FINDLEY, J. D. and BRADY, J. V. Blood pressure and heart rate changes in a continuously programmed environment. *Proc. 77th a. Conv. Am. Psychol. Ass.* 807, 1969.

49. GROSSEN, N. E., KOSTANSEK, D. J. and BOLLES, R. C. Effects of appetitive discriminative stimuli upon avoidance behavior. *J. exp. Psychol.* **81,** 340, 1969.

50. BULL, J. A. An interaction between appetitive Pavlovian CS's and instrumental avoidance responding. *Learning Motivation* **1,** 18, 1970.

51. BRADY, J. V. and HUNT, H. F. A further demonstration of the effects of electro-convulsive shock on a conditioned emotional response. *J. comp. physiol. Psychol.* **44,** 204, 1951.

52. BRADY, J. V. The effects of electro-convulsive shock on a conditioned emotional response: The permanence of the effect. *J. comp. physiol. Psychol.* **44,** 507, 1951.

53. BRADY, J. V. The effects of electro-convulsive shock on a conditioned emotional response: The significance of the interval between the emotional conditioning and the electro-convulsive shock. *J. comp. physiol. Psychol.* **45,** 9, 1952.

54. BRADY, J. V. and NAUTA, W. J. H. Subcortical mechanisms in emotional behavior: Affective changes following septal forebrain lesions in the albino rat. *J. comp. physiol. Psychol.* **46,** 339, 1953.

55. BRADY, J. V. and NAUTA, W. J. H. Subcortical mechanisms in emotional behavior: The duration of affective changes following septal and habenular lesions in the albino rat. *J. comp. physiol. Psychol.* **48,** 412, 1955.

56. BRADY, J. V. and CONRAD, D. Some effects of limbic system self-stimulation upon conditioned emotional behavior. *J. comp. physiol. Psychol.* **53,** 128, 1960.

57. BRADY, J. V. Temporal and emotional effects related to intracranial electrical self-stimulation. In: *Electrical Studies on the Unanesthetized Brain,* RAMEY, E. R. and O'DOHERTY, D. S. (Eds.) Hoeber, New York, 1960.

58. BRADY, J. V. Motivational–emotional factors and intra-cranial self-stimulation. In: *Electrical Stimulation of the Brain,* SHEER, D. (Ed.) Univ. Texas Press, Austin, 1961.

59. BRADY, J. V. Assessment of drug effects on emotional behavior. *Science* **123,** 1033, 1956.

60. BRADY, J. V. A comparative approach to the evaluation of drug effects upon behavior. In: *Brain Mechanisms and Drug Action.* FIELDS, W. S. (Ed.) C. C. Thomas, Springfield, Ill., 1957.

61. BRADY, J. V. Perspectives in the preclinical evaluation of behavioral drugs. *Proc. Sci. Med. Conf.* Am. Pharm. Manufact. Ass., Chicago, Ill., 1958.

62. BRADY, J. V. Animal experimental evaluation of drug effects upon behavior. In: *The Effect of Pharmacologic Agents on the Nervous System.* BRACELAND, F. (Ed.) William & Wilkins, Baltimore, 1959.

63. MASON, J. W., BRADY, J. V. and TOLSON, W. W. Behavioral adaptations and endocrine activity. In: *Proceedings of the Association for Research in Nervous and Mental Diseases.* LEVINE, R. (Ed.) Williams and Wilkins Co., Baltimore, 1966.

64. MASON, J. W., BRADY, J. V. and SIDMAN, M. Plasma 17-hydroxycorticosteroid levels and conditioned behavior in the rhesus monkey. *J. Endocr.* **6,** 741, 1957.

65. MASON, J. W. and BRADY, J. V. Plasma 17-hydroxycorticosteroid changes related to reserpine effects on emotional behavior. *Science* **124,** 983, 1956.

66. MASON, J. W., MANGAN, G., BRADY, J. V., CONRAD, D. and RIOCH, D. Concurrent plasma epinephrine, norepinephrine, and 17-hydroxycorticosteroid levels during conditioned emotional disturbances in monkeys. *Psychosom. Med.* **23,** 344, 1961.

67. BRADY, J. V. Emotion and the sensitivity of the psychoendocrine systems. In: *Neurophysiology and Emotion,* GLASS, D. (Ed.), p. 70. Rockefeller Univ. Press, New York, 1967.

68. BRADY, J. V., KELLY, D. and PLUMLEE, L. Autonomic and behavioral responses of the rhesus monkey to emotional conditioning. *Ann. N.Y. Acad. Sci.* **159,** 959, 1969.

69. BRADY, J. V., HENTON, W. W. and EHLE, A. Some effects of emotional conditioning upon autonomic and electromyographic activity. Meetings of the Eastern Psychological Association, 1970.

70. SIDMAN, M. Avoidance conditioning with brief shock and no exteroceptive warning signal. *Science* **118,** 157, 1953.

71. POLISH, E., BRADY, J. V., MASON, J. W., THACH, J. S. and NIEMECK, W. Gastric contents and the recurrence of duodenal lesions in the rhesus monkey during avoidance behavior. *Gastroenterology* **43,** 193, 1962.

72. BRADY, J. V., PORTER, R. W., CONRAD, D. G. and MASON, J. W. Avoidance behavior and the development of gastroduodenal ulcers. *J. exp. Analysis Behav.* **1,** 69, 1958.

73. PORTER, R. W., BRADY, J. V., CONRAD, D., MASON, J. W., GALAMBOS, R. and RIOCH, D. McK. Some experimental observations on gastrointestinal lesions in behaviorally conditioned monkeys. *Psychosom. Med.* **20,** 379, 1958.

74. RICE, H. K. The responding-rest ratio in the production of gastric ulcers in the rat. *Psychol. Rep.* **13,** 11, 1963.

75. SIDMAN, M., MASON, J. W., BRADY, J. V. and THACH, J. Quantitative relations between avoidance behavior and pituitary-adrenal cortical activity. *J. exp. Analysis Behav.* **5,** 353, 1962.

76. MASON, J. W., BRADY, J. V., POLISH, E., BAUER, J. A., ROBINSON, J. A., ROSE, R. M., and TAYLOR, E. D. Patterns of corticosteroid and pepsinogen change related to emotional stress in the monkey. *Science* **133,** 1596, 1961.

77. BRADY, J. V. Experimental studies of psychophysiological responses to stressful situations. *Symposium on Medical Aspects of Stress in the Military Climate.* p. XII, Walter Reed Army Inst., Res., Government Printing Office, Washington, D.C., 1965.

78. MASON, J. W. Organization of psychoendocrine mechanisms. *Psychosom. Med.* **30,** 565, 1968.

79. SCHACHTER, S. The interaction of cognitive and physiological determinants of emotional state. In: *Advances in Experimental Social Psychology*, BERKOWITZ, L. (Ed.) Academic Press, New York, 1964.

80. SCHACHTER, S. The assumption of identity and peripheralist-centralist controversies in motivation and emotion. In: *Feelings and Emotions*, ARNOLD, M. (Ed.), p. 111. Academic Press, New York, 1970.

J. psychiat. Res., 1971, Vol. 8, pp. 385–398. Pergamon Press. Printed in Great Britain.

AGGRESSIVE BEHAVIOR OF CHIMPANZEES AND BABOONS IN NATURAL HABITATS*

DAVID A. HAMBURG

Department of Psychiatry, Stanford University School of Medicine
Stanford, California 94305

RATIONALE AND METHOD

IT IS a great privilege to take part in this symposium honoring David Rioch, and I am deeply grateful to the organizers for inviting me. Most of the participants owe a profound debt to him. He has stimulated our thinking, challenged our complacent assumptions, modified our ideas, facilitated our work—in short, changed our lives for the better beyond anything we could have anticipated when we first met him.

Over the years, David Rioch has fostered a remarkable variety of research approaches to the understanding of brain and behavior. Prominent among these are studies of non-human primates in diverse environmental conditions. He recognized early that animal behavior could usefully be investigated in laboratories, in semi-natural colonies, and in natural habitats. The kinds of information available from these different approaches are largely complementary, and all are necessary if the complex roots of behavior are ever to be understood. Field studies in the natural habitat are extremely helpful in understanding the way that structure and behavior are adapted to environmental conditions. Experimental analysis is then essential to control the relevant variables.[1,2]

Several years ago, David Rioch had occasion to discuss a set of papers on the very topic of the present report, agonistic behavior in non-human primates.[3] In doing so, he called attention to "... the bearing which study of the social behavior of non-human primates has on our understanding of human groups and societies." He also placed "strong emphasis on the need for comparative studies, comparing not only different species under similar circumstances, but the same species under different circumstances (different habitats, different degrees of freedom, different experimental controls of the consequences of behavior . . .)."

He made additional suggestions regarding the focus of future research, directing attention to "(1) the situations and circumstances influencing the probability of occurrence of certain patterns of interaction (or behavioral events), (2) the cues or signals which are necessary and sufficient for initiating the events, (3) the factors which maintain and/or direct the

* This study was partly supported by NIMH Grant No. 1-F3-MH-36, 934-01 and partly by a grant from the Wenner-Gren Foundation for Anthropological Research.

course of the events to cues associated with their termination, and (4) the relationship of different events in the total social organization and in maintaining the group extant."

This framework is the one in which the present study has been undertaken. We have been mainly concerned with evidence on three classes of non-human primate behavior:

(1) What aggressive patterns of behavior are prominent in baboons and in chimpanzees? That is, what do patterns of threat and attack look like, both within the species and in relation to other species?

(2) What are the circumstances in which these patterns are likely to be observed?

(3) What are the circumstances in which these patterns are likely to be diminished or terminated? That is, what can we see of regulation or control of aggressive behavior through inter-animal communication?

The first of these questions has been dealt with in another report.[4] The present paper will deal mainly with the second question, and include some observations on the third question. This report is based partly on recent field studies that have included aggressive behavior as one part of a description of the behavioral repertoire of baboons and chimpanzees.[5-11] It is also based on a study focussed centrally on aggressive behavior, undertaken in 1968 by Eric Hamburg and myself in East Africa. The variety of chimpanzee under study was the *Pan satyrus* at the Gombe Stream Reserve in Tanzania, and the baboon species was the common olive baboon, *Papio anubis*, observed both at the Gombe and at the National Park near Nairobi, Kenya. We were fortunate to obtain over 100 hr of close range observation of chimpanzees at the Gombe; during much of this time forest-dwelling olive baboons were also present, interacting with the chimpanzees. At the Gombe, we had the privilege of access to the files of chimpanzee observation accumulated by Jane van Lawick Goodall over the years of her unique study beginning in 1960, to the extensive photographs of chimpanzee and baboon behavior accumulated at the same location by Hugo van Lawick, and to the observations of the several staff members working at the Gombe on both chimpanzee and baboon research. At the Nairobi Park, we also had over 100 hr of close range observation of savanna-dwelling olive baboons. Close range observation refers here to two or more animals within ten yards of the observer. The study centered on one troop consisting of 42 animals that had been studied earlier by DeVore and Washburn. This habitat, characterized by vast plains covered with tall grass and occasional clumps of trees, provided a marked contrast with the forest habitat of the Gombe. Thus, the same species of baboon could be observed in two markedly different ecological settings. In both species and both settings, a zoological definition of aggressive behavior was utilized.[12] "An animal acts aggressively when it inflicts, attempts to inflict, or threatens to inflict damage on another animal." We directed our attention toward any actions that clearly increased the probability of damage to other animals; in short, to threat and attack patterns, both within the species and directed toward other species.

SITUATIONS ELICITING AGGRESSIVE BEHAVIOR IN BABOONS

Baboons and their closely related species have made effective adaptations in habitats that were probably crucial in the emergence of early man.[13] The baboon–macaque group has spread widely through Asia and Africa in numbers that are large for primates, especially those of big body size. The baboons are the largest of all monkeys. Their ground-living capability is much greater than that of most other primates. Even in the savanna habitat, where large carnivores are difficult to detect in the tall grass, baboons cover several miles per day on the ground in search of food. They are often a mile from the nearest trees, which provide the ultimate safety for most primates. Thus, their ability to cope with predators is of central adaptive significance.

The baboon troop under study in Kenya consisted of both sexes and all ages. These animals spend their lives together in an intimate, semi-closed social system; in some circumstances a male may transfer from one troop to another. Inter-troop contact is associated with a relatively high frequency of vigilance and threat behavior.

In savanna-living baboons, aggressive behavior occurs in the presence of large carnivores, such as lions and cheetahs, and is differentiated by age and sex.[14] When a predator appears, the main body of the troop usually runs toward the nearest trees, while one or more adult males hold their ground. Soon a phalanx of adult males, flashing their enormous canine teeth, are interposed between the predator and the others in the troop. The carnivores rarely challenge the baboon males under these conditions.

Females are also quite capable of acting aggressively. Most threat and attack behavior on the part of females is elicited by interference with her infant. Both males and females intensively defend infants, especially if the infant is giving a distress call. When an infant has been injured, as we observed both in savanna and forest baboons, adult males threaten repeatedly. In these circumstances, with distress cries recurring from the infant, males threaten each other, female baboons, and human observers. In one sequence during which an infant was dying, the males threatened repeatedly over an hour's time, and many chases occurred. After the death of an infant, there is a clear tendency for the males to threaten the mother if she begins to move away from the dead infant. Some cases have been observed in which such threats persisted for several days after the infant's death, and apparently contributed to the mother's carrying the carcass until its was badly decomposed. We observed one baboon mother who was threatened whenever she moved more than a few feet away from her dead infant, but she was finally able to abandon it in very thick bush, out of sight of the adult males.

Threats, chases, and brief attacks by baboon mothers upon other females and juveniles occur frequently. The context usually appears to be some exploration of the mother's infant by another animal. Mothers differ considerably in their tolerance for such exploration. They are more likely to threaten the exploring animal in the infant's first few months than later in life. If the infant is treated roughly, or is carried away from the mother, or emits a scream, the mother is likely to attack the other animal. If the exploring animal has a high dominance status, it tends to be permitted more exploratory contact by the mother. High-ranking adult males may take considerable liberties with the infant. These males show much interest in infants, and are usually gentle in such contacts.

The two most dominant males in the troop we studied regarded each other with considerable vigilance but rarely fought. Ordinarily they stayed 100–200 yd apart at opposite ends of the troop. Their only serious quarrels arose over premium foods. On one occasion, a particular variety of nut was available in one tree. This tree elicited great interest throughout the troop. The two highest ranking males (Alpha and Beta) climbed the tree, watching each other closely, threatening from time to time. After 10 min of such interaction, Alpha attacked Beta and chased him over a 1000 yd at high speed. Similar encounters have been elicited in field experiments by placing a sought-after food about equidistant between high-ranking males.

The situations described so far are not the only ones that elicit threat and attack patterns in baboons, though they are particularly prominent in this respect. It may be useful here to summarize briefly all the situations eliciting aggressive behavior in baboons that we are able to observe in the two locations of study:[14,15] (1) protection of the troop by adult males against predators such as lions and cheetahs; (2) protection of infants, both by their mothers and by adult males; (3) resolution of disputes within the troop by adult males; (4) formation and maintenance of consort pairs at the peak of estrus; (5) attainment of preferred sleeping sites in the trees, particularly in the presence of predators; (6) acquisition of premium foods such as figs, nuts, and bananas, especially when spatially concentrated rather than widely distributed; (7) dominance interactions, especially in the presence of of premium foods, scarcity of sleeping sites, and females in full estrus; (8) exploration of strange or manifestly dangerous areas, a function largely of adult males; (9) contact between different troops, especially if such contact is infrequent. In all of these circumstances, the probability of overt threat behavior and of fighting is higher than in the other circumstances of baboon life. Generally, these situations involve either protection of or access to vital resources—including objects, locations, activities, and relations with other animals. Frustrations in either protection of or access to vital resources appear to increase the probability of threat or attack directed toward other available targets.

SITUATIONS ELICITING AGGRESSIVE BEHAVIOR IN CHIMPANZEES

The close biological relations of chimpanzee and man make the chimpanzee a subject of extraordinary interest for students of human behavior.[8] Yet until a few years ago there was scarcely any dependable information on the ways in which chimpanzee behavior meets adaptive requirements in natural habitats.[16–18] As this information has begun to become available, chiefly through Goodall's remarkable work, other lines of inquiry have been revealing impressive similarities between chimpanzees and man in various biological indices, including molecular characteristics of DNA, hemoglobin, albumin, cytochrome, and fibrinopeptides.

The chimp community we studied at the Gombe Stream Reserve in Tanzania consists at present of 45 animals. They live in a forested valley with open woodland at higher altitudes. Over the ridges on both sides there are other groups of chimpanzees. Very little is known about their contacts with the communities on the other sides, although such information as is available indicates that contact, when it does occur, is associated with high vigilance and aggressive displays. Methodologically, following animals through the forest consistently to get systematic, close-range observation of inter-group contact is very difficult.

This community breaks up in subgroups, most commonly 3–8 animals, and sometimes even individual animals for short periods. Composition is rather fluid, although there are certain enduring groups, particularly the unit of a mother and one or more of her offspring.

One of the characteristics of aggressive display by adult male chimpanzees is that their hair stands out, making the animals look, bigger and more impressive. (This is true of baboons as well.) In the aggressive display, a chimpanzee male often drags a large palm frond, brandishes it over his head as he runs, swings it, or even throws it in the direction of other animals—of the same species or another species.

An adult male who has been away for a day from a subgroup of chimpanzees who are his frequent companions usually makes an aggressive display when he returns. A brief absence, as in this case, elicits patterns that occur in more striking form when strangers meet.

We observed and photographed behavior suggesting that technical ingenuity in aggressive displays may be a significant part of dominance behavior in chimpanzees. Three years prior to our study, a large can had been left outside by the reserach workers. One of the young adult males had at that time incorporated it in his aggressive display. He ran at it, hit it, started it rolling, and chased it, hitting it repeatedly and so making loud noises. This action had a powerful effect on the other chimpanzees; they appeared to be quite frightened by this novel experience. Through these unusual displays, he rapidly became the most dominant male in the entire chimpanzee community, with less fighting than usually occurs in dominance changes of this kind. Three years later—with no intervening episode— we put the can back outside, at a time when this same male was about 100 ft away. Within 10 sec from the time the can was put down on the ground, he raced toward it and undertook a display utilizing the can, similar to the ones he had undertaken 3 yr earlier; all 8 chimpanzees within observation at the time ran off into the forest or went up trees. One young male climbed 40 ft and remained in the tree for 8 min after the displaying male had left the area. Such occurrences of vivid avoidance behavior in the face of male displays are common. While injuries do not necessarily occur under these circumstances, they are not rare.

At the Gombe Stream Reserve, bananas are made available from time to time as an attractive dietary supplement for both chimpanzees and baboons in one partially-cleared area where conditions are optimal for close-range observation. When bananas are available, frequent threatening occurs between males of similar rank. But such males rarely fight each other. Rather, a common pattern is that one of them will break off contact prior to fighting and attack a smaller, weaker, or less mobile animal. One such male attacked a mother who had her 10-month-old infant clinging ventrally. He gave her a severe beating, mainly with his fists and forearms. He did this to the same mother–infant pair three times within a week in similar situations of redirected aggression. On one occasion he actually knocked them out of a tree from a height of about 30 ft. Thus, the infant, though generally treated with great tolerance, is not immune to attack during intense episodes of redirected aggression. Infants may also be injured if they are unable to get out of the way of a male during a highly aggressive display.

After a dominant male has established his control of bananas or other premium foods, another chimpanzee may try to get him to share the food. An experienced female, for example, may back up to him in a lowered posture. This is called presenting, and it is common in many primate species in agonistic situations. After she reaches him, he may put his arm around her waist and give her a hug or a pat on the head.

In the same situation, another female might approach with arm extended, palm up, 'fear-face' expression, and making a distinctive panting sound ('pant-grunt'). The approach is ambivalent—several steps forward, then back, then forward again. It may take several minutes to cover about 30 ft. Again, he may pat her, hug her, or hold out his hand to be touched. Sometimes he may permit her to take a bit of banana.

The most organized hunting pattern known in any non-human primate has been described in the Gombe Stream area.[8] Typically, this occurs when an infant baboon (or colobus monkey) gets isolated up a tree. One adult male chimpanzee climbs after it, and 2 or 3 other adult male chimpanzees surround the base of the tree to fight off any adult male baboon who tries to defend the infant. If the chimpanzee catches the infant, the male in the tree and the next one up tear it apart, and 2 or 3 of these high-ranking males will begin to eat it immediately. There is intense excitement as other chimpanzees arrive and strive to get even a tiny bit of this freshly killed meat. These patterns are so vivid and distinctive that they are sometimes called 'begging behavior'. But when recently killed animals of the same species and age as the prey objects have been made available experimentally, the reaction of chimpanzees is quite different. They show interest and modest exploration, but not the excitement induced when they do their own killing. Moreover, they do not eat the carcass that they have not killed themselves. So far, there are only a few cases of this sort; future investigation into the predatory behavior of chimpanzees has considerable evolutionary interest.

The predator–prey relation is only one aspect of the complex interactions between chimpanzees and baboons at the Gombe Stream Reserve, and certainly not the most prominent aspect on a day-to-day basis. The two species clearly know each other well; they respond to each other differentially in a way that suggests recognition of individual animals, recognition of signals, and mutual accommodation. Overt competition sometimes occurs, especially in relation to premium foods. While the chimpanzees are generally dominant over the baboons in these encounters, the interactions are complex. For example, several adult male baboons may persist for several hours in harassing adult male chimpanzees who are controlling a supply of bananas. This harassment involves repeated, close-range threats, including display of the massive canine teeth. Occasional short runs to grab for a banana also occur. But the baboons rarely get more than a banana peel, at least until the chimpanzees have had an abundant intake.

In these persistent agonistic encounters over a premium food, baboons frequently break off contact with the adult male chimpanzees and attack a female or juvenile chimpanzee (who has no bananas). The latter usually defend themselves by rapidly climbing the nearest tree, striking downward with the fist, hitting at the baboon snout. Thus, it appears that redirected aggression may occur between these two primate species, as well as within each species.

It may be useful here to summarize briefly the variety of situations that elicit aggressive behavior in chimpanzees. From GOODALL's observations,[8] our own, and those of other workers,[19,9,20] it appears that threat or attack patterns are likely to occur in the following contexts: (1) competition over food, especially if highly desirable foods are spatially concentrated or in short supply; (2) defense of an infant by its mother; (3) a contest over the dominance prerogatives of two individuals of similar social rank; (4) redirection of aggression (e.g., when a low-ranking male has been attacked by a high-ranking male and immediately turns to attack an individual subordinate to him); (5) a failure of one animal to comply with a signal given by the aggressor (e.g. when one chimpanzee does not respond to another's invitation to groom); (6) strange appearance of another chimpanzee (e.g. a chimpanzee whose lower extremities became paralyzed); (7) changes in dominance status over time, especially among males; (8) the formation of consort pairs at the peak of estrus (the discovery of consort pairing in chimpanzees is so recent that this situation needs much clarification); (9) contacts between relatively unfamiliar chimpanzees; (10) hunting and killing of small animals (e.g. infant baboon, infant colobus monkey). Thus, as with baboons, many of the situations eliciting aggressive behavior involve: (1) protection, or (2) access to valued resources.

Since various biological indices suggest a particularly close relation between chimpanzee and gorilla, it is interesting to note several aggression-relevant patterns that are especially prominent in one or both of these species.[8,21-24]

1. Both chimpanzee and gorilla show more elaborate aggressive displays than any other primate species. This rich repertoire of threatening actions might well be called intimidation display. The patterns of submission and reassurance also seem to be more elaborate in these species than in other primates, and more similar to man.

2. In chimpanzees, 'technology' is more advanced than anything observed elsewhere among non-human primates. Simple tools are made according to an established tradition and used effectively. Both spherical and cylindrical objects, naturally occurring, are used in threat and attack, sometimes with considerable efficacy.[25]

3. In chimpanzees, attachments based on kinship strongly influence behavior over a large part of the life span—quite possibly all of it. Among other influences, kinship attachments tend to increase: (a) threat directed towards animals not part of the kinship subgroup; (b) protection of offspring's aggressive ventures in early life (especially male offspring) by the mother, and probably by older siblings as well.

DOMINANCE RELATIONS

In commenting on primate field stuidies of agonistic behavior, RIOCH highlights dominance relations.[3] He points out, "Most of the authors . . . have described chiefly competitive combative behavior, with emphasis on the complaints of the subordinate member, but they also emphasize the infrequency of disabling or lethal damage . . . There seems to be general agreement among all observers on the importance of this limited agonistic behavior for maintaining the hierarchical structure of the group, though the rigidity–flexibility dimension seems to vary with the species . . . All authors also agree on the finding that the dominant animals bear scars from their careers."

Dominance is assessed by observing who gives way to whom in situations of biologic relevance such as the presence of sought-after foods, females at the peak of estrus, or

P

preferred sleeping sites.[26] Thus, the high-ranking males get maximum access to preferred objects, animals, and locations.[27,28] In baboons and chimpanzees, the most dominant male has primary access and precedence over a very broad range of circumstances.[29] To the extent that any constraints are imposed on him, they seem to reflect in part the traditions of the group.[2] He appears to be the object of great interest within the group, receiving much attention including grooming.

Recent observations at the Gombe Stream Reserve have added much new information on dominance relations among chimpanzees.[8] This new information has been made possible by detailed, close range, longitudinal observations of individually-recognized animals. The partial clearing of one small area of forest, with provision of bananas as a dietary supplement in this area, may have accentuated dominance behavior because the bananas are a highly sought-after food, present here in rather short supply and in spatially concentrated arrangement. However, the relations are basically the same elsewhere in the forest. Some of the main points emerging from these recent observations are briefly summarized here. (1) Males are dominant over females. (2) Females are dominant over young. (3) Dominance relations are not strictly linear on an individual basis. They are also influenced by temporary associations, coalitions and enduring preferences. These latter are sometimes based on sibling relationships. (4) Aggressive displays by high-ranking males seem to reinforce status in relation to other adult males, but attacks and injuries to females and immature animals are not unusual during these dispalys. (5) All animals in this chimpanzee community of 45 animals respond differentially to each other in terms of dominance status; these differential responses appear to be learned during the first few years of life. (6) Attributes contributing to high dominance status include not only size and strength, but also coordination, motivation, and ingenuity (especially in the use of objects). (7) Mothers protect their offspring in aggressive encounters with other animals. Hence, the mother's dominance status has a considerable bearing on the ultimate dominance status of her offspring; this has also been observed in macaques when study conditions permitted longitudinal observation of individually recognized animals.

Since the primates in a local group respond differentially to each other from an early age, it appears that they are quick to learn dominance relations.[8] These relations, once established, tend to minimize serious fighting over considerable periods, at least on a time scale of months. Thus,[12,30] the ordering of individuals gives considerable predictability to the social system and appears to enhance stability of the group.[31] In these stable periods, status appears to be reinforced frequently by threats and, especially in chimpanzees, by elaborate aggressive displays. Subordinate animals give a variety of signals in response to such threats that seem to indicate recognition of status differences. These signals include facial expressions, tail positions, vocalizations, specific postures and gestures. Taken together, these signals may be considered deference behavior; they are most elaborately developed in chimpanzees, where a complex behavioral sequence has been described: threat–submission–reassurance.[8]

Such periods of stability are not permanent. From time to time, an individual makes persistent efforts to change his status. This is particularly characteristic of adolescent and young adult males, though it occurs in other circumstances as well. These change-of-status periods are associated with a considerable increase in overt fighting. This includes both: (1) attacks directed upward, challenging the position of a higher-ranking animal; and (2) attacks directed downward, when a challenging animal breaks off from encounters with a higher-ranking animal and attacks a smaller, weaker, or less mobile animal. The latter pattern, commonly observed in many primate species, is sometimes referred to as redirection of aggressive behavior.

Dominance relations exist not only between individuals but also between groups.[12] In baboons and in rhesus macaques, group size is correlated with group dominance. At water holes, for example, a small troop of baboons gives way to a large troop. Even the appearance of a few members of a dominant group will sometimes be sufficient to displace an entire subordinate group. In these inter-group encounters, as in inter-individual encounters, fighting is rare though threats are common. However, as Rioch's remark implies, occasional serious fighting does occur, and many animals bear scars from these encounters.[32,33] These fights are principally male activities. In inter-group as well as inter-individual dominance relations, much individual learning of group traditions evidently occurs. There is a great need for field studies that focus primarily on relations between groups.

GROOMING BEHAVIOR

Grooming—taking the fingers and lips and going down through the hair to the skin in a deliberate, repeated way—is one of the most prominent behavior patterns in non-human primates.[7,34] This activity has a grossly observable cleansing effect, removing debris from wounds, and all sorts of foreign matter from the skin and fur. However, even in laboratories where the primates are free of ectoparasites, dirt, burrs, and other foreign matter, a substantial proportion of each day is spent in grooming activities.

In both natural habitats and laboratories, there appears to be a sex difference in grooming, with females spending a larger proportion of their time grooming other animals—from early life onwards. However, both sexes appear to find the experience of being groomed intrinsically rewarding. They actively solicit grooming from other animals, and usually reciprocate when solicited by other animals. In studies where geneaological relations are known, it appears that most social grooming occurs between closely related animals.[35]

In our observations, chimpanzees show an increased intensity and duration of grooming in two situations: (1) immediately after an elaborate male aggressive display; and (2) when closely ranked, competitive males are in the presence of a highly sought-after food. The emphasis on grooming in these agonistic circumstances is consistent with other observations suggesting that grooming tends to regulate aggression and promote cohesion in strongly dominance-oriented species.[6]

Among chimpanzees, baboons, and several species of macaques, threats are rarely directed toward high ranking animals, and attacks upward are exceedingly rare. Most aggression is directed downward, i.e. toward lower ranking animals. On the other hand, grooming tends to be directed upward in several species.[26,36] Both the frequency and duration of receiving grooming are highly correlated with status. So, dominance affords priority in respect to grooming as well as to food and sex.

LEARNING OF AGGRESSIVE BEHAVIOR

Chimpanzees acquire considerable skill in using tools in agonistic encounters. Some throw stones with notable accuracy. Some wield 'clubs'. We saw a 4-yr-old male—only about one-third of the way to full maturity—attack an adult male baboon with a 10-ft palm frond, driving him off in to the forest. This young chimpanzee had watched two older siblings engaging in much the same kind of behavior over the preceding 2 yr. The infant repeated their behavior from an early point in his life, initially in a very clumsy way after observing them at length; eventually he perfected the skill and used it effectively against the formidable adult male baboon.

This observational learning of complex aggressive patterns highlights a sequence that is prominent in adaptation of primates to natural habitats; observation, imitation, practice.[37] The young have access to almost the whole repertoire of adult behavior with respect to aggression, sex, feeding, and all other activities.[38] The young observe intently, and then imitate, cautiously at first, various behavior sequences; including the aggressive patterns; in respect to the latter, male infants seem more interested than females among the chimpanzees and baboons we observed.

In field and experimental studies there is considerable evidence of learning in regard to aggressive behavior. In non-human primate societies, especially among the ground-living species, aggressive behavior is present in abundance, with many similarities in its expression and in the contexts of its occurrence. But there are variations in keeping with local conditions, even within a species. So perhaps it has been adaptive in evolution to learn easily when and how to be aggressive, flexibly in keeping with environmental conditions.

Since the human species relies upon learning in adaptation even more than these close biological relatives, the primate studies call attention to analogous processes in human infancy, childhood and adolescence. What are the crucial modes of learning for human aggressive patterns? Are there internal dispositions that affect the ease with which such patterns are learned? Are there sensitive periods of development that crucially affect later aggressive behavior? As the studies of non-human primates progress, they may help to guide research on development of behavior into lines that take account of man's biological heritage.

Several findings of non-human primate research are of special interest in relation to recent human studies: (1) differential preferences and/or facility for clearing aggressive patterns; (2) stranger contact as an instigation for agonistic behavior; (3) the potency of observational learning from models who behave aggressively.

McGrew has recently conducted studies of young children—studies that utilize the methods and findings of primate ethology.[39,40] To a substantial extent, he is able to apply behavioral categories of non-human primates directly to young children. His research has examined the introduction of new children (ages 3–5) into a nursery school group. He finds that significant changes in agonistic behavior occur with such contact between strangers. Moreover, he finds a sex difference in nursery school behavior, with males showing more agonistic and quasiagonistic behavior than females.

This early sex difference is consonant with other findings in both human and non-human primates. Several studies have recently reported human behavioral sex differences in early infancy. A comprehensive survey of sex differences in aggressive behavior, utilizing various measures at different age levels of childhood and adolescence, showed a consistent finding: boys are more aggressive than girls, especially on measures of physical (as compared with verbal) aggression.[41] Most of these studies focus on the 3–6 age range.

Another point of contact between recent research on human and non-human primates lies in the body of observation, experiment and theory on the social learning of aggressive behavior by young children.[42] In a major series of experiments with children of nursery school age, it has been shown that they learn aggressive patterns with remarkable facility by viewing models who act aggressively. Specific aggressive patterns are readily acquired by viewing actual persons or filmed persons or filmed cartoons—so long as these patterns are clearly displayed by the actors. These patterns are imitated by the child in play following exposure to the model, and persist in the child's behavioral repertoire for months after a single exposure. Such imitation is greater when the model has been rewarded in the drama than when he has been punished.

Thus, there is emerging evidence that primates readily learn aggressive patterns through observational learning in a social context, shaped by rewards and punishments in social interactions; and that males in some way come to express such patterns more forcefully than females. Recent research indicates that the early exposure of developing brain to testosterone is important in the sex difference, though the mechanism of action is far from clear.[43,44] This does not, however, suggest that testosterone establishes fixed patterns of complex behavior, unmodifiable by subsequent events. More likely, the hormone affects the brain in such a way as to facilitate the learning of aggressive patterns later in life.

For any species, some patterns of behavior are easy to learn, some fairly difficult, and some exceedingly difficult. In general, patterns that have been valuable in species survival are easy to learn. The developing primate does not imitate every action it observes. Indeed, the range of stimulation available to it in the natural habitat is very great. In some way, primates are selective about the patterns that elicit persistent imitation. One line of selectivity appears to be sex-differentiated in baboons and chimpanzees: young males tend to imitate threat and attack patterns more than do young females.[8]

Another line of selectivity has been explored experimentally to some extent. Monkeys were raised in a total isolation chamber for the first 9 months of life, during which they were exposed to various types of visual input from coloured slides.[44] These slides depicted monkeys in various activities and also depicted various non-monkey stimuli. Among the categories presented, monkey pictures elicited much more interest than non-monkey pictures. Moreover, pictures of monkeys showing a species-typical threat expression were especially potent in eliciting behavioral responses. Between $2\frac{1}{2}$ and 4 months of age, threat pictures yielded a particularly high frequency of disturbance. Similar results were obtained with the use of motion picture films in the same experimental design. This work suggests that the infant rhesus has a built-in, special responsiveness to the threatening facial expression which is characteristic of its species. Once the infant monkey's attention is powerfully drawn to threat stimuli, it can learn the conditions under which threat and attack patterns are likely to occur, and the actions likely to terminate aggressive sequences. These events are vivid in natural habitats.

These monkey experiments raise the question whether any similar period exists in human development which is distinctively sensitive for the learning of aggression-relevant orientations. One interesting possibility—especially in light of the data on stranger-contact as an elicitor of aggressive responses in non-human primates—lies in recent research on reactions to strangers in human infants.[46-49] Earlier impressions about fearful, avoidance reactions to strangers have lately been subjected to experimental scrutiny. In about half the infants studied, 'stranger anxiety' is clearly observable in the middle of the first year of life and increases well into the second year of life. Indeed, in a study of Kalahari Bushmen, Konner is finding that stranger anxiety does not reach its peak until the second half of the second year, somewhat later than in Western studies (DeVore, personal communication). In general, adult males seem to elicit stronger avoidance responses than do adult females. The combination of a strange person in a strange place is especially potent in eliciting emotional disturbance in the infant. The mother's presence tends to diminish such reactions. Altogether, these studies suggest that there may be a period of about 1 year's duration during which the human infant is quite sensitive to contact with strangers. The mother's reactions to strangers during this period probably are important in shaping the infant's responses to them. Cultural and subcultural differences may enter here as well. Its remains for future investigation to determine whether this period of stranger-sensitivity may be utilized in some circumstances to shape attitudes toward out-groups or even to foster suspicion in all future human relationships.

CONCLUDING COMMENT

In closing, I should like to underscore RIOCH's plea for the development of a discipline of social biology.[3] He says, "The studies on social behavior and group organization of primates reported . . . during recent years give promise that the need for a social biology will soon be met." Other lines of inquiry offer similar promise. Indeed, the conjunction of many established disciplines will be needed to clarify the crucial interpenetrations of biological and social processes in adaptation. Such conjunction has so far rarely been achieved. But no one has shown the way more clearly than David Rioch—in the Division of Neuropsychiatry which he built and in his own creative vision of brain and behavior.

REFERENCES

1. HINDE, R. A. and TINBERGEN, N. The comparative study of species-specific behavior. In: *Behavior and Evolution*, ROE, A. and SIMPSON, G. G. (Eds), p. 251. Yale University Press, New Haven, 1958.
2. WASHBURN, S. L. and HAMBURG, D. A. The study of primate behavior. In: *Primate Behavior: Field Studies of Monkeys and Apes*, DEVORE, I. (Ed.), p. 1. Holt, Rinehart and Winston, New York, 1965.
3. RIOCH, D. M. Discussion of agonistic behavior. In: *Social Communication Among Primates*, ALTMANN, S. A. (Ed.), p. 115. University of Chicago Press, Chicago, 1967.
4. HAMBURG, D. A. An evolutionary perspective on human aggressiveness. In: *The Field of Psychiatry: Essays in Honor of Roy R. Grinker, Sr.* OFFER, D. and FREEDMAN, D. X. (Eds.) Basic Books, New York, 1971.

5. ALTMANN, S. A. *Social Communication Among Primates*, University of Chicago Press, Chicago, 392 pp., 1967.
6. BOELKINS, R. C. and HEISER, J. F. Biological bases of aggression. In: *Violence and the Struggle for Existence*, DANIELS, D. N., GILUIA, M. F. and OCHBERG, F. M. (Eds.), p. 15. Little, Brown & Co., Boston, 1970.
7. DEVORE, I. (Ed.), *Primate Behavior: Field Studies of Monkeys and Apes*, Holt, Rinehart & Winston, New York, 1965.
8. GOODALL, J. v. L. The behavior of free-living chimpanzees in the Gombe Stream Reserve. In: *Animal Behavior Monographs*, CULLEN, J. M. and BEER, C. G. (Eds.) p. 165. Bailliere, Tindall & Cassell, London, 1968.
9. REYNOLDS, V. and REYNOLDS, F. Chimpanzees of the Budongo Forest. In: *Primate Behavior, Field Studies of Monkeys and Apes*, DEVORE, I. (Ed.), p. 368. Holt, Rinehart & Winston, New York, 1965.
10. ROWELL, T. E. Forest-living baboons in Uganda. *J. Zool.* **149**, 344, 1968.
11. ROWELL, T. E. A quantitive comparison of the behavior of a wild and a caged baboon group. *Anim. Behav.* **15**, 499, 1967.
12. WASHBURN, S. L. and HAMBURG, D. A. Aggressive behavior in old world monkeys and apes. In: *Primates: Studies in Adaptation and Variability*, JAY, P. C. (Ed.), p. 458. Holt, Rinehart & Winston, New York, 1968.
13. DEVORE, I. and HALL, K. R. L. Baboon ecology. In: *Primate Behavior: Field Studies of Monkeys and Apes*, DEVORE, I. (Ed.), p. 20. Holt, Rinehart & Winston, New York, 1965.
14. HALL, K. R. L. and DEVORE, I. Baboon social behavior. In: *Primate Behavior: Field Studies of Monkeys and Apes*, DEVORE, I. (Ed.), p. 53. Holt, Rinehart & Winston, New York, 1965.
15. RANSOM, T. Observations of baboons at the Gombe Stream Reserve. Presentations at Stanford University and University of California, Berkeley, 1969.
16. GOODALL, J. v. L. Chimpanzees of the Gombe Stream Reserve. *Primate Behavior: Field Studies of Monkeys and Apes*, DEVORE, I. (Ed.), p. 425, Holt, Rinehart and Winston, New York, 1965.
17. GOODALL, J. v. L. Mother-offspring relationships in free-ranging chimpanzees. In: *Primate Ethology* MORRIS, D. (Ed.), p. 287. Aldine, Chicago, 1967.
18. GOODALL, J. v. L. A preliminary report on expressive movements and communication in the Gombe Stream chimpanzees. In: *Primates: Studies in Adaptation and Variability*, JAY, P. C. (Ed.), p. 313. Holt, Rinehart & Winston, New York, 1968.
19. KAWABE, M. One observed case of hunting behavior among wild chimpanzees living in the savanna woodland of Western Tanzania. *Primates* **7**, 393, 1966.
20. WILSON, W. L. and WILSON, C. C. Aggressive interactions of captive chimpanzees living in a semi-free ranging environment. 6571st Aeromed. Res. Lab. Tech. Rep. No. ARL-TR-68-9, Holloman Air Force Base, New Mexico, 1968.
21. FOSSEY, DIAN. Personal communication. Miss Fossey is conducting a systematic, long-term study of mountain gorilla, utilizing close-range observation in a natural habitat.
22. REYNOLDS, V. Some behavioral comparisons between the chimpanzee and the mountain gorilla in the wild. *Am. Anthrop.* **67**, 691, 1965.
23. SCHALLER, G. B. The behavior of the mountain gorilla. In: *Primate Behavior: Field Studies of Monkeys and Apes*, DEVORE, I. (Ed.), p. 324. Holt, Rinehart & Winston, New York, 1965.
24. SCHALLER, G. B. *The Mountain Gorilla: Ecology and Behavior*, University of Chicago Press, Chicago, 1963.
25. GOODALL, J. v. L. Tool-using and aimed throwing in a community of free-living chimpanzees. *Nature, Lond.* **201**, 264, 1964.
26. BOELKINS, R. C. Determination of dominance hierarchies in monkeys. *Psychon. Sci.* **7**, 317, 1967.
27. DELGADO, J. M. R. Social rank and radio-stimulated aggressiveness in monkeys. *J. nerve. ment. Dis.* **144**, 383, 1967.
28. WASHBURN, S. L. Conflict in primate society. In: *Conflict in Society*, DEREUCK, A. and KNIGHT, J. (Eds.), p. 3. Little, Brown & Co., Boston, 1966.
29. DEVORE, I. Male dominance and mating behavior in baboons. In: *Sex and Behavior*, BEACH, F. A. (Ed.), p. 266. Wiley, New York, 1965.
30. TOKUDA, K. and JENSEN, G. D. The leader's role in controlling aggressive behavior in a monkey group. *Primates* **9**, 319, 1968.
31. SOUTHWICK, C. H. and SIDDIGI, R. The role of social tradition in the maintenance of dominance in a wild rhesus group. *Primates* **8**, 341, 1967.

32. HAMBURG, D. A. Society, stress, and aggressive behavior. Presented at WHO Symposium, Stockholm, 1970. To be published in *Society, Stress and Disease*, LEVI, L. (Ed.) Oxford University Press, New York, 1971.

33. SOUTHWICK, C. H. Aggressive behavior, of rhesus monkeys in natural and captive groups. In: *Aggressive Behavior*, GARATTINI, S. and SIGG, E. B. (Eds.), p. 32. Wiley Interscience, New York, 1969.

34. JAY, P. G. *Primates: Studies in Adaptation and Variability*, Holt, Rinehart & Winston, New York, 1968.

35. LINDBURG, D. Observations of rhesus macaque in natural habitats. Presented at Department of Psychiatry, Stanford University, November, 1969.

36. BOELKINS, R. C. Grooming, aggression, and group cohesion. Presented at American Sociological Association annual meeting, San Francisco, September, 1969.

37. HAMBURG, D. A. Observations of mother-infant interaction in primate field studies. In: *Determinants of Infant Behavior IV*, FOSS, B. M. (Ed.), p. 3. Methuen & Co., London, 1969.

38. HALL, K. R. L. Social learning in monkeys. In: *Primates: Studies in Adaptation and Variability*, JAY, P. C. (Ed.), p. 383. Holt, Rinehart & Winston, New York, 1968.

39. McGREW, W. C. Aspects of social development in nursery school children with emphasis on introduction to the group. In: *Ethological Studies of Human Behavior*, BLURTON-JONES, N. (Ed.) in press.

40. McGREW, W. C. An ethological study of agonistic behavior in preschool children. *Proc. Second Int. Congr. Primatology* 1, p. 149. Karger, Basel/New York, 1969.

41. MACCOBY, E. (Ed.), *The Development of Sex Differences*, Stanford University Press, Stanford, 1966.

42. BANDURA, A. *Aggression: A Social Learning Interpretation*, to be published.

43. GARATTINI, S. and SIGG, E. B. (Eds.), *Aggressive Behavior* Wiley, New York, 1969.

44. HAMBURG, D. A. A combined biological and psychosocial approach to the study of behavioral development. In: *Stimulation in Early Infancy*, AMBROSE, A. (Ed.), p. 269. Academic Press, New York, 1969.

45. SACKETT, G. P. Monkeys reared in isolation with pictures as visual input: Evidence for an innate releasing mechanism. *Science* 154, 1468, 1966.

46. AINSWORTH, M. D. S. and WITTIG, B. A. Attachment and exploratory behavior of one-year-olds in a strange situation. In: *Determinants of Infant Behavior IV*, FOSS, B. M. (Ed.), p. 111. Methuen & Co., London, 1969.

47. MORGAN, G. A. and RICCIUTI, H. N. Infants' responses to strangers during the first year. In: *Determinants of Infant Behavior IV*, FOSS, B. M. (Ed.), p. 253. Methuen & Co., London, 1969.

48. RHEINGOLD, H. L. The effect of a strange environment on the behavior of infants. In: *Determinants of Infant Behavior IV*, FOSS, B. M. (Ed.), p. 137. Methuen & Co., London, 1969.

49. RICCIUTI, H. N. Social and emotional behavior in infancy: Some developmental issues and problems. *Merrill–Palmer Quarterly of Behavior and Development*, 14, 82, 1969.

J. psychiat. Res., 1971, Vol. 8, pp. 399–412. Pergamon Press. Printed in Great Britain

QUANTITATIVE HEDONISM*

R. J. HERRNSTEIN

Harvard University, Cambridge, Massachusetts

LET US start by considering a pigeon in action. It flies or walks or perches quietly; it eats and drinks and tends its young; it bills and coos; it cocks its head and pecks at the ground; it scratches itself and ruffles its feathers; it fights for a place in the social order. We may be unimpressed with its repertoire compared to more interesting creatures (like people), but compared to any inanimate object, to even the most versatile computerized robot, it is vastly endowed with variety. And not only are its actions diverse, they are interwoven in ever-shifting configurations, so that no simple recounting of what has gone before can usefully summarize even one pigeon's behavior, let alone that for pigeons or creatures in general. The common assumption, however, is that there is a kind of sensible order, even if not of the type we expect in inanimate objects. We expect the pigeon to be acting in accordance with its needs and circumstances—eating, drinking, mating, fighting, roosting, and so on, as necessary to sustain itself and promote its kind. But this teleological conviction cannot serve as the underlying principle to explain how the pigeon chooses among its virtually countless alternatives for action, for it is circular. We expect the pigeon to work for what it needs, but we know, finally, what it needs largely from the testimony of what it works for.

The problem is to make sense of our intuition that action is affected by its consequences to the actor, with reward strengthening, or punishment weakening, the behavior that gives rise to them. Adaptiveness is elegantly accounted for if the pigeon does whatever is pleasurable (and therefore rewarding), avoids whatever is painful (and therefore punishing), and its pleasures and pains are so constituted that doing what comes naturally is by and large doing the right thing (pragmatically, if not morally). This is, of course, just the venerable hedonistic doctrine, which modern psychology has taken over notwithstanding its long and stormy history in philosophy. But if the doctrine is not to slip back into the circularity of which it was both accused and guilty, it must seek the concrete, functional relationships between reward and punishment, on the one hand, and the strength of behavior, on the other. Or, to use the parlance of modern psychology, the principle of reinforcement must either be stated objectively or not at all.

---

* Preparation of this paper was supported by a grant from the National Institutes of Mental Health to Harvard University.

The occasion for this article is the conviction that a precise statement of reinforcement may be at hand, growing out of the discovery that the frequencies of alternative forms of behavior occur in the same proportion as the resulting reinforcements. The meaning of this simple principle is best inferred from the experiments that substantiate it. About a decade ago, I did an experiment[1] in which hungry pigeons were trained to peck at either of 2 disks side by side on the wall of an experimental chamber measuring a foot cubed. Pecking at the disks produced some pigeon feed. The schedules of reinforcement were based on the passage of time, rather than on how hard the pigeons worked. For example, at one point, pecking at one of the disks was reinforced on the average of once in 3 min, with successive reinforcements occurring at irregular intervals ranging between 5 sec and 7 min. At other times, the average interval between reinforcements was different, but the basic procedure was the same. This schedule is called a 'variable interval' and is defined as a series of minimum inter-reinforcement times. The actual inter-reinforcement times depend on how soon the subject responds after an interval in the series times out. Because the pigeons almost always pecked rapidly as compared to the scheduled intervals of reinforcement, the difference between the minimum and the actual intervals was negligible. The schedules for the two disks were mutually independent, so that reinforcement for pecking one disk had no effect on the schedule for the other. At any given moment, there might be reinforcement due for pecking at neither, either, or both disks. Once an interval timed out for one disk, it remained so until the pigeon collected the reinforcement or until the end of the day's experimental session, which typically lasted about an hour and a half. The sole connection between the two schedules was that their average intervals were chosen to keep the maximum possible rate of reinforcements constant at 40 per hr. When, for example, the schedule for 1 disk was set at an average of 3 min (20 reinforcements per hr), the schedule for the other also averaged 3 min. When it was changed to 4·5 min (13·3 reinforcements per hr) for 1 disk, the other was changed to 2·25 min (26·7 reinforcements per hr), and so on. This rate of reinforcement does not much change the pigeon's state of hunger over an experimental session.

During the course of the experiment, a number of different average inter-reinforcement times were used for pecking at each disk. At each new value, the pigeons were given as many daily sessions in the chamber as it took for the rate of pecking to achieve day-to-day stability, usually about 1–2 months. The main finding was that each pigeon distributed its pecking at the disks in the same proportion as the reinforcements. For example, when there were 20 reinforcements per hr for each disk, pecking was equally distributed between the disks. For each new set of reinforcement frequencies, and 6 pairs over the range were tried, the pecking readjusted appropriately (see Fig. 1, right panel). The pigeons pecked at a total rate of approximately 4000 responses an hr throughout the experiment, which, given the 40 reinforcements per hr, means about 100 pecks per reinforcement. This ratio of work to pay remained constant for each disk separately and for both together at all rates of reinforcement. The findings are summarized most easily by a simple equation (in which P stands for number of pecks, R for number of reinforcements, and subscripts for left and right):

$$\frac{P_L}{P_L + P_R} = \frac{R_L}{R_L + R_R} \tag{1}$$

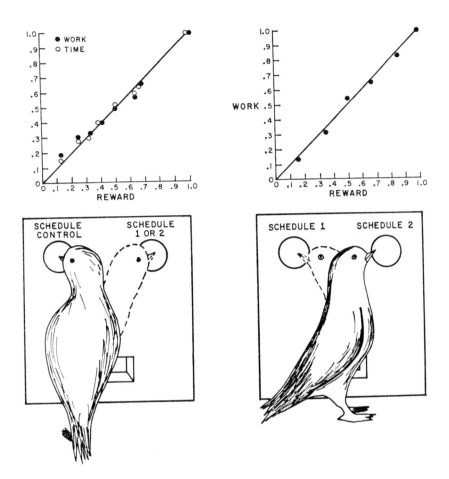

FIG. 1.   Proportion of behavior as a function of proportion of reinforcement ('reward'), for two procedures. On the left, the pigeon can switch back and forth between two schedules by pecking at the left disk (adapted from Catania, 1963). On the right, the pigeon switches simply by moving from side to side.

Although the pigeons were choosing between alternatives with uncertain consequences, this experiment and its outcome are to be distinguished from common gambling situations and the experimental studies of choice that mimic them. In ordinary games of chance, the probabilities of winning or losing are pre-set. There is, for example, 1 chance in 36 of rolling a sum of 12 on 2 honest dice, 6 chances in 36 of rolling a sum of 7, and so on. In the game of craps, the odds should be obvious to any player. In other games, for example with a slot machine ('one-armed bandit'), the odds may be obvious only to the house. But in either case, and in the typical choice experiment, the *rate* of winning (as distinguished from the *probability*) is determined by the rate of play, given the odds. If we are betting that

a sum of 12 will turn up, then the rate with which the crap-shooter throws the dice determines how fast our fortune shrinks or grows. For any given wager, the average relation
between the rate of play and the rate of winning (or losing) is a direct proportionality. In
the pigeon experiment, however, the rate of winning (i.e. reinforcement) was not much
affected by the rate of play because the underlying schedules were variable intervals. With
interval schedules, the only effect of the rate of work on the rate of pay is the difference
between the maximum possible and the actual rate of reinforcement, which was, as noted
above, negligible in the pigeon experiment. In contrast to ordinary games, an interval
schedule pre-sets the rate of winning, while the probability is an outcome of the behavior.
The faster the work on an interval schedule, the smaller the ratio of wins to 'plays,' hence
the smaller the probability of reinforcement. The relations between probabilities and rate
of winning are, in other words, diametrically opposite in classical games and interval
schedules.

In spite, then, of the superficial similarities, the pigeon experiment differs from probabilistic
situations in the underlying probability and frequency relations. Is the difference important?
In a simple game, if a subject is given a choice between alternatives that pay the same
amount, but with different probabilities, he typically chooses the better one virtually every
time and thereby maximizes his winnings. The pigeon experiment, with its variable-interval
schedules, does not have an 'optimal' solution in this sense, since winning depends on the
passage of time rather than the number of responses. Although the exclusive preference of
classical games may seem inconsistent with the graded preferences of the pigeon experiment,
it is, in fact, precisely consistent with equation (1), albeit trivially. Equation (1) says only
that the proportion of responses matches the proportion of reinforcements, which is as
true of exclusive preference as it is of the results of the pigeon experiment. It can, in fact,
be shown (but not here) that when choices have different probabilities of winning, the *only*
way to conform to equation (1) is by preferring one exclusively. In general, it can be said
that whether or not a procedure permits maximizing, the distribution of choices that differ
only in their outcome may, and most often does, conform to equation (1). The qualifications
to this bold statement are too technical (and secondary) to call for further discussion
here.[2]

The first question to ask about equation (1) is whether nontrivial confirmation requires
pigeons, or whether other creatures also distribute their behavior thus. Although much of
the relevant research has, in fact, been on pigeons, there is some on mammals. An experiment
by SHULL and PLISKOFF[3] (working at Arizona State University and the University of
Maryland) substituted rats for pigeons. In addition, the response was lever pressing instead
of disk pecking, and the reinforcer, instead of food, was electrical stimulation through
implanted electrodes of a region of the brain known to be rewarding. Nevertheless, the
distribution of responses still matched the distribution of reinforcements, in agreement
with equation (1).

SCHROEDER and HOLLAND[4] have reported a considerably more exotic confirmation of
the relation. They had undergraduates at the University of Pittsburgh looking at some dials
on a display. Two dials were on the left and 2 on the right, and any dial could show either a
deflected or a non-deflected pointer. The subject's task was to report deflections, indicating
whether they were on the right or left. The apparatus included an eye-movement camera

that kept a record of the direction of gaze. It was found that the distribution of eye movements matched the distribution of pointer deflections. In other words, when the procedure had 80 per cent of the deflections occurring on the right-hand dials, then 80 per cent of the eye movements were to the right side, and similarly at other percentages. The behavior of glancing conformed to equation (1), assuming that the subjects were being reinforced by their successes. Even in the secondary features of the results—too minor to be described here—these human subjects were in accord with the pigeons.

It has been shown that when the amount of food per reinforcement is allowed to vary, the matching relation (equation (1)) applies to the relative amounts of food rather than the relative frequencies of reinforcement. The indications from a number of experiments are that matching reflects the total effective reinforcement for each response, taking all relevant features of the reinforcer into account—its rate, amount, immediacy, and no doubt its quality, if these are allowed to vary. If this is right, it provides a basis for constructing meaningful scales of reinforcing power. For example, a hungry monkey choosing between raisins and peanuts would no doubt deviate from the matching relation if simple counts of reinforcement frequency were taken. However, analysis would show how the counts need to be transformed to restore matching. As far as reinforcement is concerned, peanuts would be equivalent to some function of raisins (or *vice versa*). Equation (1) may thus grow from description to norm, providing a means of attaching numbers to reinforcers on purely psychological grounds.

The experiments noted so far show that the matching relation holds for at least several species (including man), that the reinforcer may be at least as different as food, direct stimulation of the brain, and finding deflected pointers, and that various sorts of repetitive tasks may serve as the response. The range of applicable situations is, however, still broader than this. For example, one may wonder whether it is necessary that the response be relatively easy for the subject. Pecking a disk, pressing a lever, or moving the eyes are trivial investments for possibly sizeable gains. Perhaps, it might be supposed, if the response were more costly in psychological terms, the matching would be affected. This would be important to know, for in natural (as distinguished from laboratory) situations, the impediments to action are often substantial. It seems, however, that matching describes even very demanding responses, as in a study by HOLZ,[5] of Smith, Kline and French Co. The pigeons in his experiment had the usual 2 disks to peck at for an occasional bit of food, but in addition each peck fired a brief surge of electric shock into the pigeon's pelvic region through permanently implanted wires. Either disk gave the same shock, but from time to time the level was changed. Sometimes the shock was mild and perhaps unfelt; at other times, it was strong enough to stop all pecking, but mostly, it was in between. As long as the pigeons continued to peck at all, the proportion of responses to each disk equalled its proportion of reinforcements, as the matching relation requires. Even though the *rate* of pecking was significantly reduced by the stronger shocks, the *proportions* continued to follow equation (1). If the shocks for the two responses had been dissimilar instead of always equal, then the matching relation would have required some other proportionality, taking into account the total effective consequence, both rewarding and punishing, of each response.

Costly responses are, then, no less amenable to equation (1) than easy ones, but Holz's experiment, like the others, used repetitive responding. It could be argued that the repetitive behavior in these experiments is highly artificial and therefore irrelevant. 'Real' behavior, it might be said, comes in a continuous stream—hard, if not impossible to quantify precisely. In one form or another, the criticism of artificiality is heard by all of us who try to make quantitative sense out of psychological phenomena. It should get a comprehensive answer sometime, but for now it must suffice to note that BROWNSTEIN and PLISKOFF[6] have shown that matching is not restricted to measures of repetitive responding. Their pigeons were given the chance to choose between blue or amber illumination of the experimental chamber. One peck at a disk changed it to amber if it was blue and vice versa. Every now and then, the pigeon (which was hungry) was given a bit of food irrespective of its behavior, but the rate of feedings depended on the color of illumination. At any moment, the pigeon could switch from one schedule of feedings to the other. Except for the lack of a response requirement, the two schedules were variable intervals running concurrently, so that it was advantageous for the pigeons to switch back and forth to collect the feedings that were coming due. When a feeding was scheduled for the color not present, it was held in reserve until the pigeon switched colors. The dynamics of the situation were therefore much like those of the original pigeon experiment showing matching, with the difference that here there were no reinforced responses to count. The numbers of color-switching responses could not, themselves, have shown matching, since there have to be as many switches to a color as there are away from it, plus or minus one. However, matching was found anyway, for the pigeons kept the proportion of time spent in a given color of illumination equal to the proportion of reinforcements obtained therein.

Animals may use time to distribute their behavior even when work is required, not just when the pay comes freely. CATANIA[7], now at New York University, has shown how amount of work (i.e. number of responses) and time at work interact in one procedure. As before, the subjects were pigeons, the response was pecking at one or the other of 2 disks, and the reinforcer was food. And also as before, the food came on a pair of variable-interval schedules. The difference in Catania's experiment was that only the pecking at the right disk was ever reinforced with food (see Fig. 1, left panel). The effect of pecking at the left disk was to control the schedule on the right by switching one for the other and back. Suppose, for example, that the two schedules are variable intervals with averages of 2 and 4 min, whose accessibility is signalled by having the right disk either red or green, respectively. When the right disk is red, a peck at the left disk turns it green and switches from the 2-min to the 4-min schedule. A peck at the left disk would now switch it back. The two schedules run concurrently, so that reinforcement may be pending on the schedule not presently accessible, in which case it is held in reserve until the switch is made. The point of the procedure (which was originated by FINDLEY,[8] now of Johns Hopkins) is to yield separate measures for amount of work and time at work for the two alternatives (and also to provide a clear measure of switching behavior). With the Findley procedure, the subject gives us, separately, the number of responses for each alternative, and a partition of the time in the chamber spent with each alternative, whereas in an ordinary choice experiment (also shown in Fig. 1), the partition of time can only be estimated indirectly. As the chart shows, both work and time matched the relative reinforcement. If the pigeon was receiving 50 per cent of its reinforcement from each schedule, then it switched back and forth between them equally often. If, however, the reinforcement from one schedule was only 25 per cent of the total, then switching to that alternative must have been at one third the rate as switching away from it. Because the time and the work (on the right disk) were both divided in accordance with the reinforcement, it is self evident that the actual rate of pecking, which is the ratio of work and time, must have been constant.

It is, however, possible to put work and time into direct opposition and see what happens to matching then. The answer for one such case was found by not using variable-interval schedules for both alternatives. Instead, pecking at the left disk was reinforced on the usual variable interval, while pecking on the right disk was reinforced probabilistically, on what is called a 'variable-ratio' schedule. On the right, the *nth* response was reinforced and *n* varied irregularly from reinforcement to reinforcement. Thus, for example, a variable ratio averaging 50 may sometimes reinforce the first or second response after the preceding reinforcement and sometimes only the 200th or 300th. The reciprocal of *n* is, in other words, the probability of reward. The pigeon's situation was comparable to being in a gambling casino with two slot machines, one paying off in the usual way (the variable ratio), and the other spontaneously getting 'hot' at unpredictable intervals of time and staying that way until played (the variable interval). On the interval schedule, the rate of reinforcement was essentially independent of the rate of pecking, while on the other, reinforcement and pecking were directly proportional.

The reason for examining this unusual, perhaps unique, set of conditions is that momentary rates of pecking on ratio schedules are faster than those on interval schedules at any rate of reinforcement within the customary range of values, so that matching *cannot* hold for both amount of work and time spent working. Consider, for example, equal reinforcements from left and right. Since the momentary rate of pecking on the right (ratio schedule) is higher than that on the left (interval schedule), the pigeon cannot allocate both its time and its responses equally. If time were shared equally, there would be more pecks at the right disk than at the left; if responses were shared equally, there would be more time spent at the left than at the right. This opposition between work and time prevails at all distributions of reinforcement. When local rates of work differ, as they did in this experiment, matching cannot describe both work and time, but only one or the other (or, of course, neither). For each of the 10 pigeons studied, matching described the amount of work. Each pigeon found for itself just the right balancing off of time and work so that equation (1), interpreted as simple number of responses, was obeyed throughout the range of reinforcement frequencies. But it would be inappropriate to conclude that equation (1) always refers to number of responses, as the experiment by BROWNSTEIN and PLISKOFF[6] shows. Their pigeons matched time, instead of work, to reinforcement, and CATANIA'S[7] as noted in Fig. 1, matched both. The best general conclusion as of now is that it is the distribution of *behavior* that is governed by the distribution of reinforcement, but the quantity of behavior is sometimes best estimated by time, sometimes by response count, and sometimes perhaps otherwise. It could reasonably be argued that in any situation, the suitable measure of behavior is the one that conforms to equation (1) (or its corollaries).

There was a peculiarity of the findings in this last experiment too persistent to be overlooked. Figure 2 shows that the experimental points are not uniformly distributed along the diagonal, which is the locus of matching. For this procedure, location along both coordinates, not just the ordinate, is governed by responding. The abscissa is the relative frequency of reinforcement, but the frequency of reinforcement on a ratio schedule is proportional to the frequency of responding, so that the abscissa is not an *independent* variable in the usual sense. By responding more or less rapidly on the ratio schedule, the pigeon can shift the relative frequency of reinforcement from 1·0 all the way to 0. It is therefore noteworthy that for every pigeon, and for a large number of different values of both schedules, the almost invariable finding has been that whenever the variable-interval alternative is preferred, it is preferred virtually exclusively, in contrast to the variable ratio, for which preferences have been intermediate more often than they have been exclusive. If we were to play the slot machines the way the pigeons most often pecked the disks, we would have to play the conventional machine either not at all or at least half the time.

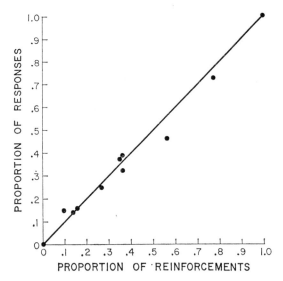

Fig. 2.   The proportion of responses to the variable-interval alternative when the choice is between variable-interval and variable-ratio schedules of reinforcement.

Essentially never would we play it without preferring it. Since the graph plots the variable-interval alternative (the other is its complement), preference for the variable interval is anything above 0·5 on the ordinate and preference for the variable ratio is anything below 0·5. The one point between 0·5 and 1·0 represents 2 cases out of 50 (5 points for each of 10 subjects). At all other tested values of the two schedules, the distribution of responding left a gap between 0·5 and 1·0 (non-inclusively) for the variable-interval alternative. This curious asymmetry between preference for interval and ratio schedules, may have broader ramifications than we can as yet state, for it was a genuine surprise even though it is not inconsistent with equation (1).

To conclude this brief résumé of matching, we should take note of some secondary procedural variations. It has been shown that matching holds for 3 and 4-choice procedures about as well as for two. There may be a limit, but for pigeons, 4 choices are not too many. When there are more than 2 choices, matching describes the various subsets as well as the total. For example, with 4 choices, there is matching for each pair of alternatives, each triad, and for all four. In fact, matching is shown even when the alternatives are sampled randomly 2, 3, or 4 at a time. Next, matching is found whether behavior is sampled continuously, as in the experiments described so far, or discretely, as in the typical probabilistic experiment. Instead of an experimental session in which behavior can occur freely at any moment, the subject may be given a pair of alternatives to choose from, an opportunity to make a single choice, and then have the alternatives withdrawn for the duration of what is usually called the 'intertrial interval.' Such experiments usually fix the probabilities of pay-off and find maximizing, with all the responses going to the better bet. However, variable-interval schedules may be adapted to a discrete-trial format and maximizing in the usual sense is no longer applicable. Instead, responding then conforms to equation (1) non-trivially, which is to say throughout the range of relative reinforcement frequencies. Several experiments (by NEVIN[9] of Columbia University and by me) have shown that matching with discrete trials does not depend on a sequential strategy of choices. In my experiments, the pattern of responding was essentially random, with successive choices independent of the one before and dependent only on the over-all frequencies of reinforcement. NEVIN's results[9] deviated from randomness, not so as to account for matching, but in addition to it.

If it is taken as proved that choice conforms to matching, the next step brings us to simple amount of behavior. On purely logical grounds, matching restricts sharply the range of possible relations between behavior and reinforcement measured as simple frequencies.[10] In other words, one may ask what is the function (or functions) relating the rate of reinforcement to the rate of responding such that, when the function is concatenated across several response alternatives, it predicts matching. And if we solve this logical problem, we must turn to the data to see if, in fact, a single account makes sense of both behavior and choice, which is to say, both absolute and relative responding.

To be concrete and relevant, let us assume that pecking at the left disk in principle obeys the same functional relations as pecking at the right. This is not to say that pecking is always the same at both locations, for there may well be factors operating at one location that are not operating at the other in any given situation. It is, simply, to say that the factors affecting responding at one location are, in principle, applicable to responding at any location, otherwise there would need to be different laws for different locations. The mathematical implications of this simple principle of symmetry are richer and more varied than might have been supposed, but they are also more complex than appropriate for recounting here.[10] Instead, I shall show that, given symmetry, the absolute rate of pecking at each alternative can obey one or the other of two simple functions and still produce matching when concatenated. The simpler of the two principles is a direct proportionality between responding and reinforcement, as follows:

$$P = kR \qquad (2)$$

If each of the two alternatives were to obey this proportionality, and if each had the same value of k (which is to assume comparable responses), then matching would be the result (subscripts referring to left and right):

$$\frac{P_L}{P_L + P_R} = \frac{kR_L}{kR_L + kR_R} = \frac{R_L}{R_L + R_R} \tag{3}$$

The second principle is a direct proportionality between responding and *relative* reinforcement, as follows:

$$P_L = \frac{kR_L}{R_L + R_R} \tag{4}$$

It, too, can readily be shown to imply matching across a pair of comparable alternative responses:

$$\frac{P_L}{P_L + P_R} = \frac{\dfrac{kR_L}{R_L + R_R}}{\dfrac{kR_L}{R_L + R_R} + \dfrac{kR_R}{R_L + R_R}} = \frac{R_L}{R_L + R_R} \tag{5}$$

The data unambiguously favor equation (4) over equation (2). Equation (2) implicitly says that no matter how many alternatives there are, the responding for each is dependent only on the reinforcement therefrom. Equation (4), on the other hand, says that reinforcement for either alternative affects the responding to both. Thus, increasing the reinforcement for the left disk should cause inverse variations in the responding to left and right, with the left rising and the right falling. And this is just what happens, as the 'contrast' effect certifies. It has been shown many times that when there is more than one alternative, any change in reinforcement affects all responses in the directions prescribed by equation (4).

Is equation (4) right quantitatively or just qualitatively? Before attempting to answer this question, we should generalize the prospective law to take account of any number of alternative sources of reinforcement. With the denominator as total reinforcement and the numerator as reinforcement conditional upon the response in question, equation (4) becomes:

$$P_1 = \frac{kR_1}{\sum_{i=0}^{n} R_i} \tag{6}$$

The simplest case is when there is only one defined alternative. In spite of first appearances, however, it should not be assumed that, k aside, numerator and denominator cancel when only one form of responding is being explicitly reinforced, for there are likely to be other sources of reinforcement anyway. Consider, once again, a pigeon pecking a disk for food. It is evident that no matter how important the food is, the pigeon may still move about the chamber, touch this edge or that corner with its beak, cock its head in an attitude of listening, ruffle its feathers, shake its foot, scratch the floor and itself, and so on. The pigeon carries within itself some residual capacity for entertainment—additional re-inforcement, in other words, which must be included in the denominator. As a practical matter, the denominator will exceed the explicitly programmed reinforcement by some amount, but by how much can only be inferred. Equation (6), then, calls for two parameters to be set: one is the constant k, and the other is the inferred extraneous reinforcement, which has been symbolized as R_0.

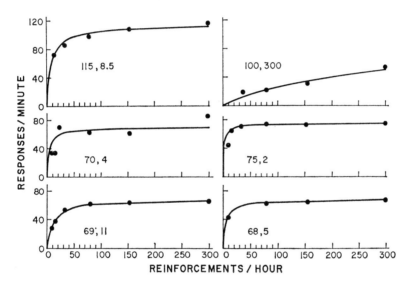

FIG. 3. Rate of pecking as a function of rate of pay, for 6 pigeons (adapted from Catania and Reynolds, 1968). The numbers are parameter values for the smooth curves, which plot equation (6).

The graphs in Fig. 3 test equation (6) thus interpreted with data from pigeons on standard variable-interval schedules programmed on a single disk. The 6 pigeons in this experiment by CATANIA and REYNOLDS[11] worked on several different variable intervals over a period of months. Rate of responding was allowed to stabilize before moving on to the next value of the schedule. Although for each pigeon, the rate of work increased with the rate of pay, the large individual differences seemed at the time to preclude any simple and general statement of the relation. The fit of points to curves, however, suggests a happier conclusion. The curves plot equation (6) with the parameters as shown, k (responses per minute) first and R_0 (reinforcements per hour) second. Five of the 6 pigeons had parameter values reasonably close to each other; the sixth had a much larger value of R_0, although it, too, approximated the predicted function. Such aberrant subjects are uncommon, but this pigeon is by no means unique in this regard. In terms of the present analysis, the pigeon at the upper right may be said to have been distracted, which is to say that its R_0 contained a source of reinforcement uncommonly large, albeit unknown to us. Not only does equation (6) fit the data in general, but the individual differences are handled by adjustments in the parameters.

Other data from single-response situations have similarly substantiated equation (6), and will not be further considered here. It remains to be shown that equation (6) handles the absolute frequency of responding to the individual alternatives in choice procedures.

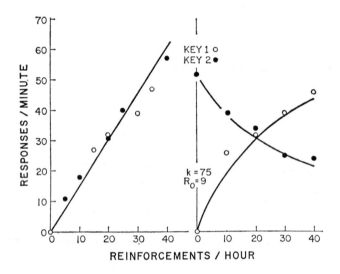

FIG. 4.   Rate of pecking at the alternatives in two versions of a two-choice procedure (adapted from Catania, 1963). Both panels plot equation (6) as a smooth curve, with parameters as shown.

A representative experiment is the one by CATANIA[7] already partly summarized in Fig. 1, where the relative measures of responding and reinforcement were plotted to exemplify matching. In Fig. 4, the absolute frequencies of responding at the two alternatives are shown for two stages of the experiment.   In stage 1 (on the left) the rates of reinforcement for the two schedules were picked so that the maximum possible rate, summing across the two alternatives, was always 40 per hr. The behavior was allowed to stabilize at a pair of values, then another pair summing to 40 was imposed for a while, and so on. Because the sum was constant, and because it may be assumed that R_0 was also constant, the

denominator in equation (6) (i.e., $\sum_{i=0}^{n} R_i = R_0 + R_1 + R_2$) becomes itself a constant.

Equation (6) with a constant denominator says that responding should be directly proportional to its reinforcement, a prediction that is well borne out by the points in the left panel.

In stage 2 (on the right), the reinforcement was not held constant for the two schedules taken together. Instead, reinforcement for one schedule ('Key 2') was held at 20 per hr while varying from 0 to 40 for the other ('Key 1'). Fitting these values into equation (6) produces the rising curve for Key 1 and the falling curve for Key 2, plotting both as a function of the reinforcement on Key 1 (reinforcement on Key 2 was constant at 20 throughout). Except for one deviant point out of ten, data and theory virtually coincide. For the two stages of the experiment, a single pair of parameter values sufficed, values that are incidentally of about the same magnitude as in Fig. 3. Other experiments similarly confirm equation (6). In fact, there is so far no clearly contradictory finding (to my knowledge) out of more than 50 different experiments. This is, of course, not to say that only one interpretation, let alone one equation, has been accepted by all investigators.

An equation that accounts for such a mass of data is a pleasant novelty in psychology, perhaps worth some further thought. Equation (6) says that responding and reinforcement are related by a constant of proportionality k, which varies from individual to individual and no doubt also from one form of behavior to another. Reinforcement, however, is not measured absolutely, but as a ratio between the reinforcement conditional upon the response and total reinforcement. Contrary to intuition, responding may therefore be more or less indifferent to the reinforcement it produces. If the response's reinforcement is a large part of the total reinforcement, which is to say that the reinforcement ratio in equation (6) is close to 1·0, then responding will stay close to the value of k. And conversely, if the response's reinforcement is only a small fraction of the total reinforcement, then the response will be quite sensitive to variations in its reinforcement, in the limiting case being directly proportional to it. Exactly offsetting these differences in sensitivity are differences in stability. If the response's reinforcement is a large part of the total reinforcement, the response is not only insensitive to its own reinforcement, but also largely impervious to fluctuations in other reinforcers. When, finally, the response is sensitive to variations in its own reinforcement because it controls only a small fraction of the total reinforcement, it is by the same token unstable, for it will be powerfully affected by changes in other reinforcers, which may not be under experimental control.

The literature on the input–output dynamics of reinforcement is notably deficient in interesting quantitative relations. After more than 70 years of research, we know that creatures work for gain, but only in qualitative terms. Equation (6) suggests that our ignorance is not just owing to ineptitude, for it predicts uninteresting results for the usual, well-controlled experiment. It is hard to fault psychologists for taking pains to guarantee that the behavior they observe is, in fact, important to the subject. Hungry animals are taught to work for food, thirsty animals for water, cold animals for warmth, and so on. Nor would it seem wrong to keep the distractions to the subject at a minimum. But a ravenously hungry animal working for food in an otherwise impoverished environment is a prescription for little if any contact with the dynamics of reinforcement, if equation (6) is right. The behavior will hover around the value of k as the experimenter futilely varies together the numerator and denominator of a fraction so close to 1·0 that the variation has little effect. In practice, the fraction will be less than 1·0, so that there is some sort of increasing monotonic relation between work and pay, but it is likely to be too shallow and too different from subject to subject to foster a conclusion or even a respectable theory. Equation (6) shows why the dynamics of reinforcement are best studied in experiments in which no single response controls the overwhelmingly dominant reinforcer—as, for example, in the choice experiment described at the beginning of this paper. However, it also shows what to expect in less optimal circumstances.

The account stops here, for the point of the paper would be little aided by a further recital of confirmatory findings. A longer account might have shown how this formulation can handle choice among dissimilar responses (for which the constant k may not be presumed equal) or how it treats situations in which reinforcement depends not only on the occurrence of some response but also on the presence of particular stimuli. But even though there is more to tell than contained herein, there are many experiments yet to be done, for research has only recently fanned out from the original paradigm of a hungry pigeon pecking a disk for food. If the principle of reinforcement seems as non-predictive as ever in its grander applications, there is reason to hope that mainly facts are lacking now, not concepts. We have begun to predict both simple rate of work and choice as we have ascertained the quantities called for by equation 6 and its corollaries. Finding the quantities is often harder than it sounds, for it requires a list of reinforcers and their magnitudes measured on a common scale, but once found, they do the job expected of them. In practical terms, it will be a good while before our analysis overtakes the complexity of behavior in the natural environment—even a pigeon's, not to mention a man's. Nevertheless, it seems that we are at last making scientific sense of our most venerable intuition about the springs of action, which the hedonistic doctrine must surely be.

REFERENCES

1. HERRNSTEIN, R. J. Relative and absolute strength of response as a function of frequency of reinforcement. *J. exp. Analysis Behav.* **4,** 267, 1961.
2. HERRNSTEIN, R. J. On the law of effect. *J. exp. Analysis Behav.* **13,** 243, 1970.
3. SHULL, R. L. and PLISKOFF, S. S. Changeover delay and concurrent performances: some effects on relative performance measures. *J. exp. Analysis Behav.* **10,** 517, 1967.
4. SCHROEDER, S. R. and HOLLAND, J. G. Reinforcement of eye movement with concurrent schedules. *J. exp. Analysis Behav.* **12,** 897, 1969.
5. HOLZ, W. C. Punishment and rate of positive reinforcement. *J. exp. Analysis Behav.* **11,** 285, 1968.
6. BROWNSTEIN, A. J. and PLISKOFF, S. S. Some effects of relative reinforcement rate and changeover delay in response-independent concurrent schedules of reinforcement. *J. exp. Analysis Behav.* **11,** 683, 1968.
7. CATANIA, A. C. Concurrent performances: reinforcement interaction and response independence. *J. exp. Analysis Behav.* **6,** 253, 1963.
8. FINDLEY, J. D. An experimental outline for building and exploring multi-operant behavior repertoires. *J. exp. Analysis Behav.* **1,** 113, 1962.
9. NEVIN, J. A. Interval reinforcement of choice behavior in discrete trials. *J. exp. Analysis Behav.* **12,** 875, 1969.
10. NATAPOFF, A. How symmetry restricts symmetric choice. *J. math. Psychol.* **7,** 444, 1970.
11. CATANIA, A. C. and REYNOLDS, G. S. A quantitative analysis of the responding maintained by interval schedules of reinforcement. *J. exp. Analysis Behav.* **11,** 327, 1968.

J. psychiat. Res., 1971, Vol. 8, pp. 413–422. Pergamon Press. Printed in Great Britain.

THE BEHAVIORAL ANALYSIS OF APHASIA*

MURRAY SIDMAN

Department of Neurology, Massachusetts General Hospital, Boston, Massachusetts

MANY disciplines claim language as their domain, and each approaches language with its own concepts and methods—behavioral, linguistic, cultural, logical, etc. Since central-nervous-system lesions do not constitute the empirical operations upon which these disciplines base their theories, the effects of such lesions provide an independent test of the theoretical formulations. All disciplines seem to accept the notion that aphasia is a major theoretical testing ground. Even if CNS lesions do not appear in the theoretical statements, such lesions must cause language to 'fracture' along lines that are consistent with the theoretical classifications.

Two major problems, however, have hindered the integration of aphasic deficits with theoretical formulations of language: The definition of language, itself; and the methods of examining and classifying aphasic deficits. The first problem has been an unnecessary hindrance, not because language is easy to define but because it need not be defined in order to study the phenomena of aphasia. Such definition has been a problem only because it has influenced the way we examine aphasic behavior, and has determined the kinds of observations we are willing to accept. The phenomena of aphasia can be classified empirically, without biasing the observations by preconceptions of what language 'really' is. The data will then be available to any theory.

The methodological problems are more serious. Few aphasiologists have felt it necessary to describe their test conditions, procedures, materials, or even the behavior of the patients. For example, we often find the patient's deficits classified as 'expressive' or 'receptive', as 'recognition' or 'comprehension' disorders, etc., without any specification of the actual task or of the responses required of him; we find the writing of one set of words from dictation compared with the reading of another set of words from text, and, added to these confusions, no indication of the behavior that was required to demonstrate 'reading'; we find responses to spoken sentences compared with responses to single printed words; some examiners tell the patient that he responded correctly, and others give the patient no feedback at all. The list could go on indefinitely; anyone who has attempted seriously to survey the literature on aphasia is familiar with the inevitable frustration.

* This research was supported by Grant NS 03535 from the National Institute of Neurological Diseases and Stroke, and by the Joseph P. Kennedy, Jr., Laboratories of the Neurology Service, Massachusetts General Hospital. Colleagues in these studies have been J. Leicester, J. P. Mohr, P. B. Rosenberger and L. T. Stoddard.

Rather than add yet another set of theoretical suppositions and concepts, we have attempted in our studies of aphasia to provide the kind of operational specificity that would make our data useful to anyone. We have used the characteristic stimulus materials and responses of traditional aphasiology, so that we might avoid refining out of existence the very phenomena that give this field much of its fascination, and have simply added a few elementary considerations of scientific common sense. The methods are not, of course, free of preconceptions, but these are quite simple and explicit. Their justification, or lack of it, can be judged by their analytic power and consistency.

STIMULUS–RESPONSE RELATIONS

Let us start with the word, 'hat', a simple stimulus that has at least the potential of being language. Some of the many forms the stimulus, 'hat', may take are listed on the left side of Table 1. It may be a word in visual text; an auditory word, pronounced or spelled; a tactile word, felt but not seen; or an object or picture in any of several varieties or forms.

TABLE 1.   SEVERAL FORMS OF THE STIMULUS, 'HAT' AND SEVERAL TYPES OF
APPROPRIATE RESPONSES

Stimulus: *Hat*	Responses
Visual word, upper case	Oral pronunciation
Visual word, lower case	Oral spelling
Visual word, script	Oral synonym
Visual objects	
Visual pictures	Written naming, upper case
	Written naming, lower case
Auditory word, pronounced	Written naming, script
Auditory word, spelled	Written synonym
Tactile word, upper case	Matching to visual or tactile word, u.c.
Tactile word, lower case	Matching to visual or tactile word, l.c.
Tactile word, script	Matching to visual or tactile word, script
Tactile object	Matching to auditory word, pronounced
	Matching to auditory word, spelled
	Matching to visual or tactile objects
	Matching to visual pictures

Appropriate responses to these stimuli are listed on the right side of Table 1—various types of naming, writing, and matching. No single one of these stimulus–response relations can be taken as evidence for language: A parrot can repeat pronounced words; a dog can be taught to do many of the matching tasks; a person who speaks only French can copy the printed English word. But when one of the stimuli, for example, the pronounced word, can give rise appropriately to all of the listed responses, and when all varieties of the stimulus can give rise to the same response, for example, oral pronunciation, we approach language more closely. An additional step is taken when each of the listed stimuli can be shown to control all the listed responses. Finally, when corresponding forms of other stimuli, for example, cat, hay, hut, etc., can be shown to control a corresponding list of responses, it is difficult not to conclude that we are dealing with some aspect of language.

The main point of this analysis is to show that we can specify a large segment of language behavior simply in terms of a set of stimulus–response relations. The approach does not necessarily encompass everything that might be called language. Yet to deny that the specified set of stimulus–response relations constitutes language, on the ground that it fails to deal with concepts, grammatical or syntactical relations, memory, learning, or development, etc., would be to ignore a large and important, if limited, class of language behavior. The appropriate question is whether the stimulus–response classification is meaningful; in the present context, does it permit us to chart lines along which behavior fractures in aphasia?

That the answer turns out to be, 'yes' should not surprise us, for many basic observations in aphasia are of deficient stimulus–response relations. A single stimulus controls many responses; a single response is controlled by many stimuli; and CNS disease need not break down all relations in which a particular stimulus or response participates. In Fig. 1, for example, S is a written word that controls reading aloud (S–R_1), copying on paper (S–R_2), and pointing to a picture (S–R_3). A cerebral lesion that leaves S–R_1 and S–R_2 intact but destroys S–R_3 is often said to leave the patient with the ability to read the word without knowing its significance. If the lesion leaves S–R_3 intact but destroys the other S–R relations, we have the condition of Broca's aphasia.

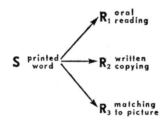

FIG. 1.   Schematic representation of three stimulus–response relations, each of which shares the same stimulus.

The following scheme for testing utilizes a manageable number of elements from Table 1. Sample stimuli, at the left, provide initial input to the patient in any of three modalities, vision, hearing, or touch; he processes the samples according to the demands of each task. In simultaneous matching (top line), pressing the sample exposes a second set of input stimuli, the choices; the final response in the sequence is to press a choice that corresponds to the sample. Delayed matching has the same initial input and final output as simultaneous matching, but a time delay intervenes between sample press and appearance of choices; choices appear without the sample, which the patient must remember. Naming and writing have the same initial input as matching; the output differs. A complete description of the procedures and their automation may be found elsewhere.[1] This scheme permits us to evaluate four types of response to a single stimulus, for example, to a printed 3-letter word;

or a single response to several different stimuli, for example, oral naming of visual, auditory, and tactile words. It is possible, then, to observe the elementary but vital precautions of maintaining input constancy while varying the responses required of the patient, and maintaining response constancy while varying the input.

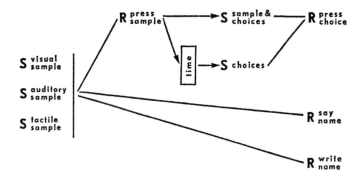

FIG. 2.   Summary of test procedures as described in text.

IDENTITY VS. NONIDENTITY TASKS

Figure 3 shows the nearly complete test profile of a single patient whose deficits had become relatively stable after a severe head injury 5 yr earlier. He had undergone a left temporal craniotomy and evacuation of a subdural hematoma, and also had a right temporal burr hole placed.* The patient had a permanent right hemiplegia, hemianopia, severe aphasia, and amnesia. His test profile is arranged to facilitate two types of analysis. First, each of the four types of response, simultaneous matching, oral naming, writing, and delayed matching, can be examined individually as a function of different stimulus materials and sample stimuli. Second, specific sample stimuli, for example, visual, tactile, or auditory letters can be examined as a function of the type of response that was required of the patient.

Before examining the test scores in any detail, it will be advantageous to take account of the differences emphasized by the solid black and the gray bars. Solid black indicates 'identity' tasks; gray indicates 'nonidentity' tasks. The distinction is as follows:

Take simultaneous visual–visual matching of letters. This is an identity task because the sample letter and the correct choice are exactly the same. The patient can match a letter without recognizing it as a letter, even without having seen it before. Tactile–visual matching may be a second type of identity task. Having learned that tactile and visual stimuli, although physically different, may be equivalent, the patient can match a tactile to a visual letter without having experienced the letter before in either modality.

The same considerations apply to trigrams, 3-letter words, pictures, colors, and digits, the identity matching tasks for these materials being indicated by solid black bars. Note that in simultaneous matching, the patient performed all the identity tasks nearly perfectly.

---

* The study of this patient was made possible through the cooperation of Dr. D. Frank Benson, Boston Veterans Administration Hospital.

So long as the patient can discriminate and match any physical stimulus aspect, for example, shape, area, color, or angularity, he need have no behavior that is uniquely common to a particular sample and choice. He cannot, however, match a letter seen to a letter heard without having learned a name or some other response that is uniquely common to that particular visual letter and to its auditory counterpart; auditory–visual matching is 'nonidentity'. Similarly, each of the following is a nonidentity matching task: matching of words with pictures, and *vice-versa*; color names with colors and vice versa, digit names with digits, and vice versa; and digits with dots. The patient was not deficient in all of these simultaneous matching tasks, but all of his serious deficits were in nonidentity matching (gray bars).

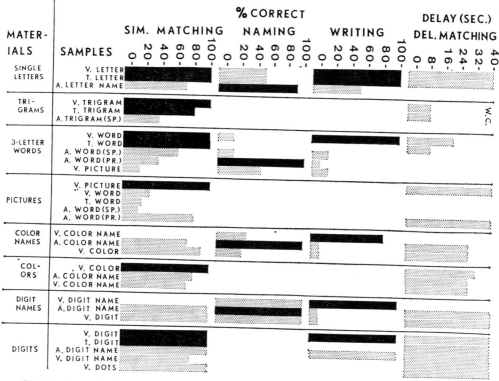

FIG. 3.   Example of a test profile. '*Materials*' indicates the choice stimuli in the matching tasks, as well as the product of the naming and writing tasks, in response to each of the indicated sample stimuli. *V.*—visual; *T.*—tactile; *A.*—auditory.

Certain naming and writing tasks constitute additional identity classes. For example, auditory–naming may involve only repetition. A patient who can imitate sounds will be able to name a dictated letter even if he has neither heard nor spoken it before. He may also copy a visual letter without having seen or written it before. Tactile–writing may also be an identity task; a patient who can draw tactile samples may copy a tactile letter he has never felt or written before.

By contrast, the patient could not do nonidentity naming and writing tasks by imitation, copying, or form equivalence, but only by virtue of learned mediating responses. The patient's scores on the naming and writing tasks, like simultaneous matching, reflect the identity–non–identity distinction. Those naming tasks that could be done by mere oral repetition, and those writing tasks that could be done by copying the samples, were nearly perfect; all deficits were in the nonidentity tasks.

Delayed matching must be regarded as a nonidentity task, even with identity materials. Sample and choice are never available for simultaneous comparison, and the patient must respond to the sample with some behavior that permits him to bridge the delay. In support of this, we may note that even some of the identity matching tasks broke down when changed from simultaneous to delay (trigrams, 3-letter words, colors).

The identity–nonidentity distinction, reflected in the patient's test scores, provides a necessary control in the study of aphasic deficits. For example, even while the patient had trouble naming visual and tactile letters, he matched and copied those same letters perfectly. Even while he had trouble matching and writing dictated letters, he was able to repeat them orally. Each input, visual, tactile and auditory letters, was involved in at least one intact stimulus–response relation. Therefore, none of his problems with letters could be classified as input deficits. Similarly, output deficit with letters could be ruled out because there was at least one adequate performance with each of the three types of response: matching, naming, and writing.

The identity performances provide the same type of control for each of the test materials. The patient's deficits, therefore, cannot be classed as input or output and must, by exclusion, fall into a relational category; they indicate deficient input–output relations. These relational deficits were not confined to any particular stimulus modality, stimulus material, or response. The patient's naming and writing deficits were not simply expressive; his matching deficits were not simply receptive. Inputs were deficient only when related to certain types of output, and outputs only when related to certain input stimuli.

Without going into all the interesting details of the patient's test profile, we can summarize the following major characteristics. Eliminating the identity tasks (solid black bars) from consideration, since they have served their control function, we see, with the exception of certain tasks involving numbers: relational writing deficits that cut across stimulus materials and modalities; relational naming deficits that cut across stimulus materials and modalities; and relational matching deficits that appear largely confined to tasks that involve visual letters and words as samples or choices. Delayed matching requires further clarification, and has been discussed elsewhere.[1]

The classification along the lines of empirical stimulus–response relations does reveal orderly categories of behavioral deficit in aphasia. The case presented here is not unique, nor is this the only deficit constellation the methods are capable of revealing. Some additional findings, and their implications for the study of language, will now be discussed.

LETTERS AND WORDS

The separate analysis of performances on identity tasks serves as a control for input and output deficits, and permits the identification of relational deficits. Relational deficits are a unique product of a stimulus–response analysis. Language, too, is a relational process. It is neither a particular type of input nor is it merely speech or any other single output, but is a process that includes many types of input, output, and their interrelations. But it would not be profitable to equate language deficit with the relational category, for this deficit category is not a unitary entity. Different nonidentity performance profiles among stimulus materials, input modalities, and output responses illustrate its multifaceted nature.

A particularly interesting example is the difference some patients show when analogous performances with letters and words are compared. Relational deficits that involve either letters or words might, with some justification, be considered language deficits. Yet not only may a patient's performances with these two materials differ, but the simpler-appearing materials, letters, may actually be associated with the more severe deficits. Because words are longer than letters, contain several letters as elements, and come from a larger stimulus population, one might reasonably expect more severe deficits with words than with letters; this expectation justifies the comparison of absolute test scores across the two different stimulus materials, a practice that is otherwise likely to lead to misleading conclusions.

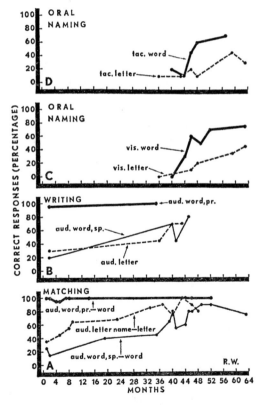

FIG. 4. Test scores as a function of time. Each frame shows the patient's scores for a given response: matching, writing, or naming; each curve is labelled with the type of stimulus to which the patient responded. The curves in frame *A, Matching,* show the sample and choice stimuli, the latter always visual.

An illustrative patient is a boy who suffered an occlusion of the left middle cerebral artery, with right hemiparesis and complete loss of oral speech.[2] Tested frequently over the next five years, his deficits evolved in a most interesting way. The heavy black curve in Fig. 4 shows his nearly perfect performance in matching auditory-pronounced 3-letter words (dictated) to visual-word choices (printed). The same task with single letters, dictated samples to be matched to visual choices (broken-line), was, however, severely deficient at first, and improved only slowly over the next four years. When the samples were the dictated words, spelled rather than pronounced, to be matched to the same visual words, the patient's performance was also grossly deficient, and improved only slowly.

Comparable deficits were observed in writing. The patient was able from the beginning to write the dictated-pronounced words, but had great difficulty writing dictated single letters and dictated-spelled words (Fig. 4).

During the first 3 yr, before the patient was capable of any oral speech, the selective matching and writing deficits with letters were assumed to be specific auditory–visual intermodality deficits (the patient performed well on the identity tasks, visual and tactile matching and writing of letters, and auditory–auditory matching). But this assumption was premature, as was demonstrated when oral naming began to appear during the fourth year. With both visual (Fig. 4C) and tactile (Fig. 4D) samples, the patient improved more rapidly in naming words than in naming single letters.

Thus the distinction between word and letter deficits generalized across the three input modalities, vision, hearing and touch, and across the three output responses, matching, naming and writing.

One might have been tempted to classify responses to words and letters both as language, with, perhaps, words being more prone to deficit because of their greater complexity. But this patient's generally more severe deficits in response to letters than to words indicate clearly that the category, language, is too gross. The stimulus–response analysis, unprejudiced by preconceptions of what language 'really' is, can uncover types of deficit specificity for which any theory of language must find a place.

THE PRESUMED PREREQUISITES FOR SPELLING

In the literature on aphasia, one often finds statements about ancillary mental or internal processes that are presumed to underlie the observed performances. The type of analysis proposed here, because of its operational specificity, can often be useful in checking the adequacy of such formulations.

For example, spelling is sometimes characterized as a performance that requires mental transformations of spelled words into written form, and then the 'reading' of these written words (images). Such a view is subscribed to by NIELSEN[3] and has been most explicitly stated by GESCHWIND,[4] whose writings are otherwise noteworthy for their empirical specification: "In order to comprehend a word spelled out loud, the listener must transform it into written form and then 'read' it. Conversely, to spell orally one must transform the spoken word into its written form and then 'read' the letters one by one." (p. 278).

This conception was checked by examining certain relevant test scores of a patient who has been extensively described elsewhere[1]. The data are from weeks 7 and 8 post-stroke. Figure 5 deals with the comprehension of dictated-spelled words. We see first (Bar *A*) that the patient was relatively proficient at pronouncing dictated-spelled words; Bar *B* shows equal proficiency in matching the spelled words to pictures, demonstrating that the patient comprehended the spelled words; Bar *C* shows that he could match dictated-spelled words to printed words. He could respond in several appropriate ways to the spelled words.

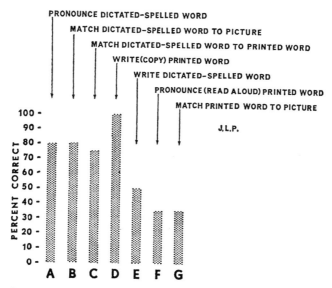

FIG. 5. Test scores on spelling comprehension and presumed related tasks.

But although his printed-word input was intact (Bar *D*), the patient was deficient in demonstrating explicitly the first of the tasks held to be necessary for spelling comprehension —writing the dictated-spelled words (Bar *E*); he was only poorly able to transform spelled words into written form.

Even if we were to suppose that his poor writing was merely apraxic or paragraphic, and that his internal writing, or imagery, was intact, the patient showed also that he could not explicitly perform the second of the presumed necessary mental tasks (Bar *F*); he was deficient at reading the written words aloud. Bar *G* shows that he was also deficient in comprehending the written words.

The patient could comprehend oral spelling, but was unable with the same words, to perform the tasks held to be necessary for spelling comprehension.

What of the converse task, oral spelling? Figure 6 shows that the patient could spell pronounced words aloud (Bar *A*), comprehend pronounced words (Bar *B*), and match pronounced to printed words (Bar *C*). But he was deficient in the first of the tasks held necessary for oral spelling, transcribing the pronounced words into written form (Bar *D*). The second of the presumed necessary tasks, reading the written letters one by one, was not tested directly with the 3-letter words, but was tested with trigrams; the patient was grossly deficient at this task (Bar *E*). He was also deficient, as we have seen before, in reading aloud and comprehending the written words (Bars *F* and *G*).

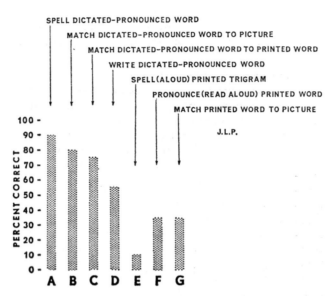

FIG. 6.　Test scores on oral spelling and presumed related tasks.

The patient could comprehend spelled words and could spell orally, but was unable to demonstrate the supposedly necessary underlying processes. He was deficient in writing dictated-spelled and pronounced words, in reading aloud and spelling from text, and even in comprehending written text. It might be proposed that the overt performances described above could have been deficient while their internal counterparts were still intact. Acceptance of such a proposal would, of course, remove the study of language and aphasia from the domain of all sciences. Here, preconceived mentalistic conceptions of a language process proved amenable to specific analysis by means of relevant stimulus–response relations. An alternative proposal, therefore, is that all such mentalistic conceptions be translated into testable form and, if not translatable, that they be abandoned.

REFERENCES

1. SIDMAN, M., STODDARD, L. T., MOHR, J. P. and LEICESTER, J. Behavioral studies of aphasia: Methods of investigation and analysis, *Neuropsychologia* (in press).
2. ROSENBERGER, P. B., MOHR, J. P., STODDARD, L. T. and SIDMAN, M. Inter- and intra-modality matching deficits in a dysphasic youth. *Archs Neurol.* **18**, 549, 1968.
3. NIELSEN, J. M. *Agnosia, Apraxia, Aphasia,* 2nd ed. Hafner, New York, 1962.
4. GESCHWIND, N. Disconnexion syndromes in animals and man. *Brain* **88**, 237, 1965.

J. psychiat. Res., 1971, Vol. 8, pp. 423–438. Pergamon Press. Printed in Great Britain.

SHORT-TERM STORAGE AND LONG-TERM STORAGE IN RECALL*

MURRAY GLANZER

New York University, New York, New York

OVER the past ten years major changes have taken place in the study of memory. These changes are:

(1). Renewed and broadened interest in memory. Until recently there was very little interest in the field. That little interest was concentrated narrowly on a limited range of rote-learning tasks. At present the field is one of the most active areas of research in psychology. It includes the consideration of memory in a variety of laboratory tasks directed at memory *per se*, in higher order cognitive functioning and in clinical situations. The results from each of these approaches stimulate and inform the others. Even within the laboratory tasks focussed on memory, *per se*, a much wider range of tasks is used than was used previously—probe tasks, distractor tasks, running memory tasks.

(2). Emphasis on the short term aspects of memory. Much of the current work is concerned with memory in situations in which the subject is presented with an item a single time and is tested a few seconds later. A major discovery during this period has been that such simple short term situations can give very clear and reliable information about the nature of the information processing carried out by the subject.

(3). Establishment of a number of powerful and stable relations with respect to these tasks. The work on a range of these memory tasks has resulted in convergence on a general model for recall. According to this model, recall is a process that involves two or more distinct storage mechanisms. A number of investigators[1-4] have developed this model in varying degrees of complexity. Only a relatively simple aspect of the model will be considered here and that with special reference to free recall. The generality of the statements made will, however, also be indicated.

The work that will be outlined below exemplifies this development in the field of memory research. It is particularly appropriate to outline the author's work at this time since the work was started at the Walter Reed Army Institute of Research, under the sponsorship of Dr. David McKenzie Rioch.

THE MODEL

The model will be outlined informally here in a series of assertions. There is at present a large body of data to support these assertions. Some of the supporting data will be surveyed in subsequent paragraphs.

---

* This paper was written under R01HD04212 between the National Institute of Child Health and Human Development and New York University.

S

The basic elements of the model are shown in the flow diagram of Fig. 1. An item enters the system, first going through preliminary processing, at a 'sensory' level. This processing includes storage of the input information over very short periods of time, e.g. half a second or less. Some of the details of this stage have been examined by SPERLING[5] and others. This part of the processing will not be considered further here.

In the subsequent discussion the term 'item' will be used to stand for the term 'information about the item'. There is no implication that the item is a concrete entity that is being transported whole in the system.

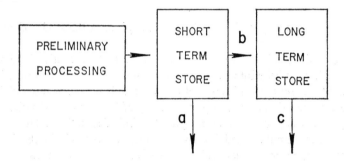

FIG. 1.   Flow chart of the processing of items in free recall.

The item, that is, information about the item, next appears in short-term store (STS). It stays there for varying periods of time depending on the experimental conditions. These will be detailed below. Originally it was hypothesized that items left STS simply because of the passage of time. This hypothesis is one variant of the 'decay' theory of forgetting. It is clear now that items do not simply decay or fade from STS as a function of time. They are displaced by the entry of subsequent items. Data on this point will be discussed below.

When an item has entered STS it can either stay or drop out of the system. The loss of the item is indicated by the arrow labelled a. During its stay in STS a representation of some or all of the information about the item may be registered in long-term store (LTS). This transfer of information to LTS is indicated by the arrow labelled b in the figure.

Transmission of information to LTS does not imply removal of that information from STS. An item can be represented in both stores at the same time. Arrow c represents LTS information being lost or becoming inaccessible.

The STS is very limited in its capacity. Most experiments indicate a capacity of 2–3 items. The LTS is not limited in this way. It can, under optimal conditions, contain an unlimited number of items. It is, however, limited in the number of items it can accept within a given period of time. Each item that is transmitted to LTS requires some processing time. Therefore, if the amount of time is limited, a limited number of items will be registered in LTS.

Access to information in STS is relatively direct. Access to information in LTS is relatively indirect. This is seen in the temporal characteristics of responses in recall. Items from STS appear early at a fast rate. Items from LTS appear at a slower, steadier rate.

A number of details could be added to this picture for a fuller model of recall. They are merely indicated here.

(1). Various types of store may be distinguished in STS according to the sensory mode through which the items are presented.

(2). The LTS that is outlined in the figure is a very extensive, complex system. Only a minuscule part of that system will be considered here.

(3). There are a variety of activities carried out by the subject either to maintain an item in STS or to facilitate its transfer to LTS. The term rehearsal has been used to refer to both of these activities:

The serial position curve

In the case of free recall, a major reason for assuming the flow and the separate storage mechanisms shown in Fig. 1 lies in a very prominent and reliable characteristic of free recall—the serial position function. When probability of recall of an item is plotted as a function of the position of the item in presentation, a bimodal curve is obtained. Subjects are most likely to recall the end items, next most likely the beginning items, and are least likely to recall the middle items of the list. Examples of serial position functions are found in Fig. 2.

Since the beginning and end of the serial position curve respond differently to a range of experimental variables, the positions are considered to represent output from different storage mechanisms. A major part of the end peak is considered to consist of output from STS. The early sections of the curve are considered to consist solely of output from LTS.

There are two main methods of separating the output from STS and LTS. One is the interaction method, the other is the subtraction method.

The interaction method

The interaction method consists of imposing variables on the free-recall task and observing differential effects on the serial position curve. If the curve is raised or lowered in all positions except the last few, the variable is considered to affect LTS primarily. An example of the application of this method is found in an experiment by GLANZER and CUNITZ.[2] Lists of twenty words each were presented to groups of subjects at one of three different rates—one word every 3 sec, 6 sec or 9 sec. The resulting family of curves in Fig. 2 shows a separation according to rate across all positions except the last few. The interpretation of this interaction of rate and serial position is, that presentation rate affects only LTS. An interaction effect of this type is found with almost all the classic rote-learning variables. The serial position curves are almost identical with those shown in Fig. 2.

1. *Rate of presentation.*[2,6,7] See Fig. 2.

2. *Word frequency.*[7,8] Words of higher normative frequency are recalled more easily than words of low frequency. This effect holds as indicated above for all of the serial position curve except the end peak.

3. *List length.*[6,9] As the length of the list increases all but the end peak declines.

4. *Mnemonic or associative structure.*[10] The same interaction appears when the recall of lists containing associated or mnemonically related words is compared with the recall of unrelated words. The curves for such lists are shown in Fig. 3.

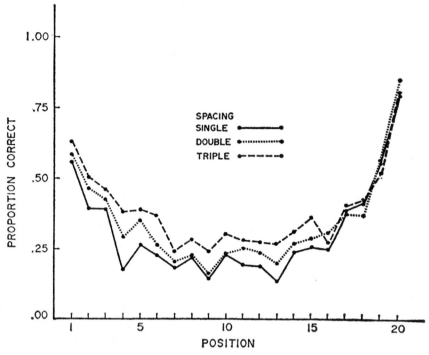

FIG. 2. Serial position curves for three different rates of presentation, single (3 sec), double (6 sec), triple (9 sec). (After GLANZER and CUNITZ[2].)

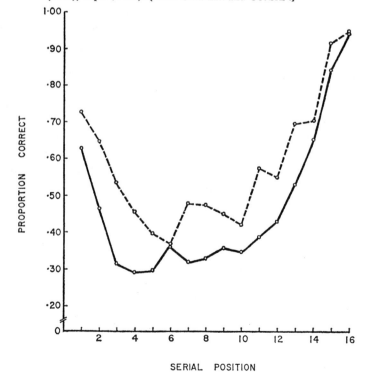

FIG. 3. Serial position curves for high (broken line) and low (solid line) mnemonic or associative structure. (After GLANZER and SCHWARTZ[10].)

5. *Concurrent task load.*[11,12] If subjects have to carry out a secondary task, e.g. card sorting or addition of numbers, in the intervals between the presentation of list items, the probability of recall of the list items is lowered. The more difficult the concurrent task, the greater this effect. Figure 4 shows the results for an experiment in which subjects added 1, 4 or 7 to given numbers during the list presentation.[12]

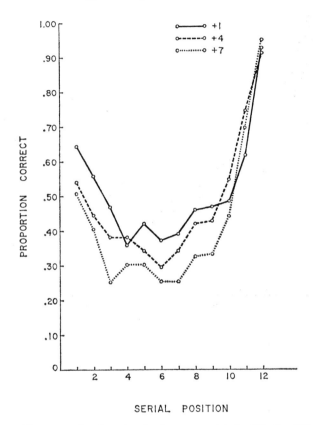

FIG. 4. Serial position curves for three levels of concurrent task difficulty. (After SILVERSTEIN and GLANZER[12].)

The interaction effects obtained above indicate that presentation rate, word frequency, list length, mnemonic structure and concurrent task load affect only LTS. They do not affect STS.

Subtraction method

The subtraction method gives a cleaner separation of LTS and STS than that given by the interaction method. The method is based on an operation that affects only the end peak.

It is assumed that the end peak consists of output from both STS and LTS. The operation that affects only the end peak is a post-list delay task. GLANZER and CUNITZ[2] gave subjects free recall lists. After each list the subject had to wait 0, 10, or 30-sec before being permitted to recall. During the 10 and 30-sec delays they carried out a simple counting task. The results are shown in Fig. 5. With a 30-sec delay task, the serial position curve flattens out completely.

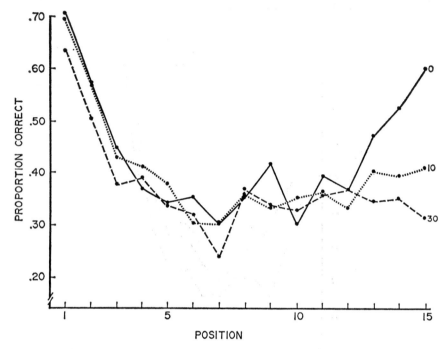

FIG. 5. Serial position curves for three delay periods—0, 10 and 30 sec. (After GLANZER and CUNITZ[2].)

All of the STS output is eliminated. The same effect was found by POSTMAN and PHILLIPS.[9] Other examples of delay and no-delay serial position curves are found in the work of RAYMOND.[7]

The delay effect furnishes the basis of a powerful technique for estimating the amount of output from STS and the amount of output from LTS. This technique was first presented by RAYMOND.[7]

Output from LTS is identified with the output obtained after a delay task. Thus, the 30-sec delay curve at the bottom of Fig. 5 is identified as output from LTS and the probability, P_i (D), that an item in list position i is recalled after delay is equated with the probability, P_i (LTS), that the item is in LTS.

$$\hat{P}_i \text{ (LTS)} = P_i \text{ (D)} \qquad (1)$$

The probability that an item is in STS cannot, however, be estimated directly. It is assumed that an item can be in both STS and LTS until the delay imposed by either subsequent list items or the post-list task removes it from STS.

This gives the following equation for recall P_i (ND) in the no-delay condition:

$$P_i \text{ (ND)} = P_i \text{ (STS)} + P_i \text{ (LTS)} - P_i \text{ (STS} \cap \text{LTS)} \qquad (2)$$

By further assuming that the probability of an item being in STS is independent of its being in LTS, the following equation holds:

$$P_i \text{ (STS} \cap \text{LTS)} = P_i \text{ (STS)} \cdot P_i \text{ (LTS)}$$

This gives then the following equation for the estimation of the probability that an item is in STS.

$$\hat{P}_i \text{ (STS)} = \frac{P_i \text{ (ND)} - P_i \text{ (D)}}{1 - P_i \text{ (D)}} \qquad (3)$$

A closely related equation was developed and applied by WAUGH and NORMAN[4] using a different estimate of P_i (LTS).

The subtraction method has been applied in a number of studies. An example may be found in a study by GLANZER and SCHWARTZ.[10] In this experiment, the subjects were given lists containing associated words, e.g. house, shack; mutton, veal; sleep, slumber, etc.

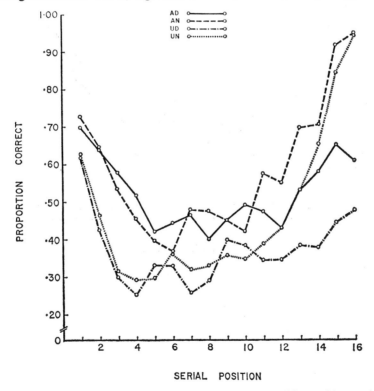

FIG. 6. Serial position curves for the delay and no-delay conditions with associated and unassociated items. AD = Associated Delay; AN = Associated No-Delay; UD = Unassociated Delay; UN=Unassociated No-Delay. (After GLANZER and SCHWARTZ[10].)

The associated pairs were placed at random through the lists, occupying half the list positions. The lists formed in this manner were followed either by a delay task or no delay. The delay and no-delay curves are shown in Fig. 6. The associated and unassociated words in the no-delay condition give the two curves with marked end peaks. These curves are the same as those that appeared in Fig. 3 showing the interaction noted there. The curves for the delay condition do not show this interaction. They are parallel across all positions. There is some evidence of an end peak, indicating incomplete elimination of STS. This is not of importance here.

By subtraction of the values for corresponding points, according to equation (3), the values for the estimated amounts of STS are obtained. These values are plotted in Fig. 7.

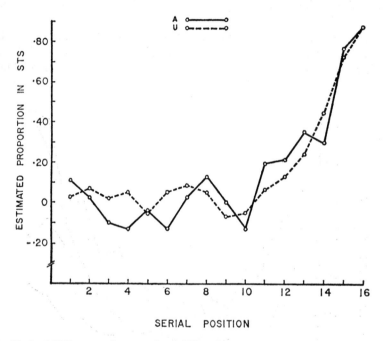

FIG. 7.   Derived STS curves for associated (A) and unassociated (U) items. (After GLANZER and SCHWARTZ[10].)

The delay curves in Fig. 6 indicate that mnemonic structure has a marked effect on LTS. The curves in Fig. 7 indicate that it has no effect on STS.

RAYMOND[7] has applied the subtraction method to the following variables: rate of presentation, normative frequency of list items and words versus nonsense syllables. In all cases a pattern of results like that in Fig. 6 and Fig. 7 was obtained. The variables affected LTS but did not affect STS.

The removal of items from STS

The delay task used to eliminate the contents of STS may have its effect in several ways. Several alternatives were studied in a series of experiments.[13] The alternatives were the following:

(1). Information load or difficulty of subsequent activity, i.e. the delay task.

(2). Similarity of items involved in subsequent activity.

(3). Number of items processed during subsequent activity.

(4). Passage of time.

The experiments involved the variation of each of the variables listed above. The results of experiments on information load and similarity indicated that those factors were not important. The final experiment in the series tested the effect of two factors, namely, number of items and time. In that experiment, both the duration of the delay task and the number of items in it were varied. Twelve-word lists were used. After each list there was either a 2-sec or a 6-sec delay. During the delay period the subject read aloud either 2 or 6 words. This design permits the separation of the effects of passage of time and number of items. The results are shown in Fig. 8. The number of items has a clear effect in eliminating items from STS, i.e. lowering the end peak. The length of the delay period has no effect.

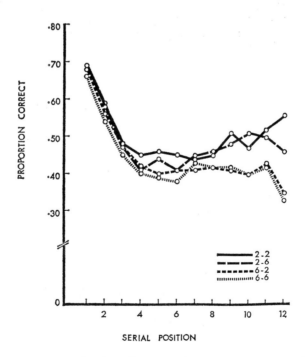

FIG. 8. Serial position curves for four delay conditions—2–2, 2 words read in 2 sec; 2–6, 2 words in 6 sec; 6–2, 6 words in 2 sec; 6–6, 6 words in 6 sec. (After GLANZER *et al.*[13])

The results of these studies and others indicate that STS is a mechanism that is sensitive to almost nothing except the number of items passing through it. These successive items displace items previously entered in STS.

Many details about the functioning of STS have been worked out over the past few years. For example, there are data that support the idea that if an item is in STS and a repetition of that item occurs, only one of the two representations is held in STS. From this it follows that it is advantageous to repeat an item only after giving a number of intervening items, i.e. after the first representation has cleared STS. This distribution effect has been demonstrated.[14]

It has also been shown that repetition of items can be imposed on the subject in a way that lowers the probability of recall. Rapid repetition of the item by the subject in the interval between successive items blocks appropriate types of rehearsal in STS. This in turn lowers the amount registered in LTS but does not affect the amount held in STS. This effect was demonstrated by GLANZER and MEINZER[15] using the interaction method.

The picture that emerges on the basis of this work is that the STS functions as both an input buffer and operating register. It accumulates short series of input information and permits the carrying out of the operations necessary to register the information in LTS. These operations include making use of structural characteristics of the sequence, e.g. redundancy, and organization of the sequence on the basis of other stored information.

There is not the space here to go into the details of both STS and LTS functioning as developed in the literature. Instead, the general applicability of the model as presented so far will be argued for in the following sections. The argument will consider generality across laboratory memory tasks, generality across subject populations and relevance to clinical performance.

Generality across laboratory tasks

The model outlined above is not restricted to the free recall task. It also applies to the following tasks which are widely used in the laboratory study of memory.

1. *Distractor tasks.* In these tasks, a single item or series of items is followed by a delay task. Frequently the series of items is a sequence of three consonants which the subject has to recall in order. The delay task may be anything from reading numbers or letters to carrying out complex mental operations. The length of the delay task may be varied.

2. *Probe tasks.* A series of items is followed by probes as to specific items. In a sequential probe task the subject is usually given a sequence of items, is then presented with one item and is asked to recall the following item. In paired associates the subject is given a sequence of paired items, is then given the first element of the pair, the stimulus term, and is asked to recall the second, the response term.

3. *Fixed-order recall tasks.* A series of items is presented, all of which are to be recalled in order. The sequence is usually longer than that used in a distractor task. This is also called a serial-recall task or memory-span task. It is very often used in clinical testing.

Results with these tasks, in general, show the same relations found in the free-recall task. Only one of these parallel results, results on presentation rate, will be described in any detail here.

MURDOCK[11] gave subjects a sequence of five paired associates. He varied the rate at which these pairs were presented. After the fifth pair was presented, the stimulus term of one of the five pairs was given to the subject, who then had to recall the response term. A plot of the probability of recall shows that the later items have an advantage over the earlier ones. There is a pronounced end peak. Moreover, when the curves for different rates are compared, the early sections of the curves are separated according to presentation rate but the end peaks merge, as in free recall.

Similar equivalences appear for the variables discussed above—length of list,[1,11,16] spacing of repetitions,[17] delay.[18-20] The references above include work on the three types of tasks listed above—distractor tasks, probe tasks and fixed-order recall tasks. It is simple to show that the model applies equally well to this range of laboratory tasks.

Generality across subject populations

The distinction between STS and LTS holds for a wide range of subjects. Examination of this range is informative as to the functioning of memory.

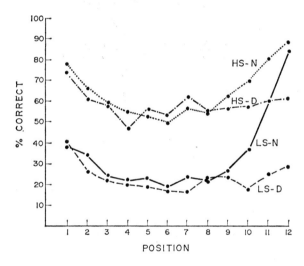

FIG. 9.   Serial position curves for high scoring (HS) and low scoring (LS) subjects on delay (D) and no-delay (N) free recall. (After RAYMOND[21].)

1. *Different levels of mnemonic skill.* RAYMOND[21] plotted the serial position curves for subjects who scored high and those who scored low in free recall. The serial position curves for these two groups with immediate recall show the standard interactive pattern seen in earlier figures. The two no-delay curves are shown in Fig. 9. Also in that figure are shown the serial position curves for each group with a 30-sec delay task. Again a pattern seen earlier appears. The end peaks have disappeared and the two curves are parallel to each other. Application of equation (3) gives the estimated amount in STS for each serial

position. The amounts are plotted in Fig. 10. This application of the subtractive method shows that the difference between the high scoring and low scoring subjects is entirely in LTS.

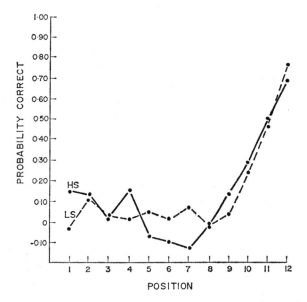

FIG. 10.   Derived STS curves for high scoring (HS) and low scoring (LS) subjects. (After RAYMOND[21].)

2. *Different levels of intelligence.* ELLIS[22] compared the performance of retardates with college students of the same age. Both groups were given a nine-item probe task. The serial position curves for the two groups show an interaction of mental age with serial position. The curves are separate with the normals higher across all positions except the last few. There the curves merge. The interaction method shows here that the difference between the groups is in the amount registered in LTS.

3. *Differences in age.* CRAIK[23] compared the free recall of two groups of subjects, age 22 and 65. He used a subtraction technique to estimate the effects of age on STS and LTS, and found that it affects only LTS. The older subjects show lower amounts in LTS. STS stays constant.

A recent study[24] makes a parallel comparison at a younger age level. Two groups of children, one 5 years old, the other 6; were given free recall lists that varied in length from two to seven items. The results for all list lengths are shown in Fig. 11.

The effect of list length, noted earlier, can be seen by comparing the six sections of the figure. As list length increases, recall of early positions declines. The final positions are relatively unaffected. More relevant here, however, is the effect of age. There is an interaction of age with serial position. The early sections of the matched curves differ. The final sections do not differ. The interaction method indicates that an increase of age in children is correlated with an increase in the amount held in LTS. STS stays constant.

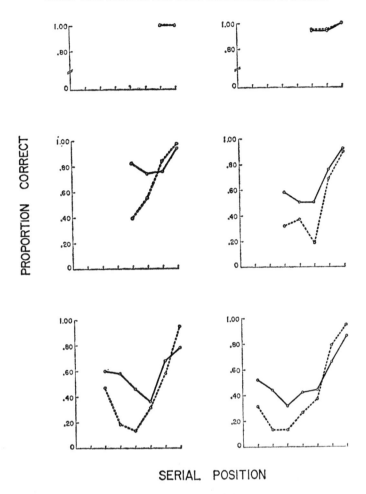

FIG. 11.   Serial position curves for 5-yr-old (broken line) and 6-yr-old (solid line) children with lists of length 2, 3, 4, 5, 6, and 7 words. (After THURM and GLANZER[24] 1971.)

Relevance to clinical performance

The distinction between LTS and STS is of importance in the case of certain memory disorders. MILNER[25] presented evidence that bilateral lesions in the hippocampal area left both LTS and STS unimpaired but blocked registration of new material in LTS. The patients could recall information that they had acquired before the lesion occurred. They could perform normally on immediate memory tasks. A distraction, however, disrupted this performance. New material, moreover, could not be learned.

DRACHMAN and ARBIT[26] studied 5 patients with known or presumed bilateral hippocampal lesions. They found that these patients' immediate memory span for short sequences of items was not impaired. They were, however, unable to learn longer sequences even after many repetitions. Their LTS contained less new information than normal. Their STS was unimpaired. SHUTTLEWORTH and MORRIS[27] cite 7 cases of their own and 29 cases of other investigators that show the same pattern of performance and disability. On the basis of these cases they propose a multiple-storage-mechanism model of memory.

There is one characteristic of the performance of these patients that is important. In addition to the impairment in the learning of new material, there is a retrograde amnesia that is widespread at first but becomes more and more limited as recovery from the lesion progresses. This characteristic is not included in the two-storage model as currently phrased.

BADDELEY and WARRINGTON[28] bring together this clinical work with the laboratory work. They studied the performance of six amnesic patients. Four were identified as alcoholics suffering from Korsakoff's psychosis, one had had a right temporal lobectomy, and one may have suffered a cerebrovascular injury. The performance of this group was compared with that of control subjects on free recall, probe tasks, distractor tasks, fixed-order recall tasks and others.

The results from several of the tasks are unclear. The results from the free recall task, however, are particularly clear and relevant. Both delay and no-delay free recall of ten-word lists were tested. In the no-delay condition the amnesic subjects exhibit a serial-position function that is lower than that of the normal control subjects in all but the last few positions. Clinical condition interacts with serial position. In the delay condition, the amnesics give a serial position curve that is lower than that for the controls across all serial positions. There is no interaction. BADDELEY and WARRINGTON[28] apply the subtraction method to their data and show that the differences lie wholly in LTS. There is no difference in STS.

CLOSING STATEMENT

The work outlined above covers only a small part of the current information concerning recall and the distinction between LTS and STS. It might seem from the outline, that any effective variable, other than number of subsequent items, will affect only LTS. There are, however, two variables that have an effect specific to STS. Both variables seem at present to indicate that STS has a special role in the processing of speech. One variable is the sense modality of the input material. Auditory presentation gives higher recall than does visual presentation.[29] This effect is, however, limited to the amount held in STS. The other variable is grouping. If material is presented to the subject in regular groups there is an increase in the amount recalled.[30] Again this effect is restricted to STS.

The main points emphasized in this paper are (1) that the area of memory is one that includes a considerable range of performance, including clinical behavior, and (2) that methods allowing a productive analysis of this performance have been developed. Moreover, reliable functional relationships have been established that furnish a basis for a fuller understanding of memory.

SUMMARY

Work over the past ten years has converged on a multiple-storage model of memory. Some of the details of the model and some data relevant to it are described. Methods for the separation of short-term and long-term storage are presented. Also presented are data concerning the generality of the model and its applicability to the study of clinical disorders.

REFERENCES

1. ATKINSON, R. C. and SHIFFRIN, R. M. Human memory: A proposed system and its control processes. In: *The psychology of learning and motivation: Advances in research and theory*, SPENCE K. W. and SPENCE J. T. (Eds.), Vol. II, p. 890, Academic Press, New York, 1968.
2. GLANZER, M. and CUNITZ, A. R. Two storage mechanisms in free recall. *J. verb. Learn. verb. Behav.* **5**, 351, 1966.
3. MURDOCK, B. B., JR. Recent developments in short-term memory. *Br. J. Psychol.* **58**, 421, 1967.
4. WAUGH, N. C. and NORMAN, D. A. Primary memory. *Psychol. Rev.* **72**, 89, 1965.
5. SPERLING, G. The information available in brief visual presentations. *Psychol. Monogr.* **74**, (Whole No. 498), 1960.
6. MURDOCK, B. B., JR. The serial position effect of free recall. *J. exp. Psychol.* **64**, 482, 1962.
7. RAYMOND, B. Short-term and long-term storage in free recall. *J. verb. Learn. verb. Behav.* **8**, 567, 1969.
8. SUMBY, W. H. Word frequency and serial position effects. *J. verb. Learn. verb. Behav.* **1**, 443, 1963.
9. POSTMAN, L. and PHILLIPS, L. W. Short-term temporal changes in free recall. *Q. Jl. exp. Psychol.* **17**, 132, 1965.
10. GLANZER, M. and SCHWARTZ, A. Mnemonic structure in free recall: Differential effects on STS and LTS. *J. verb. Learn. verb. Behav.* in press.
11. MURDOCK, B. B., JR. Effects of a subsidiary task on short-term memory. *Br. J. Psychol.* **56**, 413, 1965.
12. SILVERSTEIN, C. and GLANZER, M. Difficulty of a concurrent task in free recall: Differential effects on STS and LTS. *Psychonom. Sci.* 1971.
13. GLANZER, M., GIANUTSOS, R. and DUBIN, S. The removal of items from short-term storage. *J. verb. Learn. verb. Behav.* **8** 435, 1969.
14. GLANZER, M. Distance between related words in free recall: Trace of the STS. *J. verb. Learn. verb. Behav.* **8**, 105, 1969.
15. GLANZER, M. and MEINZER, A. The effects of intralist activity on free recall. *J. verb. Learn. verb. Behav.*, **6**, 928, 1967.
16. JAHNKE, J. C. Serial position effects in immediate serial recall. *J. verb. Learn. verb. Behav.* **2**, 284, 1963.
17. PETERSON, L. R., WAMPLER, R., KIRKPATRICK, M. and SALTZMAN, D. Effect of spacing presentations on retention of a paired associate over short intervals. *J. exp. Psychol.* **66**, 206, 1963.
18. JAHNKE, J. C. Delayed recall and the serial position effect of short-term memory. *J. exp. Psychol.* **76**, 618, 1968.
19. PETERSON, L. R. and PETERSON, M. J. Short-term retention of individual verbal items. *J. exp. Psychol.* **58**, 193, 1959.
20. TULVING, E. and ARBUCKLE, T. Y. Sources of intratrial interference in immediate recall of paired associates. *J. verb. Learn. verb. Behav.* **1**, 321, 1963.
21. RAYMOND, B. Factors affecting long-term and short-term storage in free recall. Unpublished doctoral dissertation, New York University, 1968.
22. ELLIS, N. R. Memory processes in retardates and normals: Theoretical and empirical considerations. In: *International Review of Research in Mental Retardation*, ELLIS, N. R. (Ed.), Vol. 4, p. 1. Academic Press, New York, 1970.
23. CRAIK, F. I. M. Two components in free recall. *J. verb. Learn. verb. Behav.* **7**, 996, 1968.
24. THURM, A. T. and GLANZER, M. Free recall in children: Long-term store versus short-term store. *Psychonom. Sci.* **23**, 175, 1971.
25. MILNER, B. Amnesia following operation on the temporal lobes. In: *Amnesia*, WHITLY, C. W. M. and ZANGWILL (Eds.), p. 109, Butterworths, London, 1966.
26. DRACHMAN, D. A. and ARBIT, J. Memory and the hippocampal complex. *Archs Neurol.* **15**, 52, 1966.
27. SHUTTLEWORTH, E. C. and MORRIS, C. E. The transient global amnesia syndrome. *Archs Neurol.* **15**, 515, 1966.
28. BADDELEY, A. D. and WARRINGTON, E. K. Amnesia and the distinction between long- and short-term memory. *J. verb. Learn. verb. Behav.* **9**, 176, 1970.

29. MURDOCK, B. B., JR. and WALKER, K. D. Modality effects in free recall. *J. verb. Learn. verb. Behav.* **8,** 665, 1969.
30. GIANUTSOS, R. Free recall of grouped words. Unpublished doctoral dissertation. New York University, 1970.

J. psychiat. Res., 1971, Vol. 8, pp. 439–444. Pergamon Press. Printed in Great Britain.

LINGUISTIC ASPECTS OF AMNESIA AND CONFABULATION

Edwin A. Weinstein

Department of Neurology, Mount Sinai Medical School, New York, New York

I have chosen the topic of amnestic-confabulatory state because it illustrates the multi-disciplinary, operational approach to the study of behavior characteristic of David Rioch's influence upon neuro-psychiatric research at the Walter Reed Army Institute of Research. My introduction to this somewhat unique point of view began shortly after the end of World War II when I walked into one of his lectures at the William A. White Institute of Psychiatry in New York anticipating a description of the behavior of the decerebrate cat, only to learn about the banking system of the Knights Templar. This perhaps apocryphal story may also serve as an introduction to one of the classical eponymic syndromes in neuro-psychiatry, the amnestic-confabulatory state or Korsakow syndrome. Since the original description, in the late nineteenth century, subsequent authors have maintained the concurrence of the phenomena of amnesia, confabulation, disorientation for place and time and mood changes, notably apathy. However, interpretations have varied widely reflecting the many schools of thought in neurology, psychology and psychiatry.[1] Early writers were concerned with the mechanisms of memory; registration, retention, and recall. Later observers were impressed with the passivity and lack of concern shown by patients and attributed the disturbance to lack of drive and motivation. Kral[2] suggested that the patient, as a result of his brain injury was unable to integrate sensory perceptions and affective components into a personally meaningful experience. A recent study of Talland[3] attributed the behavior to a premature closure of activation in which the patient fails to maintain the searching and matching operations essential to normal remembering. Psychoanalytically oriented writers have emphasized the wish-fulfilling and other symbolic aspects of confabulation.[4]

In this paper, I shall present the amnestic-confabulatry syndrome from the standpoint of language, with particular reference to language as an index of interaction in the environment and as a mode of adaptation to stress. The material comes from the study of 150 subjects with acute closed head injuries and another ten with ruptured aneurysms of the Circle of Willis who were followed from the acute onset through the stages of clinical recovery.[5-7]

The patients were male military personnel hospitalized at the Walter Reed General Hospital. Their ages ranged from 18 to 58 with a mean age of 25·4 yr. All patients expressed

T

a marked amnesia and/or confabulation for a period of at least one week. All had evidence of brain damage as an initial loss of consciousness or confusion. Most patients had bloody or xanthochromic spinal fluid or other signs of brain laceration. The majority of the subjects who had experienced trauma had been in automobile accidents. Subjects were interviewed at least once or twice a week for periods up to 6 months and the results recorded verbatim.

AMNESIA

While the dictionary definition of amnesia is loss of memory, in clinical usage it applies to a particular type of memory loss. It refers to the verbal statement that one does not remember an event or period of time with which one should be familiar; such as why the patient is in the hospital, the kind of work he does, where he lives and whether he is married. The sole evidence for amnesia is the patient's verbal statement and there are no objective tests that are diagnostic of amnesia. The term is not used to characterize poor performance on a test battery. Actually, amnesic patients may perform quite well on standard memory tests and may have no difficulty reproducing previously learned acts. For example, a soldier who, following a head injury states that he does not remember having been in the Army may exhibit an excellent knowledge of military protocol.

Following head injuries, the content of the retrograde amnesia* most commonly concerned the accident itself. The period of retrograde amnesia ranged from a few seconds or minutes to months or years as patients stated that they did not remember anything for a week before the accident or did not recall having joined the Army. An extended retrograde amnesia, however, transcends the physical event or the period of chronological time. Thus, the patient who says that he does not remember his accident also may not know where it occurred or the origin and destination of the automobile trip. He may not remember the make of his car even though he has owned the vehicle for several years. When a patient states that he does not remember anything that happened on the 'day' of the accident, the 'day' is not a chronological unit of 24 hr but a social or metaphorical expression like a 'bad day' or 'a day of reckoning'.

Amnesia also involves an attitude toward the event. Very few patients who have been knocked unconscious remember the actual impact. Yet, while a patient does not recall the actual impact he is not regarded as amnesic because when he is asked what happened to him he says that he was in an automobile accident. It is only when he is queried for details that he will say he does not remember the impact. The amnesic patient, on the other hand states that he does not know or does not remember what happened when asked why he is in the hospital and it takes a number of questions before the patient states "they told me I was in an accident". Similarly he may say that he does not know where he is, even though the name of the hospital is in plain sight. Nor does the amnesic patient generally express

---

* Retrograde amnesia is the period of time prior to the loss of consciousness that the patient states he cannot recall. There is little or no relationship between the severity of the injury, the duration of unconsciousness and the stated length of retrograde amnesia. This contrasts with the duration of the anterograde amnesia which correlates well with the length of the period after the accident during which the patient was disoriented.

concern over his obvious injuries and their consequences. For him, the fact of being in a hospital bed with a bandage on his head and perhaps a cast on his leg does not constitute a pattern of relatedness in his environment that includes the feeling of his having been injured. Amnesia involves not only the recall of the past but a loss of relatedness in the current and anticipated aspects of the environment.

With clinical improvement, the amnesia becomes more selective and provides a language in which a patient can represent symbolically certain problems and relationships. Such problems include physical disabilities, intellectual deficits, the prospect of discharge from military service and the loss of status consequent to incapacity. Thus a patient initially may not remember having been in the Army. As he improves, he may volunteer that he remembers having been in service but not the work that he did or the rank that he held. In this sense, amnesia can be regarded as composing not only what cannot be remembered but also what is remembered. With further recovery and the clearing of amnesia, such problems are represented in more referential fashion. For example, the soldier who formerly did not remember the rank he held expressed his concern that he would be separated from the service. One of our patients initially did not remember if he were married and did not recognize his wife. Subsequently, he recalled his marriage but complained that he could not remember in what church the ceremony had been performed. When he recalled the church, he expressed the fear that his wife would leave him. She obtained a separation shortly after he was transferred to a Veterans Hospital.

What is perceived as the main problem and the language in which it is represented were found to be related to what had been significant sources of identity. Patients with amnesia for military service were usually career soldiers, described as having been conscientious and efficient in their work. The man who had an amnesia for his marriage was described as having been very dependent on his wife and family. When the relationship among amnesic content, current problems and patterns of social relatedness was recognized, it became evident why amnesia could be so selective and why a patient could pick out some apparently insignificant detail to 'disremember'.

An interesting feature of amnesia is the 'last memory' prior to an accident forming the temporal boundary of the retrograde amnesia. Such a memory was often a symbolic representation of a current problem. For example, the 'last memory' of a patient with a severe visual loss was of getting a new lens for his camera several months before the accident. Such memories may be actual events, they may be incidents displaced in place or time, they may be condensations of several events or they may be confabulations. A remarkable 'last memory' occurred frequently among patients involved in accidents in which there had been a fatality. This was the recollection of having 'gone to sleep' of having 'passed out'. These observations suggest that the stated duration of retrograde amnesia following loss of consciousness depends on the intensity of the patient's feeling of non-involvement and how far back in time he goes to select an adequate symbol to represent the current situation.

Confabulation

Confabulation may be defined as the fictitious narration of some past event or events and, in brain injured subjects, it is most commonly elicited by questioning the patient about his injury or disability. Confabulation may be associated with amnesia, or it may precede or follow amnesia. Like amnesia the confabulation refers not only to the past but to the current situation and its anticipated consequences. What is ostensibly a designation of a past event is also to some degree a metaphorical representation of current problems. For example, a patient with an ocular palsy resulting from a ruptured aneurysm told a story of having been punched in the eye in a fight. The choice of metaphorical content is also determined by the symbolic themes that have, in the past, provided the patient with significant channels of social relatedness and sources of identity. Most commonly, the symbolism involves the family. A patient with a ruptured aneurysm claimed that he had come to the hospital to visit his sick wife. After automobile accidents, members of the family are frequently implicated and the putative injuries ascribed to a brother or son bear a striking resemblance to the patient's own. Confabulations about work and occupation also occurred. Paratroopers injured in a car wreck confabulated that they had been hurt in a jump. An officer whose intellectual deficits following a head injury had disqualified him from further service, told a story about having engaged in "counter intelligence activities." Other categories of confabulation were those of violence and death, minor illnesses and play and sports. Confabulations about violence involved having been in a fight or stories about people, usually poorly identified, being killed. Confabulations about minor illness and sports were generally part of a denial of disability as when a patient with a paretic limit denied that the limb was weak and said he had sprained his ankle in a football game. Confabulations about work and occupation were generally elaborate and lengthy while those of sports and minor illness were brief. In general the more elaborate the confabulation, the less apt it was to explicitly deny injury and disability.

The accounts of premorbid personality obtained from relatives and colleagues indicated that patients who represented their problems in confabulations about work, were work-oriented people whose occupations had provided them with an important basis of identity and a sense of purpose. Those whose confabulations involved a close relative were generally described as strongly family-oriented. A patient who confabulated that his injury had occurred from being pushed downstairs in a fight at a country club came from a family much preoccupied with money and social position. Confabulations about physical violence occurred in persons who had lived in a social environment in which violence or the anticipation of violence by others had been a major mode of communication.

Patients with well developed confabulations are generally bland and passive and, like the amnesic patient, they do not overtly express worry and concern over their condition. They maintain their fictitious stories despite cues, corrections and the obvious disbelief of their auditors. Few confabulations are bizarre and wholly unbelievable and the patient gives his account in a matter of fact manner. In confabulations about work, especially, the patient supplies technical details and expressions which lend verisimilitude to the story. Although a well-developed confabulation is generally maintained consistently in successive interviews, patients may not confabulate in all situations. One of our patients while confabulating in the formal interview, told his young sister the true version of his accident.

Events, which are in themselves true, may be used metaphorically and so serve the purpose of a confabulation. For example, a patient who had become sexually impotent, as a consequence of a ruptured intracranial aneurysm, in telling of the onset, invariably included the detail that someone had tried to revive him by pouring cold water on his genitals.

Other analogs and sequelae of confabulations are idioms, clichés, euphemisms and humor. An excellent example of the use of humor is provided by a physician who wrote an account of his experience of having suffered a severe brain injury. In his narrative, written several years after his accident, he used colorful metaphors and flowery idioms in referring to the anatomical aspects of the head injury including such expressions as "enfeebled encephalon" and "the convoluted tenant of my calcific casque".[8]

The content of confabulation may also correlate with other aspects of behavior. After apparent recovery and the disappearance of confabulation, the theme may become a dominant feature of personal relationships. After giving up a confabulation about a family member, the patient may become obsessively concerned with the health of that person. Over strict and intolerant attitudes toward the patient's children may follow a confabulation about children. Subjects who use language of violence to describe their disabilities show a high incidence of somatic complaints and emotional disturbance. The language includes confabulations of death, expressions like 'smashed' and 'tore up' and references to blood and explosions. These patients complain of headaches, insomnia and catastrophic dreams and a considerable number develop classical manifestations of conversion hysteria. The conversion motor and sensory signs appear in a portion of the body which has been the site of local impact or in which there is some organic loss. Such hysterical features may be regarded as the gesture that accompanies the verbal representation of the disability.

Comment

This presentation of amnesia and confabulation as patterns of language is a useful way of describing disturbances in perception, set, memory, affect, time sense and personality in a unitary framework and indicating a relationship among neurological, psychological and social factors. Under the conditions of the study, brain damage provided a necessary condition for the existence of the behavior. However, it is not the only etiological factor. Patients with similar brain pathology may show different clinical pictures and certain features of the syndrome, particularly the retrograde amnesia, show little or no correlation with the severity of the brain damage. Also, any explanation must take into account the fact that amnesia and confabulation occur in persons with normal brain function.

Amnesia is so commonly associated with confabulation, not because confabulation is a way of filling in memory gaps or compensating for memory loss, an explanation found in textbooks, but because they are comparable phenomena. (Actually, the great majority of neurological patients with severe memory loss do not confabulate.) In a sense, amnesia is the confabulation of loss of memory and the patient's statement that he does not remember an event is a way of talking about the event. In amnesia and confabulation, the language is an index of a relationship in the environment. The patient denies or does not recognize the existence of an actual experience and maintains the validity of a fictitious event. This contradiction may be resolved if the language is analyzed from the standpoint of metaphor, or in terms of the experiential symbolic mode as opposed to the literal or referential definition of a symbol. In a referential sense, the amnesic, confabulatory patient does not know or does not remember what happened to him because the symbol is not an element in a socially organized pattern. Under the conditions of brain dysfunction, and stress, the meaning of the symbol depended less on its physical referent than on the way it fitted into a personal identity system. Similarly, in the absence of structural brain changes, one adapts to stress by perceiving selectively the events of the environment and organizing them into socially relevant units through which one gains a sense of causality and predictability compatible with expectations based on past experience. The effect of the brain damage is to make the symbolic patterns more highly condensed, more rigid and less dependent on reinforcement by members of the social group. With improvement of brain function, the sequelae of confabulation, such as humor, clichés and anecdotes gain much of their effect from the response of the patient's auditors.

REFERENCES

1. RAPAPORT, D. *Organization and Pathology of Thought*. Columbia University Press, New York, 1951.
2. KRAL, V. A. The amnestic syndrome. *Mschr. Psychiat. Neurol.* **132**, 65, 1956.
3. TALLAND, G. A. *Deranged Memory: A Psychonomic Study of the Amnesic Syndrome*. Academic Press, New York, 1965.
4. BETLHEIM, S. and HARTMANN, H. Ueber Fehlreactionen bei der Korsàkowschen Psychose. *Arch. Psychiat. Nerv Kramkh* **72**, 257, 1924.
5. WEINSTEIN, E. A., KAHN, R. L. and MALITZ, S. Confabulation as a social process. *Psychiatry* **19**, 383, 1956.
6. WEINSTEIN, E. A., MARVIN, S. L. and KELLER, N. J. A. Amnesia as a language pattern. *Archs gen. Psychiat.* **6**, 259, 1962.
7. WEINSTEIN, E. A. and LYERLY, O. G. Confabulation following brain injury. Its analogues and sequelae. *Archs gen. Psychiat.* **18**.
8. LA BAW, W. Denial inside-out. Subjective experience with anosognosia in closed head injury. *Psychiatry* **2**, 174, 1969.

J. psychiat. Res., 1971, Vol. 8, pp. 445–478. Pergamon Press. Printed in Great Britain.

THE NEW BIOLOGY OF SLEEP

Harold L. Williams*†

Department of Psychiatry, University of Oklahoma Medical Center, Oklahoma City, Oklahoma

Since the mid-1950's, the rate of scientific publication on sleep and its neural and behavioral correlates has risen from a few articles a year to something like sixty articles a month and there is no hint that we are approaching asymptote. It seems remarkable that so much effort has been expended by so many disciplines on an extremely complex biopsychological state (or states) the functions of which remain entirely unknown. Several factors are responsible for the astounding growth of this field of study. Along with advances in electrophysiological, biochemical, pharmacological and behavioral technology which were achieved in the decades of the 1950's and 60's, there emerged a conviction that sleep was not simply a passive state, a resting state somewhere near the lower pole of a continuum of vigilance. Instead sleep was seen as a complex, constantly changing, but cyclic succession of active psychophysiological phenomena, and furthermore, it was soon realized that its phenomenology, and possibly its mechanisms, were similar if not identical among humans, the other mammals and birds. Neurobiologists were challenged by the remarkably long-term processes implicated by sleep research, and behavioral scientists by the realization that the transition from waking to sleep was not a natural boundary for behavioral investigation, that sleep was not an empty state psychologically. The demonstration by Dement and Kleitman[1] that the periodic occurrence of vigorous ocular activity in the presence of EEG desynchrony was associated with vivid visual dreams, and the immediate confirmation by Dement[2] of similar periodic bioelectric patterns in the cat stimulated the interest of investigators from nearly every discipline of the behavioral and biological sciences. Perhaps implicit in this multidisciplinary investigation of the states of sleep is the hope that an understanding of its biological and behavioral mechanisms may clarify, even resolve, the ancient controversies over mind and body.

This paper summarizes part of the work which encouraged the view that sleep is an active function of the brain, composed of at least two states, controlled by different but

* I wish to thank my colleagues, Boyd K. Lester, Joe D. Coulter and William Griffiths, for their help in thinking through and preparing this paper, and for their permission to use data, interpretations and concepts from projects which they have supervised. Lester and Griffiths are responsible for the cancer studies, and Coulter and Griffiths for the amino acid load and reserpine work.

† Address reprint requests to: Harold L. Williams, Ph.D., Department of Psychiatry, University of Oklahoma Medical Center, 800 Northeast 13th Street, Oklahoma City, Oklahoma 73104.

linked neurochemical systems, and temporally programmed in a relatively predictable sequence. The periodic phenomena of sleep and waking, and their alterations by sleep deprivation, drugs, psychological illness and aging are programmed on a long time scale which implies biochemical processes different from those recommended for millisecond neurochemistry, and the search for such mechanisms has only begun. Evidence has accumulated for both man and animals implicating the biogenic amines in the induction, maintenance and succession of the states of sleep, and some positive conclusions as well as controversial interpretations arising from these studies will be reviewed here.

SLEEP AS AN ACTIVE STATE

In 1924, and again in 1925, Hess[3,4] argued that sleep is not a passive state of the brain, but a positive vegetative function to be classed with such related activities as respiration, circulation, temperature regulation and digestion, the common function of which is regulation of the internal milieu. He asserted that sleep is not simply a state of quiescence, a a let down from waking, for many of the symptoms of sleep such as active contraction of the eyelids, increased tone of the rectal sphincter, the miotic pupil, the presence of the Babinski reflex in adolescents and adults,[5] the curled-up sleeping positions in cat and dog, and the standing positions of birds and horses are manifestations of chronic activity in the relevant musculature, and therefore of active control by the central and autonomic nervous systems. Since the 1950's, a plethora of studies of micro and macular electrical activity in the brain have failed to find sleeping neurons (see, for example, Creutzfeldt and Jung;[6] Murata and Kameda;[7] Evarts;[8] Evarts et al.[9]). It is now clear that sleep is not characterized by a general decline in bodily and brain activity. Instead, it differs from waking in a qualitative manner. It is represented by a redistribution of functions, a re-organization of the brain rather than a drop from waking to sleeping activity.

The idea that sleep is an actively induced process received support with Hess[10,11] finding that sleep can be induced by electrical stimulation of certain structures in the brain. He showed that low frequency (about 4 per sec), low voltage, rounded DC pulses delivered through thalamic placements, located between the Vicq d'Azyr and Meynert tracts in the lower two-thirds of the massa intermedia, $1 \cdot 5$–$3 \cdot 5$ mm from the midline induced a sequence of behaviors culminating in sound, long-lasting sleep in the non-anesthetized cat. Shortly after the onset of stimulation, his so-called 'elite cases' would begin circling movements as if searching for a proper place to lie down, then lie down in prone position with forepaws folded beneath the body. Following this, the eyelids drooped, the nictitating membranes protruded, the pupils contracted, the animal curled up, and went to sleep. He could be aroused by sensory stimuli. Stimulus trains delivered through electrodes located lateral to the medial thalamus caused some but not all of the symptoms of sleep. Hess' observations have since been confirmed by a number of investigations (e.g. Akert et al.;[12] Hess, Jr. et al.[13]). One important aspect of these findings is that they implicate the medial thalamus specifically as a hypnogenic area. Possibly, as Koella[14] has suggested, the thalamus is the 'head ganglion' for the organization of sleep. Despite the well-established role of non-specific thalamic structures in the modulation of sleep spindles and recruiting responses, the latter proposal has not been popular. The search for the neural mechanisms of sleep has been focused primarily on brain stem and limbic structures.

Hess' demonstration that sleep could be induced by electrical stimulation of the brain had little impact on theorists who viewed sleep as a passive state. One reason for this was the finding that sleep, or at least some of its symptoms, could be induced by electrical or chemical stimulation of the cortex, thalamus, subthalamus, hypothalamus, mesencephalon, pons, cerebellum, medulla, spinal cord and sensory nerves. Furthermore, since the undisturbed cat sleeps about two-thirds of the time anyway, it was alleged that Hess' conclusions were not valid. KLEITMAN[15] (p. 502) wrote " . . . there is not a single fact about sleep that cannot be equally well interpreted as a let-down of waking activity," and BREMER[16] doubted the existence of subcortical inhibitory mechanisms acting upon the cortex. In the light of modern neurophysiological studies in which no significant degree of cortical inhibition has been found during sleep, and in which plausible neural systems for the active induction of sleep have been identified, the pioneering work of Hess is being re-evaluated.

The identification of the regions in brain initiating the state of sleep, and the position of the passive theorists as well, were advanced by BREMER's[17] first studies of the EEG of the brain of cats after mid-collicular decerebration. This *cerveau isolé* preparation showed an EEG pattern of slow activity typical of one phase of sleep. Furthermore, the pupils were constricted and the nictitating membranes covered the eye as in normal sleep of the cat. In this preparation, only the first three cranial nerves (olfactory, optic and oculomotor) remain connected with the brain. Bremer showed that strong olfactory stimulation would produce EEG arousal, and concluded that the brain was asleep rather than comatose. When a transection was made through the caudal medulla (encephale isolé) a more or less normal wake–sleep pattern was seen. Bremer concluded that the greater number of sensory inputs to the brain stem of the latter preparation accounted for the difference in wake–sleep patterns, and that sleep was due to deafferentiation of the brain.

In 1949, MORUZZI and MAGOUN[18] showed that repetitive electrical stimulation of the midbrain reticular formation was effective in transforming a slow-wave sleep pattern to a low amplitude fast wave pattern typical of the waking state. The period of EEG activation so obtained usually outlasted the period of stimulation, and the EEG desynchrony was usually accompanied by behavioral arousal.

Damage to the midbrain reticular formation causes prolonged sleep. Such lesions occur in encephalitis lethargica, where the lesion is often found in the central gray of the midbrain. LINDSLEY[19] showed that experimental lesions in the midbrain reticular formation caused a prolonged state of somnolence, while lesions in the specific sensory pathways did not cause EEG sleep. Thus, the integrity of the reticular formation is required for EEG and behavioral wakefulness.

In their original study, Moruzzi and Magoun suggested that the ascending influence from the reticular formation acted on the non-specific thalamic nuclei to interfere with their pacemaker activity. This was shown by the fact that recruiting waves excited from the thalamus could be blocked by stimulation of the reticular formation. It is also possible that the reticular system can exert direct inhibitory influence on the cortex, and finally, in addition to ascending reticulo-cortical influences, corticofugal actions on the reticular formation are now well established.

Reduction of activity in a tonic activating system is certainly one way that sleep can come about, and in this sense, the passive theories of sleep induction are sustained. But it appears, also, that sleep and waking are influenced by an active sleep-producing mechanism. The soporific effect of electrical stimulation of the massa intermedia of the thalamus and other parts of the diencephalon could result from inhibition of the reticular system of the midbrain, and the reticulo-cortico-reticular loop also permits active inhibition of the reticular activating system by means of feedback from the cortex. But active suppression of the reticular activating system can arise from the lower brain stem. Lesions in the mid pons cause an EEG arousal pattern, while lesions a few millimeters higher at the rostro-pontine level result in EEG sleep.[20,21] This suggests that a mechanism present in the caudal regions of the reticular formation can induce sleep by inhibiting the rostral portions of the reticular formation. Magnes et al.[22,23] elicited widespread bilateral synchronization of the cortical EEG by low-frequency stimulation of the region of the nucleus of the solitary tract, whereas high-frequency stimulation of the same brain-stem site caused desynchronization of the EEG, again suggesting that structures in the caudal brain stem participate in the active induction of sleep.

Thus it is now evident that there are structures in the lower pons and medulla that are capable of synchronizing cortical rhythms and inducing or sustaining behavioral sleep, their presence having been demonstrated both by transection and stimulation. Apparently these systems act by damping or modulating more rostral regions of the midbrain reticular formation.

REM SLEEP

The experiments mentioned above and many others convinced most neurophysiologists that there are brain mechanisms capable of the active induction of sleep. This view was further encouraged by the discovery that sleep consists of at least two distinct, successive stages—NREM (non-rapid eye movement), forebrain or slow-wave sleep; and REM (rapid eye movement) paradoxical, hindbrain, activated, desynchronized or fast sleep. NREM or slow-wave (SW) sleep is characterized by EEG slow waves and spindles and in man is usually classified into stages 1, 2, 3 and 4,[1] differentiated primarily on the basis of EEG frequency and amplitude. In SW sleep, cardiorespiratory activity is steady, and of lower frequency than during quiet waking. The skeletal musculature is greatly but not completely relaxed, and the eyes are relatively motionless. Upon awakening from this stage, subjects are likely to report that they were 'thinking' rather than 'dreaming'. In normal mammals, SW sleep always precedes REM sleep, after which both states alternate with waking in a more or less predictable sequence.

The low-voltage, variable frequency EEG of REM sleep resembles the waking EEG, especially in the cat. In man, the average EEG frequency is slower than during waking ranging from 4 to 10 Hz. During REM sleep, in the presence of relative EEG activation, the body becomes completely relaxed, loss of muscle tone in the neck of the cat and the submental region in man being profound. It is now understood that this is a true paralysis, caused by inhibitory effects on the spinal anterior horn cells.[24] Cerebral blood flow is greater during REM sleep than during waking.[25] Heart rate, respiration and blood pressure become highly variable, particularly during the bursts of rapid eye movements,[26] and the penis is in a state of tonic erection.[27] When awakened from REM sleep, the subject is likely to report vivid visual dreams.

The states of sleep each have two different phenomenological aspects, classed as phasic or tonic, which can become dissociated in certain drug states and other conditions. Phasic events during SW sleep include bursts of non-specific electrodermal activity, 14 Hz spindles, K-complexes and brief periods of EMG suppression. Phasic phenomena during REM sleep precede and accompany the bursts of conjugate eye movements, and include, in the cat, high-voltage EEG spikes which originate in the pons, and can be recorded from the reticular formation, the lateral geniculate and the occipital cortex. These PGO spikes occur at a fairly constant daily rate in the cat[28] about 14,000 per day, and they always precede REM sleep by a half minute or so. So far, PGO spikes or their representation have not been identified in the human EEG.

Neural mechanisms of REM sleep

Animal experiments with depth recording have revealed that the cortical desynchrony of REM sleep is associated with characteristic electrical patterns in other parts of the brain. For example, a synchronized, 4–6 Hz theta rhythm is found in the hippocampus of the cat,[29] the dog,[30] the rodents,[31] the opossum[32] and man,[33] and a 6–8 Hz rhythm is reported for the pontine reticular formation of the cat[14] (p. 18). A remarkable series of studies by MICHEL JOUVET and his colleagues made use of the hippocampal theta rhythm in their search for the brain areas responsible for REM sleep, e.g.[34–37] They found that with a transection through the rostral border of the midbrain, caudal indicators of SW sleep disappeared but REM sleep identified by eye movements and atonia was preserved. Furthermore, more caudally placed transections failed to eliminate the observable symptoms of REM sleep until the brain stem was transected at the lower border of the pons. The localization of a REM trigger in the pons was confirmed by a series of coagulation studies in which complete destruction of the *nucleus reticularis pontis caudalis* eliminated REM sleep. The otherwise intact cat continued to have SW sleep with normal periodicity. It is not yet certain whether it is possible to trigger the REM state by stimulation of the pontine center. Several investigators have reported that they could induce REM sleep by stimulating this or nearby areas.[38–41] However, KRIPKE et al.[42] were unable to replicate this effect in the monkey.

Most investigators agree that the center for the initiation of REM sleep is in the pons, but the route by which the cortex is desynchronized is not certain. JOUVET'S group first thought that limbic pathways were involved[36] but lesions and transections of the suspected limbic structures and pathways have failed to eliminate cortical desynchrony during REM.[43,44] Thus, the mechanism may be very diffuse, or it might be humoral rather than neural.

The phasic and tonic features of REM sleep appear to be organized in separate structures. JOUVET found that bilateral destruction of the locus coeruleus would abolish the tonic atonia of the REM state,[45] but the neural basis of the phasic components probably includes the lateral vestibular nuclei[46] and oculomotor control regions as well as the pontine centers.

THE NEED FOR SLEEP

Apparently, there is a biological need for each kind of sleep. When a human or other mammal is selectively deprived of REM sleep, there is a systematic tendency for this state to appear at shorter and shorter intervals, and when, subsequently, undisturbed sleep is allowed, a rebound occurs to higher than average levels. Meanwhile, SW sleep is virtually unaffected, and furthermore, deprivation of the latter stage does not affect REM.[47]

The normal occurrence of SW sleep at the beginning of sleep suggests that it may have important biological priority, and studies of total sleep deprivation support this notion. During recovery from sleep loss, human subjects first show excess SW sleep, whereas REM rebound is delayed until the second recovery night.[48,49] When normals are deprived specifically of stage 4 (the high-voltage phase of SW sleep) they subsequently show stage 4 rebound, but no alteration of stage REM.[50]

These data support the view that the two kinds of sleep are organized by different neurological systems, and indeed this inference is sustained by the fact that with various drugs, specific brain lesions, aging, pregnancy and other conditions, either stage of sleep can be suppressed without altering the other.

Quantitative aspects

There has been remarkable uniformity among published studies concerning the quantitative characteristics of the stages of sleep. The sleep of normal young men, adapted to the laboratory, is composed of about 23 per cent stage REM, with an estimated maximum range of 12–35 per cent.[51] Aging is associated with some loss of REM sleep, and a dramatic disappearance of high-voltage SW sleep. Newborn mammals, especially those whose central nervous systems are incompletely developed at birth, also have high proportions of REM sleep, and little or no SW sleep.[52] During a night of sleep in normal young adults, the time of occurrence of the first and succeeding epochs of stage REM is also quite stable. The first REM period begins about 100 min after the onset of sleep (first sleep spindle of stage 2) and REM recurs about every 100 min thereafter. The first period of REM sleep tends to be shortest, often lasting no longer than five or six minutes, while later periods of REM may last as long as thirty to sixty minutes. Most of the REM time occurs in the last third of the night while most high-voltage SW sleep is found in the first third of the night. In the laboratory cat, REM sleep periods occupy about 15 per cent, while SW sleep accounts for about 42 per cent of the 24-hr day, summing to a total sleep time of about 13 hr and 40 min.[53] As JOUVET[28] has pointed out, the extraordinary stability of sleep parameters in man and animals makes it possible " . . . to consider slow-wave sleep and paradoxical sleep as a quantitative index of the inner most mechanisms of the brain. This advance has made it possible to study the sleep states in relation to qualitative alterations in brain function such as result from drug injection or limited brain lesion, or in relation to data obtained through biochemical analysis" (p. 34).

In summary, it appears that sleep is an active state of the nervous system, consisting of at least two qualitatively different phases which are probably controlled by sequentially linked but distinct brain organizations. In normal humans and other mammals the time of occurrence, duration and order of these stages is systematic and subject to quantification. The long time course of their cycles and their slow recovery after chemical, physiological or psychological challenge suggests that humoral factors other than those involved in short-term neural mechanisms are involved in their modulation.

SOME POSSIBLE BIOCHEMICAL SUBSTRATES

The experimental investigation of hypnogenic substances began with the studies of PIÉRON[54] and LEGENDRE and PIÉRON[55,56] who withdrew cerebrospinal fluid from experimentally fatigued dogs and injected it into the fourth ventricle of non-fatigued recipient dogs which promptly showed signs of drowsiness and sleep. Dogs treated with cerebrospinal fluid from non-fatigued animals showed no such effects. SCHNEDORF and IVY[57] confirmed these results but questioned their validity because it was found that in both groups of animals, body temperature rose and cerebrospinal fluid pressure was elevated. More recently, KORNMÜLLER and his colleagues[58] and MONNER et al.[59] using pairs of cats or abbits whose circulation was crossed, produced sleep in recipient animals by using Hess' method of thalamic electrical stimulation in the donor. MONNIER and HOSLI[60,61] dialized venous blood from sleeping and waking donors and found that dialysate from a sleeping rabbit put an alert recipient to sleep, while dialysate from an alert donor aroused a sleeping animal.

These experiments and others suggest that during sleep deprivation or sleep, a factor is present in the cerebrospinal fluid or in blood which induces sleep in animals treated with these fluids or their extracts. Unfortunately, we have no idea what this hypnogenic substance may be. Monnier's work suggests that it is a small dialysable molecule. One possible candidate, acetylcholine, was tested in the studies of Schnedorf and Ivy, but they found no evidence of this substance in the cerebrospinal fluid of fatigued dogs. Nevertheless, HERNANDEZ-PEON's[62] chemical stimulation studies in cats appear to implicate acetylcholine as a synaptic transmitter in the hypnogenic system.

Recent research suggests that certain amines and other organic chemicals found in the central nervous system can induce sleep. For example, JOUANY et al.[63] reported that gamma-hydroxybutyrate (GHB) induces natural sleep in cats, and JOUVET et al.[64] found that doses of 200–500 mg/kg of 4-butyrolactone or sodium 4-hydroxybutyrate administered i.p. to cats induced a state of unresponsiveness in which, however, the eyes remained open and the nictitating membrane was not relaxed, and that 50 mg/kg of 4-butyrolactone would cause the rapid onset of REM sleep. Unfortunately, neither WINTERS and SPOONER[65] nor METCALF et al.[66] were able to confirm these findings in cats or humans, respectively. Interest in these related chemical substances was stimulated primarily by the fact that gamma aminobutyric acid has been found in the brain, but the conflicting evidence from different laboratories permits no interpretation of its possible role in the control of sleep.

Recent studies suggest that the induction and maintenance of the stages of sleep (and waking) are controlled at least in part by biogenic amines, specifically, serotonin and norepinephrine. However, there are contradictory data, and conflicting opinions concerning which of these neurohumors is associated with what stage of sleep. Serotonin (5-HT) which occurs naturally in the brain[67] may be involved as a transmitter substance in the central nervous organization of trophotropic functions[68,69] and as will be shown, it does seem to be a possible candidate as a hypnogen. For example, in 1965 and 1966, KOELLA[70] and KOELLA et al.[71] found that serotonin injected by intracarotid route in the cat induced a biphasic change of the EEG consisting of an initial arousal pattern lasting from a half-minute to two minutes which was followed by prolonged hypersynchrony. This sequence was accompanied by first a decrease, and then a prolonged increase in recruiting responses, and by pupillary dilation followed by constriction. Other studies by this group implicated the fourth ventricle, specifically the area postrema, in this serotonergic effect. Surgical destruction of this extra-blood–brain-barrier region prevented the 5-HT effect, and local application of 5-HT on the area postrema induced cortical hypersynchrony. Koella suggested that 5-HT acted upon receptor sites in the area postrema, and that this stimulating effect was transmitted by dendrites to neurons in the nucleus of the solitary tract. As mentioned earlier, the hypersynchronizing properties of the solitary tract nucleus were demonstrated by MORUZZI[72] and his colleagues. Several investigators have found that i.v. or i.p. injection of the precursor of serotonin, 5-hydroxytryptophan (5-HTP) (which crosses the blood–brain barrier), could induce a state resembling slow-wave sleep, e.g.,[73] but JOUVET[74] reported that large doses of 5-HTP in cats cause suppression of REM sleep for 5 or 6 hr. In 1964, MATSUMOTO and JOUVET[75] found that high doses of reserpine (0·5 mg/kg) caused prolonged insomnia in cats, with SW sleep absent for about 2 days, and REM sleep eliminated for 2–4 days or more. When reserpine was followed by an injection of 5-HTP, SW sleep reappeared immediately, but REM sleep was apparently not observed. In contrast, when reserpine was followed by dihydroxyphenylalanine (DOPA), a precursor of norepinephrine (NE), REM sleep was restored. Thus, there was a hint that serotonin might be involved in the control of SW sleep whereas the catecholamines might be necessary for REM sleep.

The substance p-chlorophenylalanine (PCPA) depletes animal tissues, more or less selectively, of serotonin, apparently by inhibition of the enzyme, tryptophan hydroxylase. JOUVET[28] found that a single injection of PCPA (400 mg/kg) in the cat had no notable effect for 24 hr, but following this there was a sudden decrease in both states of sleep and a period of insomnia which persisted for the next 36 hr, after which there was a slow recovery of both stages of sleep. The decrease and recovery of SW sleep was found to be correlated with the decrease and recovery of serotonin in cerebral tissue. WEITZMAN and his co-workers[76] partially confirmed these results in monkeys. Total sleep was reduced subsequent to PCPA administration, but this was due principally to inhibition of SW sleep, the absolute reduction in REM sleep being small. CLARA TORDA[77] found that repeated doses of PCPA selectively depleted 5-HT from the brain of the white rat, leaving NE intact, and that both stages of sleep were eliminated following PCPA. She also confirmed and extended Jouvet's results by showing that EEG indicators of SW sleep could be reinstated immediately after small amounts of serotonin were injected into either the third or lateral ventricle.

The fluorescent technique developed by FALCK[78] and FALCK et al.[79] has made it possible to map serotonergic and noradrenergic terminals throughout the brain stem. Serotonergic neurons, with their yellow fluorescence, are found in high density in the Raphé region of the medulla, pons and mesencephalon.[80,81] JOUVET[82] showed that after destruction of the nuclei of Raphé, the cat was awake constantly for about 2 or 3 days. The lesion also resulted in depletion of brain serotonin. Very scanty anatomical evidence suggests that the serotonergic neurons of the Raphé system may be acting on diencephalic or telencephalic structures rather than on the mesencephalic reticular formation.

As mentioned earlier, Jouvet believes that NE is necessary for REM sleep to occur. His findings with reserpine and DOPA in cats would seem to support such a view, and he has other evidence to bolster this notion. For example, he found that cauterization of the locus coeruleus of the pons, a region rich in NE-containing neurons, eliminated the tonic muscle relaxation which normally accompanies REM sleep.[82] The lesion did not, however, affect the phasic (PGO spike) components of REM. There are a number of difficulties with the NE concept. Among them is the finding that the precursors of NE (or NE itself) injected into the brain cause EEG arousal and behavioral activation rather than sleep, e.g.[77] Norepinephrine can be selectively depleted from body tissues either with alpha-methyl-paratyrosine which blocks synthesis of DOPA from tyrosine, or with Disulfiram which inhibits dopamine-beta-hydroxylase, thus blocking NE synthesis. Using this technique, MARANTZ and RECHTSCHAFFEN[83] depleted cerebral NE in rats to about half the normal value, but found no effect on either stage of sleep. CLARA TORDA,[77] with repeated doses of alpha-methyl p-tyrosine or Disulfiram, was able to reduce NE levels in the rat cerebrum to about one per cent of normal levels. Sleep EEG measures, based exclusively on cortical and hippocampal leads, suggested increased SW sleep and decreased REM. The presence of some REM sleep (i.e. cortical desynchrony and hippocampal theta) in the NE-depleted brain implied that NE alone was not required for the occurrence of that state. In the same series of studies, Torda depleted rat brains of both 5-HT and NE, after which she was able to induce both EEG states of sleep with various combinations of the two monoamines. These experiments and others convinced Torda that " . . . the various phases of the sleep-wakefulness cycle depend on the relative concentrations of serotonin and norepinephrine (and/or related substances) released at their pertinent intracerebral sites of action" (p. 807).

SEROTONIN IN MAN

L-Tryptophan

Several investigators who agree that serotonin probably has something to do with the control of SW sleep believe that it also modulates REM sleep. This notion is based primarily on work with humans. OSWALD et al.[84] found that 5 of 16 normal adults given 5–10 g of L-tryptophan (amino acid precursor of 5-HT) orally at bedtime tended to enter REM sleep abnormally soon after sleep onset, while lactose, L-tyrosine or DL-methionine did not cause this effect. In two REM responders, studied over many trials, L-tryptophan invariably shortened REM-onset latency except when methysergide, an effective central and peripheral 5-HT blocking agent, was used. The effect of 5-HTP was not as consistent as that of L-tryptophan, but now and then appeared to produce the same early onset of stage REM.

Tryptophan is rapidly absorbed from the gut (see, for example, Fig. 1, prepared from OSWALD's Table 1,[84] p. 392), and like 5-HTP, it quickly reaches the brain, causing a rapid rise in the 5-HT content of brain regions in which it is normally present.[85-87] Thus it could be expected to have fairly rapid central effects. HARTMANN[88] gave oral doses (6–10g) of L-tryptophan to normal adults and found a small by significant increase in REM sleep. However, he did not find the earlier onset of REM that Oswald had recorded. MANDELL et al.[89] reported a large increase in REM sleep after i.v. injection of 5-HTP.

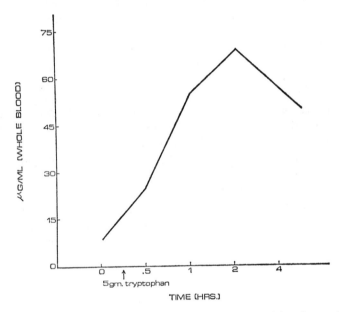

FIG. 1.   Average uptake of L-tryptophan in blood of four young adults after oral ingestion of 5 g. (Prepared from OSWALD's[84] Table 1, p. 392.)

It has been observed that patients with idiopathic narcolepsy frequently move directly from waking to REM sleep, a phenomenon which has never been observed in normal humans or animals.[90] EVANS and OSWALD[91] administered 5 g of L-tryptophan orally to several narcoleptic patients 15 min before bedtime. The average duration of their initial REM period was doubled from about 14 to about 30 min.

In a series of rat studies, HARTMANN[92] also found an effect, not on REM sleep itself, but on the normally stable REM-to-REM cycle. A tryptophan-loaded diet increased the frequency of REM epochs, whereas a diet free of tryptophan lengthened the period of the cycle. As will be seen, similar effects are found in man.

Since none of the investigators of amino acid effects had examined the entire sleep profile, we undertook a replication and extension of the Oswald and Hartmann studies in human subjects. After three baseline nights, two doses, 7·5 g each of L-tryptophan and L-phenylalanine, were administered in apple sauce to eleven subjects at intervals of one week, with baseline sessions in the middle of and following the end of each series. The subjects were aware that amino acids were being studied, but were not told which substance was administered on a given night. On baseline nights, they received apple sauce, but of course, this does not constitute a placebo for these evil tasting compounds. Later, we devised a placebo composed primarily of sweetened chocolate, and ran the tryptophan study again, on eight more subjects. The results were the same as those to be reported here.

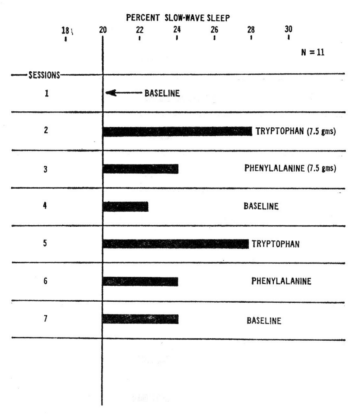

FIG. 2.   Effect of oral doses (7·5 g) of L-tryptophan and L-phenylalanine on SW sleep (stages 3 & 4) in 11 young adult males. Sessions are one week apart, with amino acids administered a half hour before bedtime.

Figure 2 indicates that both of the amino acids tended to increase the per cent of SW sleep, defined here as stages 3 and 4, but this trend was significant only for L-tryptophan. SW sleep increased from a baseline level of 20·0 per cent to a treatment level of 28·2 per cent. Per cent time awake declined with tryptophan (Fig. 3) as did time to sleep onset (first 14 Hz spindle of stage 2) and the frequency of brief arousals, each of these effects being significant beyond the 0·01 significance level (zero mu t test). Although tryptophan had no

U

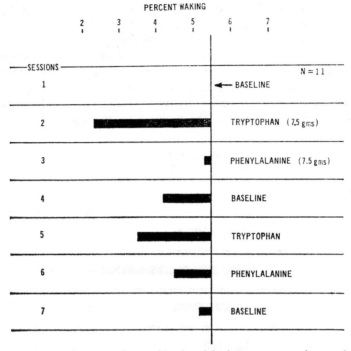

Fig. 3.   Effect of 7·5 g of L-tryptophan and L-phenylalanine on per cent time awake in human volunteers.

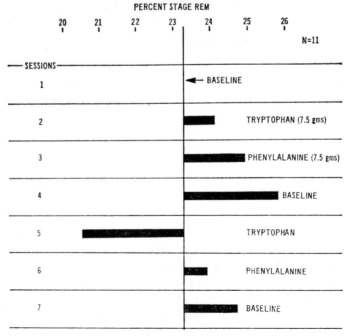

Fig. 4.   Effect of 7·5 g of L-tryptophan and L-phenylalanine on per cent stage REM.

general effect on the total amount of REM sleep (Fig. 4), or the latency of REM onset, it did (as in Hartmann's rats) reduce the time from REM epoch to REM epoch from a baseline average of 97–91 min after tryptophan (Fig. 5). Two of the 11 subjects did show increases in per cent stage REM as well as decreases in latency of the first REM epoch on each night of tryptophan load. Each of those subjects also showed an increase in the amount of SW sleep. One of the two latter subjects submitted to four more tryptophan and four more baseline nights over a period of three months. For this subject, tryptophan load was consistently associated with increases in the amount of SW sleep, but the amount of REM sleep varied unsystematically around baseline levels. Nevertheless, he did show a reliable tendency for early onset of REM sleep under tryptophan load. Phenylalanine had no systematic effects on any of the sleep variables studied.

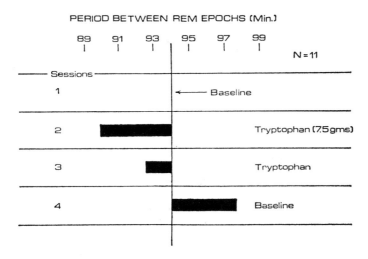

FIG. 5.   Effect of 7·5 g of L-tryptophan on the period of the REM-to-REM cycle.

L-tryptophan had other interesting effects on human behavior. Less than 20 min after its ingestion, our subjects began to complain of drowsiness. In fact several of them went to sleep as electrodes were being applied. They noticed mild feelings of disorientation and drunkenness, and some of them reported that the state resembled a psychedelic trip. OSWALD and his coworkers[84] observed these same phenomena both with L-tryptophan and with 5-HTP, and noted also that the conversation of their subjects tended to become lewd. Oswald mentions that SMITH and PROCKOP[93] had observed similar behavior after tryptophan and that tryptophan administered to dogs can provoke spontaneous ejaculation.[94]

Our results encouraged the tentative conclusion that tryptophan, and perhaps serotonin, are involved primarily in the mechanisms controlling SW sleep. When there were effects on REM sleep they seemed to be on the ultradian cycle, the biological clock which organizes REM periodicity, rather than on the REM state itself.

Since doses of L-tryptophan between 5 and 10 g had uncovered about two out of ten subjects who appeared to be 'REM responders' in Oswald's sense, we decided to repeat the study with a tryptophan load increased to 12 grams. The plan of the study was similar to the 7·5 g experiment except that we now had a placebo. Thus, after an adaptation night which was discarded, each of eight subjects was given 12 g of L-tryptophan, mixed with the chocolate placebo, on two occasions, one or two weeks apart, a half hour before bedtime. In this study, each night of tryptophan load was followed by a non-medication

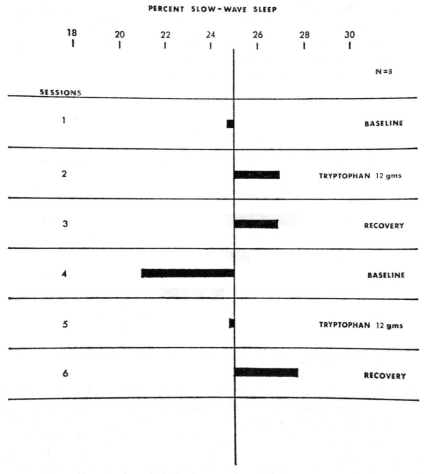

FIG. 6. Effect of high load (12 g) of L-tryptophan on SW sleep (stages 3 & 4) in 8 young adult males. Baseline and tryptophan load nights were a week apart, and recovery sessions were the successive nights following tryptophan load. Note rebound tendency on recovery nights.

recovery night. The placebo was administered on baseline and recovery nights, and our subjects were not able to detect the difference. Under high tryptophan load, sedation effects in the first half hour appeared to be more intense, and feelings of euphoria, drunkenness and disorientation were greater than for the smaller tryptophan load. However, the effects on sleep may have been qualitatively different with the 12 g dose. Fig. 6 shows a trend toward increased SW sleep on the tryptophan session, at least with the first dose, but the effect across subjects was not systematic, and, of course, not statistically significant. There was, however, a systematic and significant rebound effect on the recovery session. With a larger dose of tryptophan, each subject showed a dramatic increase in the amount of REM sleep (Fig. 7). On the average, REM sleep increased from 96 min on baseline-placebo

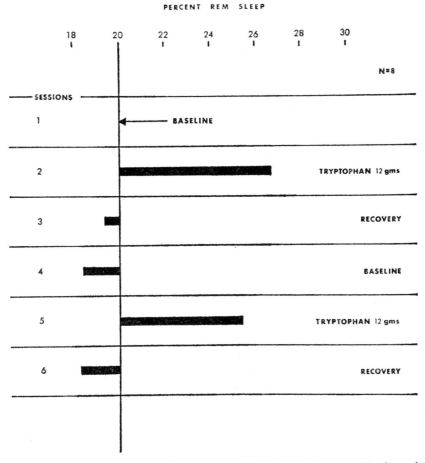

FIG. 7. Effect of high tryptophan load on per cent REM sleep in 8 volunteers. The dose-related increase in REM sleep is apparently due to a decrease in the period of the REM-to-REM cycle.

nights to 125 on tryptophan nights, and reverted to 88 min on the recovery night, the tryptophan effect being significant beyond the 0·001 level (zero mu t test). Data analyses for this latter project are not complete, but preliminary tallies strongly suggest that this effect (like that found with the lower dose of tryptophan) resulted from acceleration of the REM-to-REM cycle rather than lengthening of the REM epochs. Under high tryptophan load, the latency of onset of REM sleep was variable between subjects, and the average change from baseline was not statistically significant. However, two subjects had zero latencies, entering REM sleep immediately after a minute or two of stage 1, and one had a REM onset latency of 5 min. These figures are far below the cutoff for normal subjects, estimated by Oswald to be about 45 min.

These results indicate that in humans, alterations in sleep caused by tryptophan (and possibly by serotonin) are dependent on dose. Moderate loads of the amino acid cause a reliable increase in SW sleep, shortening of the period of the ultradian REM-to-REM cycle, and sedation. With a larger dose the sedation effect again appears, but the change in SW sleep is delayed until the recovery night, 24 hr later. The amount of REM sleep is greatly increased, probably because of a reduction in the period of the REM-to-REM cycle, as if the demand for stage REM now has precedence over the demand for SW sleep. It is reasonable to speculate that in man, at least, serotonin is involved in the mechanisms controlling both kinds of sleep. The administration of L-tryptophan has been shown to increase both the absolute amount of serotonin[87] and its turnover.[95] Perhaps the rate at which REM sleep is triggered is a function of rate of turnover of free serotonin in pontine sites. JOUVET proposed such a mechanism,[28] suggesting that " . . . the action of a deaminated metabolite of 5 HT might be involved in the triggering of paradoxical-sleep mechanisms" (p. 38). This hypothesis was based partly on the fact that certain of the more potent mono-amine oxidase inhibitors which prevent the catabolism of 5-HT (and also NE) lead to an increase in SW sleep and to total suppression of REM sleep. Perhaps, then, monoamine oxidase is necessary to the passage from SW to REM sleep.

Reserpine

The effect of reserpine on sleep is interesting both from a biochemical and clinical perspective. The drug interferes with storage of the biogenic amines and depletes the brain of both serotonin[96] and the catecholamines.[97] As was mentioned earlier, Jouvet found that a single large dose (0·5 mg/kg) of reserpine caused prolonged insomnia in cats, but that SW sleep could be restored in the reserpinized cat with 5-HTP, and REM sleep with DOPA. HOFFMAN and DOMINO,[98] in a carefully controlled dose-response study, confirmed this reserpine effect for the cat and showed that the decrease in both stages of sleep was a function of dose. Considered together with the L-tryptophan effects reviewed earlier, these results are consistent with the notion that SW sleep is mediated by serotonergic mechanisms.

In *Macaca mulatta*[99] and in man,[88,98] moderate to large doses of reserpine caused dose-dependent increases in the amount of stage REM, and decreases in the latency of onset of the first REM epoch. In man, these effects were especially large on the recovery night following medication. The different dose–response effects of reserpine in cats and man may be due to species differences in metabolism of the monoamines. For example, PSCHEIDT et al.[100] reported that in primates, drugs which inhibit monoamine oxidase, potentiate both brain serotonin and norepinephrine, while in cats the MAO inhibitors increase only serotonin.

Our studies examined the effects of single and repeated doses of reserpine (1 mg) on the amount and distribution of the EEG stages of sleep in man. In Experiment 1, 10 paid young adult males served as subjects, and went through our usual baseline (placebo) treatment, recovery and final baseline procedure. Reserpine was administered orally about

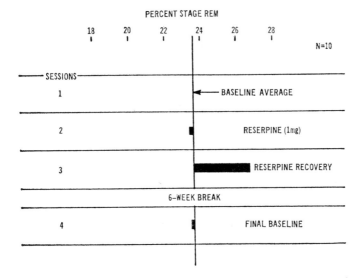

FIG. 8.   Effect of a single dose of reserpine (1 mg) on per cent stage REM in 10 normal adults. The sharp increase on the reserpine-recovery night is due to a decrease in the period of the REM-to-REM cycle.

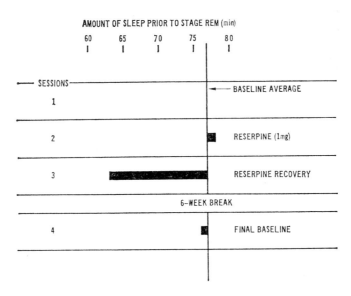

FIG. 9.   Decrease on the post-medication recovery night in latency of REM onset with a single dose (1 mg) of reserpine.

a half hour before bedtime. The drug caused no systematic changes in EEG sleep profiles on the night the dose was given. However, as can be seen in Fig. 8, on the following (recovery) night there was a substantial increase in stage REM. Nine of the ten subjects showed this effect. Along with this increase, there was a decrease in time to onset of the first REM epoch (Fig. 9), and in the average time from REM epoch to REM epoch. On the average, REM increased by 17 min on the recovery night, whereas there was a sharp decrease in the amount of SW sleep (Fig. 10). The acceleration of the ultradian REM-to-REM cycle resulted in a significant increase (from about 4 to about 5) in the number of REM epochs for the recovery night. There were no significant changes in other EEG stages. The Pearson correlation of -0.50 between change scores for stage REM and stage SW was not quite significant with this small sample, but suggests a tendency within subjects for REM to increase at the expense of SW sleep.

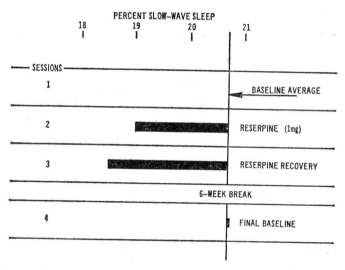

FIG. 10.   Decrease in per cent SW sleep on both the medication and recovery nights with 1 mg of reserpine.

In Experiment 2, ten young males were given oral doses (1 mg) of reserpine on three successive nights, the fourth night being a recovery session. This repeated dose study confirmed and extended the results of Experiment 1. The figures presented here are based on data from the first six subjects, but they are representative of results found for all 10. As in Experiment 1, there were no systematic changes in sleep scores on the first medication night, but beginning on the second drug night, the per cent stage REM rose, and continued to rise through the third drug night, then reversed toward, but did not reach, baseline (Fig. 11). By the third medication night, the average gain in stage REM ($N = 10$) was 30 min and the average REM level remained 18 min above baseline on the post-medication session. Stage SW decreased after the first drug night and remained below baseline on the recovery night (Fig. 12). Kendall's Coefficient of Concordance (W) computed for the

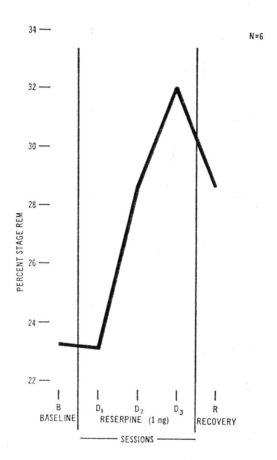

FIG. 11. Systematic increase, and partially sustained rise, in per cent stage REM during and after the three successive nights of reserpine (1 mg per session) medication. The increase in stage REM is due to acceleration of the REM cycle.

baseline and medication sessions was significant beyond the 0·01 level, and per cent stage REM remained significantly higher, whereas per cent SW sleep was significantly below the baseline average during the post-medication recovery session.

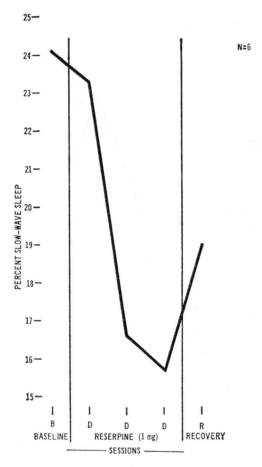

Fig. 12. Systematic and partially sustained decrease in SW sleep (stages 3 & 4) during and after three successive doses of reserpine (1 mg).

As expected from the single-dose study, reserpine again reduced the latency of onset of the first epoch of stage REM, although the effect was somewhat irregular (Fig. 13) and shortened the intervals between successive REM epochs (Fig. 14). From the baseline average ($N = 10$) of 94 min, latency of the first REM epoch decreased 21 min by the second and 34 min by the third medication night. Although the average REM latency remained low on the recovery session it was not significantly shorter than the baseline average. From a baseline mean ($N = 10$) of 106 min, the time between epochs of stage REM decreased by about 20 min on the third drug night and showed no sign of reverting to

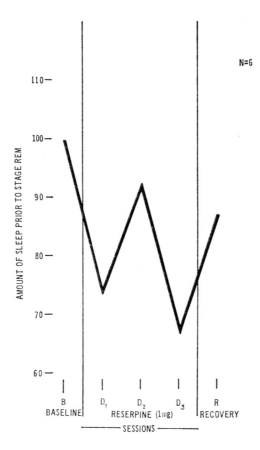

FIG. 13. Irregular but generally declining latency of onset of stage REM during and after reserpine medication.

control levels on the post-medication session. As in Experiment 1, the average duration
of REM epochs was not altered by reserpine. The increase in per cent stage REM can be
accounted for entirely by decrease in the period of the REM cycle, and the resulting increase
in frequency of REM epochs. The latter score rose from 3·6 during baseline to 5·2 on the
third drug night, remaining at 5·0 on the post-medication session, changes which were
significant beyond the 0·05 confidence level (sign test).

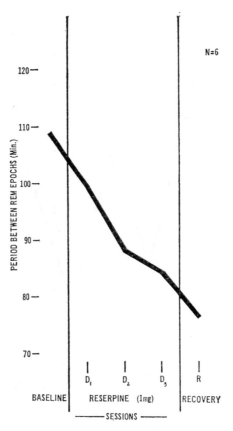

FIG. 14. Systematic acceleration (decreases of the period) of the REM-to-REM cycle, during
and after reserpine medication.

Clearly, in man, the effects on sleep of clinical doses of reserpine, and high loads of
tryptophan, are very similar. Both accelerate the ultradian period of the REM cycle, both
reduce the latency of REM onset, both have well-known sedation effects. Yet, in one
sense, their effects on serotonin levels in brain and other tissues are opposite. Reserpine
depletes while tryptophan increases the supply of this monoamine. However, in a second
aspect, their effects on serotonin are probably similar. Through different mechanisms,
each compound apparently causes increased synthesis and turnover of 5-HT. As was
mentioned earlier, L-tryptophan, as a 5-HT precursor which easily passes the blood–brain

barrier, enhances serotonin pools, and potentiates turnover. Reserpine depletes both 5-HT and catecholamine pools, but when their levels are reduced, turnover rate almost certainly increases. Apparently synthesis is controlled by a feedback mechanism, the function of which is to achieve a steady state. (See NEFF and COSTA[101] for NE, and TOZER et al.[102] for 5-HT). Each of the two treatments affected the rate at which stage REM was triggered, but not the duration of its epochs. It is as if the ultradian clock were a cumulative counter with an automatic reset, counting the rate of synthesis of some serotonin by-product which, with reserpine medication or tryptophan load, and the resulting increase in serotonin turnover, developed a systematic bias.

CATECHOLAMINES IN MAN

It is possible, but highly unlikely, that serotonin levels, monoamine oxidase and some catabolic biproduct of serotonin turnover are sufficient mechanisms for the induction and maintenance of both states of sleep. However, there is some evidence that norepinephrine has a critical role in REM sleep, at least for its tonic aspects. JOUVET[82] found that large doses of reserpine administered to cats dissociated the EEG components of REM sleep. Thus, PGO spike activity became continuous in the reserpinized animal, and this was accompanied by discrete lateral eye movements and small twitches of the vibrissae, ears and digits. However, the muscle atony characteristic of REM sleep was blocked for many hours. 5-HTP, injected i.v. 2–3 hr after reserpine, had two effects. First, it immediately suppressed PGO activity for 4–6 hr. Second, it induced EEG and behavioral signs of SW sleep, which reappeared periodically for 4–6 hr, after which the fast cortical PGO activity of reserpine reappeared. L-DOPA injected i.p. also had two effects. First, it enhanced the frequency of PGO activity by about 30–50 per cent. Second, it induced, after a latency of 20–30 min, brief periods of SW sleep which were always followed by behavioral and polygraphic REM sleep, with extinction of EMG and clusters of rapid eye movements. During 5 or 6 hr after DOPA injection, 2 or 3 periods of SW and REM sleep would appear, after which the reserpine syndrome reappeared. The fact that L-DOPA reinstated both SW and REM sleep in the reserpinized cat implies that the catecholamine system may be involved in the mechanisms for both states. CLARA TORDA[77] concluded that normal EEG sleep depends on the ratio between levels of 5-HT and the catecholamines.

Recently, we were afforded an opportunity to examine sleep and performance in a group of patients with inoperable malignancies who had volunteered for a study of the therapeutic effects of a low phenylalanine-tyrosine synthetic diet supplemented with vitamins. The possible therapeutic effects of such diets had been suggested in the work of CHRISTENSEN and STREICHER[103] and LORINCZ and KUTTNER.[104] It had been observed by ward physicians that several patients receiving this treatment developed severe disturbances of sleep, periods of disorientation, nocturnal confusion and visual hallucinations, all of which were reversed when the patient returned to a normal diet. Because of these observations, we undertook a series of psychiatric and sleep studies on these patients which is continuing.

Although the patients selected for dietary treatment had inoperable malignancies, their health was not deteriorating rapidly, and their physical condition was relatively good.

Three patients reported here (and by LESTER et al.[105]) were given a synthetic diet, very low in phenylalanine and tyrosine, based on a casein hydrolysate from which these amino acids had been removed. The diet was supplemented with a multivitamin preparation, and with foods known to be very low in phenylalanine-tyrosine content.

Clinical EEGs were obtained every two weeks, and mental status examinations were conducted about once a week. In five cases, various tests of short- and long-term memory were given (i.e. story recall, object recall and digit span).

EEG sleep studies were done once a week on each patient. Psychiatric case reports on three of these patients are presented in LESTER et al.,[105] and will be summarized briefly here.

Case reports

(1) Mr. M., a 66-yr-old man, was admitted to the hospital for the fourth time with a diagnosis of squamous cell carcinoma of the larynx. He had had a total laryngectomy and left radical neck dissection in 1965. Metastic lesions in the lung were found in November, 1966. He had been treated with various chemotherapeutic agents, and was admitted this time for treatment on the synthetic diet.

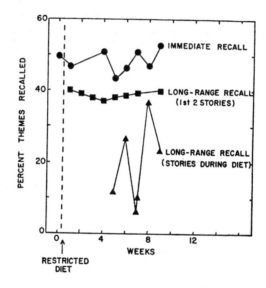

FIG. 15.   Per cent of themes recalled of several stories matched for length and difficulty. Each new story given from the fourth week of the deprivation diet was requested by title one week later. Note that immediate recall and very long-range recall (first two stories) are stable, but that one-week delayed recall during the diet is variable, and possibly impaired. The subject was a patient volunteer with inoperable cancer, treated on a synthetic diet almost free of phenylalanine and tyrosine. (Taken from LESTER et al.[105])

On initial psychiatric examination, Mr. M. was found to be alert, oriented, cooperative and active, eager to participate in the research program. Two or three weeks after starting the synthetic diet, Mr. M. began to complain of sleepiness, and his level of activity went down. After four weeks on the diet, he stopped O-T, sat in his room most of the time, and withdrew from active social contacts. Although he did not appear to be psychologically depressed, he moved about slowly, and preferred to sit quietly in his room. After 9 weeks on the diet, Mr. M. refused to cooperate in formal psychological testing, but was willing to be examined by the psychiatrist.

Figure 15 summarizes data obtained by giving serial stories, with a new one given at each recall point. The immediate recall scores indicate that Mr. M. was able to register, store and immediately retrieve a new story for the first ten weeks of the diet. Furthermore, he was able to retrieve two stories acquired at the onset of the diet (long-range recall, first two stories). Thus there appeared to be no decay of well-established verbal memories. However, his recall of stories (one-week delayed recall) given 3–8 weeks after initiation of the diet suggests that the diet may have impaired mechanisms for transfer of information from short- to long-term storage. Obviously, we need more systematic studies of memory in these patients.

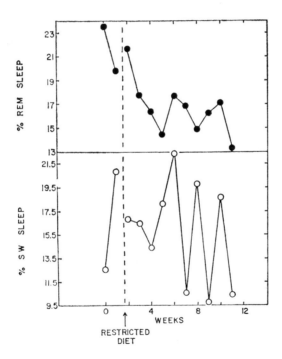

FIG. 16.   Per cent REM sleep shows a systematic decrease with phenylalanine-tyrosine deprivation, whereas SW sleep becomes highly variable from session to session. Sleep was increasingly disrupted in this and other patients. (Taken from LESTER et al.[105])

From Jouvet's (and Torda's) findings it is reasonable to anticipate that depletion of the catecholamines would result in disruption of both SW (stages 3 and 4) and REM sleep. Figure 16 shows that the diet was associated with a progressive decline in the per cent of REM sleep, and that per cent SW sleep was highly variable, but tended to decline. The absolute amounts of stages REM and SW showed identical trends. Similar effects were seen in the other five patients. As will be seen, similar effects found in other treated patients, were reversed by tyrosine supplement or by resumption of a normal hospital diet. However, when the diet was supplemented with L-DOPA (500 mg to 2 gms per day) the effects on sleep were highly variable. Higher doses of DOPA caused further disruption of sleep and long periods of insomnia, whereas lower doses (250–500 mg) were associated with transient improvement in the sleep profile.

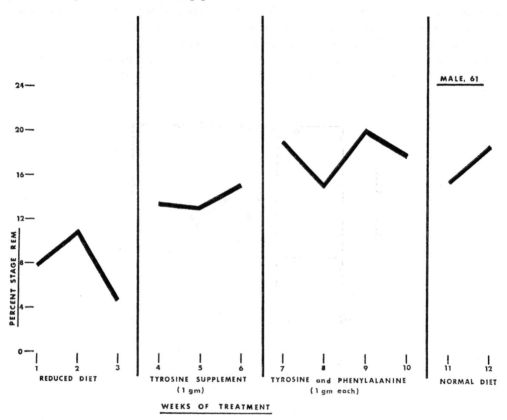

FIG. 17.   Progressive effect on REM sleep of phenylalanine-tyrosine deprivation in a patient with inoperable cancer. Note the partial reversal of this effect after tyrosine supplement, and recovery to normal levels after phenylalanine supplement. SW sleep became highly variable during dietary stress, and sleep was increasingly disrupted by periods of insomnia. (Taken from LESTER et al.[105])

(2) Mr. J. L., a 61-yr-old man, was admitted for dietary management of a metastatic renal cell carcinoma. Known metastases included a 4-by-6 cm. mass involving the right posterior eighth rib and adjacent lung. Initial clinical impression was of a normal male with lower-middle-class background, and low-normal intelligence. He could repeat six numbers forward and five backward and 11 of 27 themes of the Cowboy Story. Twenty-eight days after beginning the synthetic diet, he became increasingly irritable, restless at

night, and lethargic by day. He set his bed on fire, blaming the staff, insisting that a man in white came into his room and knocked a cigarette from his hand, and that he, the patient, had run to the door yelling after the intruder. The patient felt that someone or something was trying to 'get' him during the nights, and complained bitterly of increasing insomnia. 'When I close my eyes, it is like a TV screen in that I see all sorts of things—and know they are not really there, but become scared anyway.'

Mr. L. became less and less active during the day, he spoke slowly, and infrequently, and he appeared puzzled by the night-time events. His immediate and remote recall of new and old stories declined somewhat, but he remained oriented (during days) for time and place.

After four weeks on the diet, Mr. L's previously normal EEG showed progressive diffuse paroxysmal slowing, and low-voltage 4–6/sec activity with paroxysmal epochs of 2–4/sec high amplitude waves which lasted for 2–4 sec.

Fig. 17 shows the progressive effect of the synthetic diet on per cent REM sleep. During this period, the sleep pattern became increasingly disrupted by body movements and periods of waking, and (as in the first case) SW sleep became highly variable from night to night. Almost immediately after the diet was supplemented with tyrosine, the sleep profile improved, and stage REM increased from a low of 4 per cent to about 15 per cent. Addition of phenylalanine to the diet resulted in further improvement in sleep, and REM per cent increased to within normal limits for this age group. After tyrosine and phenylalanine were added to the diet, the patient became more active and spontaneous, and his recall of stories improved. However, two weeks after the resumption of a normal diet, Mr. L.'s clinical EEG remained abnormal. The patient died about four months after resuming a normal diet, and the brain was examined for metastatic lesions, none being found.

(3) Mrs. P., a 73-yr-old woman was admitted with a recurrent squamous cell carcinoma of the cervix. During her first psychiatric examination she moved rapidly, talked well, had a 'peppery' style, and showed no impairment of memory or orientation. One month after starting the diet, she began to complain of 'crazy' feelings in her head, and her appearance had changed. She looked much older, moved about slowly and was somewhat withdrawn. She could recall significant events on the ward, and she could recite stories acquired prior to treatment, but her immediate recall for new stories declined.

During the next two weeks she felt increasingly ill, complaining of 'sores' on her tongue, tiredness and weakness. She made few spontaneous attempts to relate to others, she was unkempt, and she remarked half jokingly that the diet was 'a human body from some of those dead people student doctors work on.' She was preoccupied with somatic complaints and she was convinced that she had seen faces on a tree outside her window. She recalled the Cowboy Story which she had learned prior to treatment but refused to attempt other stories.

After a tyrosine supplement (2 gm daily) was added to the diet, she showed rapid improvement, becoming alert, cooperative and spontaneous.

Her clinical EEG remained essentially normal except that during the eighth week on the synthetic diet, infrequent occipital spikes, enhanced by hyperventilation appeared. Fig. 18

shows the loss of REM sleep during the diet, and its brisk recovery after tyrosine supplement. As in the other cases, the sleep profile was increasingly disrupted by periods of arousal, and SW sleep became highly variable.

The other three cases so far studied all showed similar alterations of sleep and behavior. However, when L-DOPA rather than tyrosine was added to the diet, the results were not consistent.

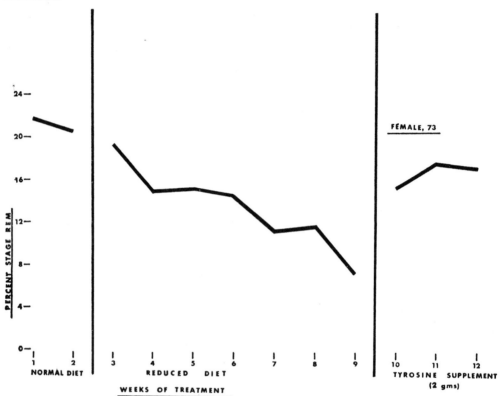

Fig. 18. Systematic decrease in REM sleep during deprivation of phenylalanine and tyrosine, reversed by tyrosine supplement. There was a slight further rise in per cent REM when this patient was returned to her customary diet. (Taken from Lester et al.[105])

Clearly, deprivation of phenylalanine and tyrosine causes a reversible syndrome which includes disruption of sleep, with a marked decline in stage REM, impaired memory, reduced activity, slowing and periods of mild disorientation. The memory deficit is reminiscent of Korsakoff's syndrome in that the patient seems able to register incoming information and act upon it, but may not be able to convert it to long-range store.

One must emphasize, of course, that the syndrome described here may have nothing to do with depletion of the catecholamines. Instead, it may be related to severe protein defficiency of the type involved in Kwashiorkor. The latter condition also produces an apathetic state and abnormalities in the clinical EEG.[106]

SUMMARY AND CONCLUSION

Despite the extraordinary research effort expended on sleep in the last fifteen years, we still know very little about this extremely complex state. For example, we have no evidence concerning its biological significance. Studies of the effects of sleep deprivation have not revealed systematic alterations in any biological mechanism from which a functional theory of sleep could be constructed. It appears, however, that we are learning something about its neural and biochemical substrates. Most neural scientists would now agree that there are active neural mechanisms for the induction and maintenance of sleep, which include among others, bulbar-reticulo-bulbar and reticular-cortical-reticular feedback loops. There would be disagreement, however, concerning the role of diencephalic structures, especially non-specific nuclei of the thalamus in this system. Koella, and other students of Hess, argue that the extremely complex syndrome of sleep involves the entire brain, organized hierarchically, in a way which differs qualitatively, not quantitatively, from the organization of waking. Where is the director of this symphony? Hess and Koella locate it in the thalamus because, they assert, the entire sleep syndrome, including biologically specific pre-sleep behaviors, is induced by low-frequency electrical stimulation in, and only in, the medial thalamic nuclei. Perhaps few would agree, but it is true that most investigators have neglected the thalamus in favor of brain stem systems in their search for the organizers of sleep.

Most investigators would agree that there are at least two great systems of sleep, REM and non-REM, which, although sequentially linked, are triggered, and sustained, by different neural mechanisms.

The long-term temporal features of the states of sleep, of the regular, almost imperturbable ultradian cycle which organizes their occurrence, and of their response to pharmacological, neurological or psychological perturbation recommends neurobiochemistry as the basic science of sleep, but examination of biochemical substrates has only begun. Techniques are still being developed for discrete microbiochemistry in living brains, and respectable biochemists are cautious about approaching the monstrous problems already implied in sleep research. Thus, studies having relevance to biochemistry are correlative rather than causative in their conception, the kind of studies neurophysiologists and psychologists, but not biochemists, are likely to undertake, when addressing a problem in chemistry.

Of the several candidates for a hypnogenic substance, serotonin enjoys the greatest popularity. Data from chicks, rabbits, rats, cats and humans indicate that its depletion is correlated with insomnia and its potentiation with sedation and sleep. Furthermore, serotonin or its metabolic byproducts is somehow involved in triggering REM sleep. Jouvet's studies of cats, Torda's studies of rats, and our (as well as Hartmann's, Oswald's, Mandell's and Domino's) studies of humans permit two guesses: First, that a certain level of free serotonin in serotonergic brain tissue is neccessary for SW sleep, and that within limits, SW sleep will increase as a function of these free levels. Second, that the rate of turnover of serotonin or some catabolic byproduct of the amine is a data base for the ultradian clock which times the periodic occurrence of REM sleep. Our reserpine and tryptophan load studies in man, and Hartmann's studies of tryptophan load and deprivation in rats, suggest that the clock is a cumulative counter with a reset mechanism which can be biased by changes in the rate of serotonin turnover.

The importance of the catecholamines, and specifically norepinephrine, in the control of REM sleep is not so certain. Percursors of NE induce arousal and waking rather than REM sleep. Specific depletion of NE from brain and body tissues may reduce but does not totally eliminate REM sleep. Surgical destruction of the NE-rich locus coeruleus eliminates tonic but not phasic symptoms of REM. In our cancer patients, deprived of phenyalanine and tyrosine, and presumably, brain catecholamines, REM sleep was dramatically diminished, and then restored with a tyrosine dietary supplement. However, this dietary stress led to a complex syndrome of apathy, withdrawal, memory impairment, nocturnal confusion and insomnia which was reminiscent of the disorders found with protein deficiency. Furthermore, the fact that therapeutic effects of L-DOPA were unreliable and inconsistent while tyrosine induced a brisk reversal of the syndrome, suggests that depletion of the catecholamines may not have been the basis for the disorder. As JOUVET[28] suggested, the REM sleep mechanism probably requires more than one biochemical key in order to operate.

REFERENCES

1. DEMENT, W. C. and KLEITMAN, N. Cyclic variations in EEG during sleep and their relations to eye movements, body motility, and dreaming. *Electroenceph. clin. Neurophysiol.* **9**, 673, 1957.
2. DEMENT, W. Occurrence of low voltage, fast electroencephalogram patterns during behavioral sleep in cat. *Electroenceph. clin. Neurophysiol.* **10**, 291, 1958.
3. HESS, W. R. Über die wechselbeziehungen zwischen psychischen und vegetativen funktionen. *Arch. Neurol. Psychiat., Chicago* **15**, 260, 1924.
4. HESS, W. R. Über die wechselbezienhungen zwischen psychischen und vegetativen funktionen. *Arch. Neurol. Psychiat., Chicago* **16**, 36 and 285, 1925.
5. BICKEL, A. Der babinski'sche zehenreflex unter physiologischen und pathologischen bedingungen. *Dt. Z. Nerv Heilk.* **22**, 163, 1902.
6. CREUTZFELDT, O. and JUNG, R. Neuronal discharge in the cat's motor cortex during sleep and arousal. *Ciba Foundation Symposium on the Nature of Sleep*, p. 131, WOLSTENHOLME, G. E. W. and O'CONNOR, M. (Eds.) Little, Brown, Boston, 1961.
7. MURATA, K. and KAMEDA, K. The activity of single cortical neurones of unrestrained cats during sleep and wakefulness. *Archs ital. Biol.* **101**, 306, 1963.
8. EVARTS, E. V. Effects of sleep and waking on activity of single units in the unrestrained cat. *Ciba Foundation Symposium on the Nature of Sleep*, p. 171, WOLSTENHOLME, G. E. W. and O'CONNOR, M. (Eds.) Little, Brown, Boston, 1961.
9. EVARTS, E. V., BENTAL, E., BIHARI, B. and HUTTENLOCHER, P. R. Spontaneous discharges of single neurons during sleep and waking. *Science* **135**, 726, 1962.
10. HESS, W. R. Der Schlaf. *Klin. Wschr.* **12**, 129, 1933.
11. HESS, W. R. Das schlafsyndrom als folge dienzephaler reizung. *Helv. physiol. pharmac. Acta* **2**, 305, 1944.
12. AKERT, K., KOELLA, W. P. and HESS, R., JR. Sleep produced by electrical stimulation of the thalamus. *Am. J. Physiol.* **168**, 260, 1952.
13. HESS, R., JR., AKERT, K. and KOELLA, W. Les potentials bioélectriques du cortex et du thalamus et leur altération par stimulation du centre hypnique chez le chat. *Rev. Neurol. Psychiat.* **83**, 537, 1950.
14. KOELLA, W. P. *Sleep: Its Nature and Physiological Organization.* Charles C. Thomas, Springfield, 1967.
15. KLEITMAN, N. *Sleep and Wakefulness.* University of Chicago Press, Chicago, 1939.
16. BREMER, F. and TERZUOLO, C. Contribution à L'étude des méchanismes physiologiques du maintien de L'activité vigile du cerveau. *Archs int. Physiol.* **60**, 157, 1954.

17. BREMER, F. Cerveau 'isolé' et physiologie du sommeil. *C. r. Séanc. Soc. Biol.* **118**, 1235, 1935.
18. MORUZZI, G. and MAGOUN, H. W. Brain stem reticular formation and activation of the EEG. *Electroenceph. clin. Neurophysiol.* **1**, 455, 1949.
19. LINDSLEY, D. B., BOWDEN, J. and MAGOUN, H. W. Effect upon the EEG of acute injury to the brain stem activating system. *Electroenceph. clin. Neurophysiol.* **1**, 475, 1949.
20. BATINI, C., MORUZZI, G., PALESTINI, M., ROSSI, G. F. and ZANCHETTI, A. Persistent patterns of wakefulness in the pretrigeminal midpontine preparation. *Science* **128**, 30, 1958.
21. BATINI, C., MAGNI, F., PALESTINI, M., ROSSI, G. F. and ZANCHETTI, A. Neural mechanisms underlying the enduring EEG and behavioral activation in the midpontine pretrigeminal cat. *Archs. ital. Biol.* **97**, 13, 1959.
22. MAGNES, J., MORUZZI, G. and POMPEIANO, O. EEG synchronization from medullary structures. *Fedn. Proc. Fedn. Am. Socs exp. Biol.* **20**, 336, 1961.
23. MAGNES, J., MORUZZI, G. and POMPEIANO, O. Synchronization of the EEG produced by low-frequency electrical stimulation of the region of the solitary tract. *Archs. ital. Biol.* **99**, 33, 1961.
24. POMPEIANO, O. The neurophysiological mechanisms of the postural and motor events during desynchronized sleep. In: *Sleep and Altered States of Consciousness*, KETY, S. S. EVARTS, E. V. and WILLIAMS, H. L. (Eds.), Chap. 17., Proc. Ass. Res. Nervous and Mental Disease, Vol. 45, Williams & Wilkins, Baltimore, Md., 1967.
25. REIVICH, M., ISAACS, G., EVARTS, E. V. and KETY, S. S. The effect of slow wave sleep and REM sleep on regional cerebral blood flow in cats. *J. Neurochem.* **15**, 301, 1968.
26. SNYDER, F., HOBSON, J., MORRISON, D. and GOLDFRANK, F. Changes in respiration, heart rate and systolic blood pressure in relation to electroencephalographic patterns of human sleep. *J. appl. Physiol.* **19**, 417, 1964.
27. FISHER, C., GROSS, J. and BYRNE, J. Cycle of penile erection synchronous with dreaming (REM) sleep. *Archs. gen. Psychiat., Chicago* **12**, 29, 1965.
28. JOUVET, M. Biogenic amines and the states of sleep. *Science* **163**, 32, 1969.
29. CADILHAC, J. PASSOUANT-FONTAINE, T. and PASSOUANT, P. Modifications de L'activité de L'hippocampe suivant les divers stades du sommeil spontane chez le chat. *Rev. Neurol. Psychiat., Paris* **105**, 171, 1961.
30. SHIMAZONO, Y., HORIE, T., YANAGISAWA, Y., HORI, N., CHIKAZAWA, W. and SHOZUKA, K. Correlation of rhythmic waves of hippocampus with behavior of dogs. *Neurol. Medicochir., Tokyo* **2**, 82, 1960.
31. WEISS, T. and ROLDAN, E. Comparative study of sleep cycles in rodents. *Experientia* **20**, 429, 1964.
32. SNYDER, F. Observation concerning REM-state in a living fossil. Report to the Association for the Psychophysiological Study of Sleep, Palo Alto, California, March, 1964.
33. BANCAUD J., TALAIRACH, J., BORDAS-FERRER, M., AUBER, J. and MARCHAND, M. Les accès épileptiques au cours du sommeil de nuit. *Rev. Neurol. Psychiat., Paris* **110**, 314, 1964.
34. JOUVET, D., VIMONT, P., DELORME, F. and JOUVET, M. Étud de la privation sélective de la phase paradoxale du sommeil chez le chat. *C. r. Séanc. Soc. Biol., Paris* **158**, 756, 1964.
35. JOUVET, M. Telencephalic and rhombencephalic sleep in the cat. *Ciba Foundation Symposium on the Nature of Sleep.* WOLSTENHOLME, G. E. W. and O'CONNOR, M. (Eds.) Little, Brown, Boston, 1961.
36. JOUVET, M. Recherches sur les structures nerveuses et les mecanismes responsables des differentes phases du sommeil physiologique. *Archs. ital. Biol.* **100**, 125, 1962.
37. JOUVET, M. Sur L'existence d'un système hypnotique ponto'limbique: Ses rapports avec L'activité onirique. *Physiologie de L'Hippocampe* (Colloques Intern. du C.R.N.S. No. 107), PASSOUANT, P., (Ed.), p. 297, C.N.R.S., Paris, 1962.
38. JOUVET, M. and MICHEL, F. Déclenchement de la 'phase paradoxale' du sommeil par stimulation de tronc cérébrale chez le chat interact et mésencéphalique chronique. *C r. Séanc. Soc. Biol.* **154**, 636, 1960.
39. FAURE, J., BENSCH, C. and VINCENT, D. Rôle d'un système mésencéphalo-limbique dans la 'phase paradoxale' du sommeil chez le lapin. *C. r. Séanc. Soc. Biol.* **156**, 70, 1962.
40. FAVALE, E., GIUSSANI, A. and ROSSI, G. Induziono del sonno profondo nel gatto mediate stimolazione elettrica della sostanza reticolare del tronco encefalico. *Ital. biol. Sper.* **37**, 265, 1961.
41. PARMEGGIANI, P. and ZANOCCO, G. Cortical and subcortical recordings during low voltage fast EEG phase of sleep in the cat. *Helv. physiol. pharmacol. Acta.* **19**, C97, 1961.
42. KRIPKE, D., WEITZMAN, E. and POLLAK, C. Attempts to induce the rapid eye movement stage of sleep in macaca mulatta by brain stem stimulation. *Psychophysiology* **2**, 132, 1966.

43. CARLI, G., ARMERGAL, V. and ZANCHETTI, A. Brain stem–limbic connections, and the electrographic aspects of deep sleep in the cat. *Archs. ital. Biol.* **103**, 751, 1965.

44. HOBSON, J. The effects of chronic brain stem lesions on cortical and muscular activity during sleep and waking in the cat. *Electroenceph. clin. Neurophysiol.* **19**, 41, 1965.

45. JOUVET, M. Neurophysiology of the states of sleep. *The Neurosciences: A Study Program*, QUARTON, G. C., MELNECHUK, T. and SCHMITT, F. O. (Eds.) The Rockefeller University Press, New York, 1967.

46. POMPEIANO, O. and MORRISON, A. Vestibular influences during sleep: I. Abolition of the rapid eye movements of desynchronized sleep following vestibular lesions. *Archs. ital. Biol.* **103**, 569, 1965.

47. DEMENT, W. Effect of dream deprivation. *Science* **131**, 1705, 1960.

48. BERGER, R. J. and OSWALD, I. Effects of sleep deprivation on behavior, subsequent sleep and dreaming. *J. ment. Sci.* **108**, 457, 1962.

49. WILLIAMS, H. L., HAMMACK, J. R., DALY, R. L., DEMENT, W. C. and LUBIN, A. Responses to auditory stimulation, sleep loss and the EEG stages of sleep. *Electroenceph. clin. Neurophysiol.* **16**, 269, 1964.

50. AGNEW, H., WEBB, W. and WILLIAMS, R. The effect of stage four sleep deprivation. *Electroenceph. clin. Neurophysiol.* **17**, 68, 1964.

51. OSWALD, I. Drugs and sleep. *Pharmac. Rev.* **20**, 273, 1968.

52. VALATX, J., JOUVET, D. and JOUVET, M. Évolution EEG des differents etats de sommeil chez le chaton. *Electroenceph. clin. Neurophysiol.* **17**, 218, 1964.

53. JOUVET, M. The rhombencephalic phase of sleep. *Progress in Brain Research—Vol. 1, Brain Mechanisms*, MORUZZI, G., FESSARD, A., and JASPER, H. H. (Eds.), p. 407. Elsevier, Amsterdam, 1963.

54. PIÉRON, H. *Le Probleme Physiologique du Sommeil*. Masson, Paris, 1913.

55. LEGENDRE, R. and PIÉRON, H. Le problème des facteurs du sommeil. Resultats D'injections vasculaires et intracérébrales de liquides insomniques. *C. r. Séanc. Soc. Biol.* **68**, 1077, 1910.

56. LEGENDRE, R. and PIÉRON, H. Du développement, au cours de L'insommie expérimentale, de propriétees hypnotoxiques des humeurs en relation avec le besoin croissant de sommeil. *C. r. Séanc. Soc. Biol.* **70**, 190, 1911.

57. SCHNEDORF, J. G. and IVY, A. C. An examination of the hypnotoxin theory of sleep. *Am. J. Physiol.* **125**, 491, 1939.

58. KORNMÜLLER, A. E., LUX, H. D., WINKEL, K. and KLEE, M. Neurohumoral ausgelöste schlafzustande an tieren mit gekreuztem kreislauf unter der kontrolle von EEG-ableitungen. *Naturwissenschaften* **48**, 503, 1961.

59. MONNIER, M., KOLLER, TH. and GRABER, S. Humoral influences of induced sleep and arousal upon electrical brain activity of animals with crossed circulation. *Expl. Neurol.* **8**, 264, 1963.

60. MONNIER, M. and HOSLI, L. Dialysis of sleep and waking factors in blood of the rabbit. *Science* **146**, 796, 1964.

61. MONNIER, M. and HOSLI, L. Humoral transmission of sleep and wakefulness II. Hemodialysis of a sleep inducing humor during stimulation of the thalamic somnogenic area. *Pflügers. Arch. ges. Physiol.* **282**, 60, 1965.

62. HERNÁNDEZ-PÉON, R. Central neuro-humoral transmission in sleep and wakefulness. *Progress in Brain Research—Vol. 18, Sleep Mechanisms*. AKERT, K., BALLY, C. and SCHADÉ, J. P. (Eds.), p. 96. Elsevier, Amsterdam, 1965.

63. JOUANY, J. M., GERARD, J., BROUSSOLE, B., REYNIER, M., ORSETTI, A., VERMUTH, C. and BARON, C. Pharmacologie comparée des sels de L'acide butyrique et de L'acide 4-hydroxybutyrique. *Agressologie* **1**, 417, 1960.

64. JOUVET, M., CIER, A., MOUNIER, D. and VALATX, J. L. Effects du 4-butyrolactone et du 4-hydroxybutyrate de sodium sur L'EEG et le comportement du chat. *C. r. Séanc. Soc. Biol.* **155**, 1313, 1961.

65. WINTERS, W. D. and SPOONER, C. E. A neurophysiological comparison of gamma-hydroxybutyrate with pentobarbital in cats. *Electroenceph. clin. Neurophysiol.* **18**, 287, 1965.

66. METCALFE, D. R., ENDE, R. N. and STRIPE, J. T. An EEG-behavioral study of sodium hydroxybutyrate in humans. *Electroenceph. clin. Neurophysiol.* **20**, 506, 1966.

67. AMIN, A. H., CRAWFORD, T. B. N. and GADDUM, J. H. The distribution of substance P and 5-hydroxytryptamine in the central nervous system of the dog. *J. Physiol., Lond.* **726**, 596, 1954.

68. BRODIE, B. B. and SHORE, P. A. A concept for a role of serotonin and norepinephrine as chemical mediators in the brain. *Ann. N.Y. Acad. Sci.* **66**, 631, 1957.

69. BRODIE, B. B. and SHORE, P. A. On a role for serotonin and norepinephrine as chemical mediators in the central autonomic nervous system. *Hormones, Brain Function and Behavior*, HOAGLAND, H. (Eds.), p. 161. Academic Press, New York, 1957.

70. KOELLA, W. P. The mode and locus of action of serotonin in its effects on the recruiting responses and the EEG of cats. *Am. J. Physiol.* **211**, 926, 1966.

71. KOELLA, W. P., TRUNCA, C. M. and CZICMAN, J. S. Serotonin: Effect on recruiting responses of the cat. *Life Sci.* **4**, 173, 1965.

72. MORUZZI, G. Synchronizing influences of the brain stem and the inhibitory mechanisms underlying the production of sleep by sensory stimulation. *Electroenceph. clin. Neurophysiol. Suppl.* **13**, 231, 1960.

73. MONNIER, M. and TISSOT, R. Action de la reserpine et de ses médiateurs (5 HTP, sérotonine et DOPA-noradrénaline) sur le comportement et le cerveau du lapin. *Helv. physiol. pharmac. Acta* **16**, 255, 1958.

74. JOUVET, M. Mechanisms of the states of sleep: A neuropharmacological approach. *Ass. Res. Nerv. Ment. Dis. Res. Publ.* **45**, 86, 1967.

75. MATSUMOTO, J. and JOUVET, M. Effets de réserpine, DOPA et 5-HTP sur les deux états de sommeil. *C. r. Séanc. Soc. Biol.* **158**, 2137, 1964.

76. WEITZMAN, E. D., RAPPORT, M. M., McGREGOR, P. and JACOBY, J. Sleep patterns of the monkey and brain serotonin concentration: Effect of p. chlorophenylalanine. *Science* **160**, 1361, 1968.

77. TORDA, CLARA. Biochemical and bioelectric processes related to sleep, paradoxical sleep and arousal. *Psychol. Rep.* **24**, 807, 1969.

78. FALCK, B. Cellular localization of monoamines. *Biogenic Amines—Progress in Brain Research*, Vol. 8, HIMWICH, H. E. and HIMWICH, W. A. (Eds.) Elsevier, Amsterdam, 1964.

79. FALCK, B., HILLARP, N. A., THIEME, G. and THORP, A. Fluorescence of catecholamines and related compounds condensed with formaldehyde. *J. Histochem. Cytochem.* **10**, 348, 1962.

80. DAHLSTROM, A. and FUXE, K. Evidence for the existence of monoamines containing neurons in the central nervous system. *Acta physiol. scand. Suppl.* **62**, 232, 1964.

81. DAHLSTROM, A. and FUXE, K. Evidence for the existence of monoamine neurons in the central nervous system. II. Experimentally induced changes in the intraneuronal amine levels of bulbospinal neuron systems. *Acta physiol. scand. Suppl.* **64**, 247, 1965.

82. JOUVET, M. Mechanisms of the states of sleep. *Sleep and Altered States of Consciousness.* KETY, S. S., EVARTS, E. V. and WILLIAMS, H. L. (Eds.) Williams & Wilkins, Baltimore, 1967.

83. MARANTZ, R. and RECHTSCHAFFEN, A. Effect of alpha methyltyrosine on sleep in the rat. *Percept. Mot. Skills* **25**, 805, 1967.

84. OSWALD, I., ASHCROFT, G. W., BERGER, R. J., ECCLESTON, D., EVANS, J. I. and THACORE, V. R. Some experiments in the chemistry of normal sleep. *Br. J. Psychiat.* **112**, 391, 1966.

85. COSTA, E. and RINALDI, F. Biochemical and electroencephalographic changes in the brain of rabbits injected with 5-hydroxytryptophan (Influence of chlorpromazine premedication). *Am. J. Physiol.* **194**, 214, 1958.

86. BOGDANSKI, D. F., WEISSBACH, H. and UDENFRIEND, S. The distribution of serotonin, 5-hydroxytryptophan decarboxylase and monoamine oxidase in brain. *J. Neurochem.* **1**, 272, 1957.

87. HESS, S. M. and DOEPFNER, W. Behavioral effects and brain amine contents in rats. *Archs int. Pharmacodyn. Thér.* **134**, 89, 1961.

88. HARTMANN, E. The effect of tryptophane on the sleep-dream cycle in man. Rep. to the Association for the Psychophysiological Study of Sleep. Gainesville, March, 1966.

89. MANDELL, M. P., MANDELL, A. J. and JACOBSON, A. Biochemical and neurophysiological studies of paradoxical sleep. *Recent Adv. Biol. Psychiat.* **7**, 115, 1964.

90. RECHTSCHAFFEN, A. and DEMENT, W. Studies on the relation of narcolepsy, cataplexy and sleep with low voltage fast EEG activity. *Res. Publ. Ass. Res. Nerv. Ment. Dis.* **45**, 1967.

91. EVANS, J. I. and OSWALD, I. Some experiments in the chemistry of narcoleptic sleep. *Br. J. Psychiat.* **112**, 401, 1966.

92. HARTMANN, E. The sleep-dream cycle and brain serotonin. *Psychonom. Sci.* **8**, 295, 1967.

93. SMITH, B. and PROCKOP, D. J. Central-nervous-system effects of ingestion of L-tryptophan by normal subjects. *New Engl. J. Med.* **267**, 1338, 1962.

94. HIMWICH, W. A. and COSTA, E. Behavioral changes associated with changes in concentration of brain serotonin. *Fedn. Proc. Fedn. Am. Socs exp. Biol.* **19**, 838, 1960.

95. ASHCROFT, G. W., ECCLESTON, D. and CRAWFORD, T. B. B. 5-hydroxyindole metabolism in rat brain (Methods). *J. Neurochem.* **12,** 483, 1965.

96. PLETSCHER, A., SHORE, P. A. and BRODIE, B. B. Serotonin as a mediator of reserpine action in brain. *J. Pharmac. exp. Ther.* **116,** 84, 1956.

97. HOLZBAUER, M. and VOGT, M. Depression by reserpine of the noradrenaline concentration in the hypothalamus of the cat. *J. Neurochem.* **1,** 8, 1956.

98. HOFFMAN, J. S. and DOMINO, E. F. Comparative effects of reserpine on the sleep cycle of man and cat. *J. Pharmac. exp. Ther.* **170,** 190, 1969.

99. REITE, M., PEGRAM, G. V., STEPHENS, L. M., BIXLER, E. C. and LEWIS, O. L. The effect of reserpine and monoamine oxidase inhibitors on paradoxical sleep in the monkey. *Psychopharmacologia* **14,** 12, 1969.

100. PSCHEIDT, G. R., MORPURGO, C. and HIMWICH, H. Studies on norepinephrine and 5-hydroxy tryptamine in various species. In: *Comparative Neurochemistry,* RICHTER, D. (Ed.), p. 401. Pergamon, New York, 1964.

101. NEFF, N. H. and COSTA, E. Application of steady-state kinetics to the study of catecholamine turnover after monoamine oxidase inhibition or reserpine administration. *J. Pharmacol. exp. Ther.* **160,** 40, 1968.

102. TOZER, T. N., NEFF, N. H. and BRODIE, B. B. Application of steady state kinetics to the synthesis rate and turnover time of serotonin in the brain of normal and reserpine-treated rats. *J. Pharmacol. exp. Ther.* **153,** 177, 1966.

103. CHRISTENSEN, H. N. and STREICHER, J. A. Association between rapid growth and elevated cell concentrations of amino acids: In fetal tissues. *J. biol. Chem.* **175,** 95, 1948.

104. LORINCZ, A. B. and KUTTNER, R. E. Response of malignancy to phenylalanine restriction. *Neb. St. med. J.* **50,** 609, 1965.

105. LESTER, B. K., CHANES, R. E. and CONDIT, P. T. A clinical syndrome and EEG-sleep changes associated with amino acid deprivation. *Am. J. Psychiat.* **126,** 71, 1969.

106. ENGEL, R. Abnormal brain wave patterns in kwashiorkor. *Electroenceph. clin. Neurophysiol.* **8,** 489, 1956.

J. psychiat. Res., 1971, Vol. 8, pp. 479–498. Pergamon Press. Printed in Great Britain.

CURRENT STATUS AND FUTURE PROSPECTS FOR RESEARCH IN PSYCHOSOMATIC MEDICINE

HERBERT WEINER

Department of Psychiatry, Montefiore Hospital and Medical Center
and
Albert Einstein College of Medicine, Bronx, New York

I. INTRODUCTION

RESEARCH in Psychosomatic Medicine in the past 30 years has had a curious and checkered history. It is a field which has been largely dominated by one man—FRANZ ALEXANDER[1]—whose intuitive and, at times, inspired formulations leave much to be desired from both a scientific and conceptual point of view. At one time, it was inundated by baroque and untestable hypotheses. Nevertheless, research in psychosomatic medicine has continued to attract investigators over the years, presumably because it addresses itself to some of the most complex problems in biology.

Psychosomatic research is concerned with the relative contributions of heredity and environment to the etiology and pathogenesis of physiological disorders, and the development of new models of the pathogenesis of disease. On another level, it attempts to explain how nonmaterial events, such as the behavioral or psychological responses to psychosocial stimuli, are translated into material, i.e. anatomical, enzymatic, autonomic or endocrine, events. Concomitantly, it seeks to elucidate the role of the central nervous system in the control and regulation of humoral, neural and even enzymatic processes.

These questions remain unanswered. However, we have gained some understanding of the factors which have impeded their resolution. For one, the methodological weaknesses of past clinical psychosomatic research have been identified. Secondly, it has become apparent that progress in this field can be achieved only if investigators keep pace with—and draw upon—the contributions of workers in related fields, such as physiology, neurobiology and genetic research.

An attempt will be made in this paper to elaborate on these assertions as they apply to three representative psychosomatic disorders, i.e. peptic ulcer, essential hypertension, and Graves' Disease.

II. METHODOLOGICAL PROBLEMS IN CLINICAL PSYCHOSOMATIC RESEARCH

The heterogeneity of the subject populations studied has emerged as a major methodological weakness of earlier research which led to hypotheses concerning the role of

479

intrapsychic conflict in the activation of specific organic processes. In studies of peptic ulcer disease, for example, the experimental population has at times included patients with gastric as well as duodenal ulcer. Admittedly, these syndromes share many features in common. But, as is well known, they also present significant differences, beyond the anatomical location of the lesion, which justify their classification as separate morbid entities, brought about by different etiological and pathogenetic mechanisms.[2] Furthermore, the sub-types which fall within these two major categories may be preceded by distinctive mechanisms. Thus, the investigator in this area is immediately faced with a major source of experimental error. He may not be studying a homogeneous disease with a uniform etiology and pathogenesis.

A second methodological problem, the lack of reliable data as to when the illness started, has crucial implications for studies of the environmental events surrounding the onset of the disease, and the subject's psychological responses to these events. No such information is available, for example, with respect to essential hypertension. As PICKERING[3] has pointed out, there is no agreement as to the dividing line between normal and elevated blood pressure; the criterion of elevated diastolic pressure shifts is purely an arbitrary one. In fact, it may be meaningless. Marked variations in blood pressure occur in persons who are thought to be hypertensive.

In addition to the heterogeneity of subject populations and the unavailability of reliable data as to the onset of disease, clinical psychosomatic research has been impeded by methodological problems which, in fact, are intrinsic to all clinical studies that employ psychological tools. Psychiatry and psychoanalysis are observational sciences at best. The human observer is a difficult instrument to calibrate, however. In addition, generalizations were often formed on the basis of single case studies; subjective inferences and objective observations were intermingled; inter-rater or test–retest reliabilities were not assessed; and hypotheses were not validated on the basis of studies of new subject populations. Finally, the categories of units of behavior which are usually observed are either not defined at all, or they are not operationally defined and there is little agreement as to what they consist of.

But the major methodological problem which has bedevilled all of psychosomatic research, regardless of the specific techniques used, stems from the fact that, in most instances, the observer is aware of the nature of his subject's illness beforehand. And the problem of experimenter bias is compounded by the fact that the subject, in turn, usually knows that his illness is supposed to have psychosocial determinants. He may, therefore, select or withhold appropriate historical material to please or frustrate the experimenter, or because he fears exposure. Proper controls may circumvent some of these problems, but they cannot solve them all. Only when subjects are selected and studied prior to the onset of disease, do many of these methodological issues fall away.

Psychological findings may be contaminated by other flaws in research design. The evolution of Alexander's original formulations regarding the personality pattern of peptic ulcer patients served to underscore the need to take socio-economic factors into account in clinical studies, as well as such factors as age, sex, intelligence, and educational background. Subjects and controls must be matched with respect to each of these variables. Obviously, it is also important to control such variables as the length of illness, the patient's age at onset, his medical history, the effects of hospitalization, and, of course, the possible effects of medication prescribed for the patient on his psychological functioning. Different kinds of control groups may have to be issued, depending on specific research goals. But, above all, each finding should be validated on a new subject and control population.

III. VALIDATION STUDIES

Only in two instances, peptic ulcer and Graves' disease, where predictor variables are available, has one major methodological weakness of retrospective studies been overcome. These validation studies had as their aim the test of Alexander's formulations concerning the occurrence of specific conflicts in subjects prior to the development of syndromes.

(a) *Peptic ulcer*

MIRSKY et al.[4] took a first major step toward the achievement of this goal by identifying the physiological condition necessary for the development of duodenal ulcer, i.e. the hypersecretion of pepsinogen. Concomitantly, he and his co-workers postulated that those individuals with the highest levels of serum pepsinogen were most likely to develop peptic ulcer disease under appropriate stress.

WEINER et al.[5] attempted to test both this postulate and Alexander's hypothesis regarding the central conflict in peptic ulcer within a controlled social setting. Serum pepsinogen was measured in 2073 U.S. Army draftees, and a group of 63 hypersecretors and 57 hyposecretors were selected for special study. At the start of basic training, each of these 120 men completed a battery of psychological tests and a gastrointestinal X-ray examination. The first examination revealed evidence of duodenal ulcer in 4 subjects, all of whom were hypersecretors. A second roentgenological examination, administered after the 120 subjects had been exposed to basic training for 8–16 weeks, further substantiated Mirsky's postulate. Five additional subjects, all hypersecretors of serum pepsinogen, had X-ray evidence of duodenal ulceration.

Although the study verified Alexander's formulations in general, the findings were not conclusive. On the basis of psychological test data only, which put Alexander's hypothesis into operation, three investigators correctly assigned 71 per cent of the 120 subjects to the hypersecretor, and 51 per cent to the hyposecretor groups. In addition, 10 of the total group of 120 subjects were selected as most likely to have had an ulcer when they began basic training, or to have developed one subsequently. These predictions were correct for 7 of the 10 subjects. There was some discrepancy, however, between the personality characteristics which were significantly associated with hypersecretion of serum pepsinogen and duodenal ulceration in this study and those hypothesized by Alexander, because Alexander's original formulations of the personality characteristics of subjects prone to or with peptic ulcer, lacked sufficient specificity.

In retrospect, this study has noteworthy limitations.. For one, obviously, the population from which these subjects were drawn would not be considered representative. It consisted of young men, drawn from a predominantly urban population, residing in the northeastern section of the United States. Ethnic and social factors may play an important role, unknown as yet, in determining serum pepsinogen levels.[6,7] Secondly, the psychological findings have not been fully validated on another population.[8] Therefore, some of the criteria developed by WEINER et al.[5] may have test–retest reliability, and some may not. In fact, when these authors retested their original subject population, they found that psychological criteria indicative of anxiety no longer discriminated between the hyposecretor and hypersecretor groups, although the other criteria did.[9]

Because of this instability of the test criteria, the study should be verified on a new population, particularly in light of recent developments in our understanding of the pathophysiology of peptic ulcer disease. The findings derived from recent studies suggest that damage to the gastric mucosa (such as ulceration and gastritis) may raise levels of serum or plasma pepsinogen. In addition, there is new evidence that individual variations both in plasma and urinary pepsinogen occur from day to day, and possibly from hour to hour. Clearly, then, single determinations of levels should be viewed with caution.[10]

But another complicating factor has now appeared. There is evidence that seven electrophoretically distinct pepsinogens can be extracted from human gastroduodenal mucosa.[11,12] Pepsinogen (Pg) 1–5 occur in the gastric body and fundus; three of these (Pg 2–4) are invariably excreted in the urine. Two additional pepsinogens (Pg 6, 7) are found in the antrum and proximal duodenum and are rarely excreted. Pg 1–4 occur in all human beings but Pg 5 does not. Its presence or absence appears to be genetically determined; when present it may be related to the etiology of peptic ulcer.[13]

On the other hand, TAYLOR[14] has published data which suggest a significant increase in frequency of occurrence of Pepsin 1 in the gastric juice of patients with gastric ulcer and a less significant increase in those with duodenal ulcer. Whether this relationship is causal remains to be determined.

These findings suggest that the relationship of pepsinogens to peptic ulcer is considerably more complex than was originally believed and that the pepsin isoenzymes relevant to peptic ulcer do not appear in the urine. Only further work can resolve this puzzle.

The predictive study by WEINER et al.[5] concerned itself with the etiology of peptic ulcer disease. If valid, the study findings mean that a high concentration of serum pepsinogen (as a criterion of gastric hypersecretion), in combination with certain personality character- istics, predispose some persons to react to a stressful environmental situation by developing a duodenal ulcer. The study does not address itself to the problem of pathogenesis. MIRSKY[15] believes that variations in the concentration of serum pepsinogen are genetically determined. He has postulated that if a high level of serum pepsinogen is present at birth, this inborn trait may influence the mother–child relationship and personality development, and thereby play a central role in determining the adult psychological characteristics specified in the study. This hypothesis has not been tested to date, but it is eminently testable by available techniques.

(b) Graves' disease

Two studies have been reported in the past 15 years which are guided by the same logic. In the general population there are subjects whose thyroid glands have a greater avidity for iodine or clear it more rapidly, yet who are not clinically hyperthyroid. This subgroup should demonstrate the same kind of conflicts (e.g. over-dependency) or show similar personality characteristics as patients who are clinically hyperthyroid. Subjects at risk should be identified prior to the onset of the illness; the psychosocial events which surrounded its onset can then be studied.

DONGIER and his co-workers[16] used the rate of decay of ^{131}I from the gland as a criterion of the more rapid clearance of iodine from the thyroid gland. They found a shorter half-life of ^{131}I in subjects with a family history of Graves' disease. Those with a faster decay of ^{131}I from the gland had the personality characteristics of patients with hyperthyroidism, although they were not clinically hyperthyroid.

WALLERSTEIN et al.[17] studied subjects in whom there is an increase locally in the thyroid gland in the uptake of [131]I. Some of these subjects had very mild symptoms of hyperthyroidism; others did not. Regardless of whether they did or did not, their psychological profiles differed from those of a control group without 'hot spots' in the gland. Note, however, that these 'hot spots' may very well be the precursors of toxic thyroid adenomata. In fact, some of these subjects, though asymptomatic, had a palpable thyroid nodule.[18] The investigators made reliable predictions of hot spots in a new population, after the development of a personality profile, and also studied patients with diffuse (not nodular) enlargements of the gland. Curiously enough, the personality profiles of subjects with hot spots and diffuse increases of ^{131}I uptake but no clinical hyperthyroidism were the same as those of clinically hyperthyroid patients.

The point is that we know today that the pathogenesis of Graves' disease with diffuse goiter, differs from the pathogenesis of toxic nodular goiter—the pathogenetic factor in the former, but not the latter, being the long acting thyroid stimulator (LATS). If Wallerstein's findings are correct, and confirm Alexander's formulations for the most part, then they clearly are not specific for Graves' disease. Futhermore, one would have to postulate that there is a common personality predisposition in all cases of hyperthyroidism, regardless of pathogenesis, and that under certain circumstances this predisposing factor, acting through one or another mechanism, produces hyperthyroidism regardless of its nature. But no such common mechanism is known. Further, Alexander's hypothesis that specific psychologic characteristics in some manner act to release thyrotropin to incite Graves' disease is open to question, in view of the fact that thyrotropin is not the pathogenetic variable. In fact, Graves' disease may occur after hypophysectomy.

IV. PSYCHOPHYSIOLOGICAL STUDIES

Early attempts to verify some of Alexander's observations and formulations in the laboratory and on human subjects were fraught by other equally noxious methodological and conceptual problems.

Very often, only a single physiological variable was used to demonstrate that the perception of psychosocial stimuli would produce the physiological changes associated with the disease under investigation. Obviously, the fact that acute elevations of blood pressure occur in normotensive or hypertensive patients in the laboratory, that subjects with a gastric fistula respond to emotional arousal by an increase in the secretion of hydrochloric acid, or that patients with hyperthyroidism as well as normal subjects showed increases in the rate of turnover of radio-iodine and autonomic arousal when viewing a 'stressful' film,[19] neither proves nor disproves that psychological factors have etiologic or pathogenic significance in the respective disease states. Such short-term changes may have nothing to do with the onset of the disease under study. The sustained changes in function in human beings which constitute the disease state itself have never been brought about in the laboratory.

Secondly, recent advances in physiology and in animal research, as summarized in the following sections of this paper, have cast serious doubt on the relevance of many of the physiological and biochemical variables studied to date.[20]

Until recently, the isolation of relevant psychological variables with high predictive value constituted still another methodological problem. We have taken important steps forward in this area, however. There is considerable evidence that the subject's perception of the experimental setting (i.e. the initial laboratory experience, and of the experimenter); the way these perceptions are interpreted and defended against; and the subject's concomitant emotional behavior, are relevant to both the mobilization and suppression of hormonal and autonomic variables. The fact that these psychological variables have been correlated with the suppression of hormonal and autonomic activity (as well as the stimulation of high levels of activity) is particularly noteworthy.

Clearly, psychophysiological research also requires skills in the evaluation of correlated behavioral and physiological change. And, chiefly as a result of LACEY's work,[21-25] there have been important advances in this area as well. Specifically, Lacey has emphasized that in evaluating cardiovascular responses, it is crucial to differentiate three manifestations of any autonomic function. Background (nonspecific or spontaneous) activity[21,26] must be differentiated from the initial or attained level of function ('tension'), and from the magnitude of change ('liability') which occurs coincident with an imposed stimulus.[22] Each of these functions must be treated independently. He has also reminded us that autonomic functions, e.g. heart rate, skin resistance, or blood pressure, show low intercorrelations, regardless of whether tension or lability scores are calculated.[23] It follows, then, that a particular stimulus may correlate with one function and not another.

LACEY is one of the few workers who have carried out repetitive tests of autonomic function on the same population of subjects.[22,24] His conclusions are not only striking, but convincing. There are individual differences in resting spontaneous activity, some of which can be correlated with specific behaviors.[21] He and others have further demonstrated that, in response to a given stimulus, many (but not all) subjects exhibit a reproducible but individual pattern of response in several physiological variables, both with regard to the 'tension' level attained and 'liability'.[23-25]

Some workers have concluded from these findings that these inherent (perhaps constitutionally or genetically determined) patterns of autonomic responses occur independent of the 'stress', no matter how complex; therefore, any attempt to find specific psychological correlates of physiological responses would be futile. Alternative hypotheses have been advanced. REISER[27] has suggested that the reproducibility of response patterns may be a function of the subject's responses to the experimenter and the experiment, rather than the specific stress situations used to elicit the response. Another hypothesis suggests itself. Many different psychological tasks and situations or physical stimuli elicit similar and perhaps inherent physiological responses in any given subject. Obviously, such a statement is not logically equivalent to the conclusion that responses occur independent of tasks or stimuli.

We know today that 'coping' and 'defensive' devices in man are critical intervening variables between the perception of the psychosocial stimulus, the psychological response (including the emotional one) to that perception, and the concomitant physiological response.[28-34] In fact, it may not be too early to suggest that these devices may be important regulators of physiological change. In any event, these coping devices and their homologues in the nervous system clearly merit further investigation.

Naturalistic studies of human subjects have also suggested that bereavement or separation may be the critical antecedents of behavioral disturbances and physiological change both in man and animals.[35-37] Profound behavioral changes in young primates are known to occur upon separation from their mothers. Yet very little is known about the mechanisms by which separation affects bodily processes. HOFER[38], and HOFER and WEINER[39] have shown, however, that on separating 14 day old rats from their mothers a profound fall in heart rate occurred; the heart rate could be restored on feeding rat milk to the pups.

Another set of findings which derive from psychophysiologic research in animals and man teaches us to look for patterned changes in several endocrine and autonomic variables. From such a pattern it may be possible to discern mediating mechanisms: e.g. BROD[40-42] showed that mental arithmetic produced changes in B.P., muscle and splanchnic blood flow, heart rate and cardiac output in normal and hypertensive subjects which differed in the two subject populations only in duration and degree. This pattern is analogous to that produced by chronic, perifornical hypothalamic stimulation in animals,[43] and is apparently mediated by brain circuits mediating the sympathetic 'vasodilator' system.[44]

Largely as a consequence of MASON's work[45] using avoidance conditioning in monkeys, we have learned to look for organized patterns of hormonal responses: Some changes in hormone levels are acutely correlated in time with this independent variable while others far outlast it.

Future work in this area might therefore be guided by a study of those variables with high predictive power—the psychosocial situation, behavioral, perceptual, adaptive, affective and defensive variables, in conjunction with a variety of relevant physiological variables, and in a longitudinal manner.

V. RECENT PHYSIOLOGICAL ADVANCES

As noted earlier in this paper, and underscored in the preceding section, lack of progress in psychosomatic research can be attributed in some measure to the fact that workers in this field have failed to keep abreast of developments in related fields. In all the diseases under review, new and important variables have been discovered, and their regulation has been linked to the C.N.S. This section will deal, in particular, with the possible relevance of hormonal variables to the etiology and pathogenesis of disease in man. Admittedly, this is not yet fully understood, but the groundwork has been laid.

(a) *Peptic Ulcer*

(1) *Gastrin*

Gastrin has recently come to the fore as a critical variable in the autoregulation of gastric secretion. There is also considerable evidence to suggest that gastrin is one of the key regulators of acid secretion: Gastrin, the vagus nerve, and histamine appear to act in synergism with regard to parietal cell stimulation and the concomitant secretion of hydrochloric acid.

Methods of sufficient sensitivity, i.e. radioimmuno-assays,[46-48] have been developed only recently to measure circulating levels of gastrin—and to demonstrate conclusively that gastrin may play an important mediating role in the Zollinger–Ellison syndrome.[47] However, we have not yet accumulated evidence of equal weight to attest to the mediating role of gastrin in peptic ulcer disease in man. In view of the fact that gastrin plays an important role in the regulation of gastric secretion, and is regulated in turn by the vagus, it might be interesting to study the effects of psychological stimuli and brain stimulation on gastric production.

(2) *Hormonal influences on gastric function*

One of the principal mechanisms by which the nervous system regulates bodily function is the release of the trophic hormones of the pituitary gland. When their influence is measured in terms of the release of adrenocortical and other hormones, abundant evidence exists that the trophic hormones are influenced, in turn, by environmental events and psychological factors.[45]

(A) *The adrenocortical hormones.* There is some evidence that the cortical hormones may be involved in the pathogenesis of peptic ulcer disease, possibly by altering the composition of gastric mucus, or be acting synergistically with certain secretory stimulants. Studies of animals who are subjected to psychological stresses while gastric and steroid secretion are being measured might elucidate the respective roles of these hormones.

(B) *Growth hormone.* The role of growth hormone in gastric function is still not fully understood. However, we do know that growth hormone influences the pancreatic hormones,[49] and may therefore affect gastric secretion indirectly.

(C) *Histamine.* As is well known, histamine is a powerful stimulant of acid secretion by the stomach, and weakly stimulates the secretion of pepsinogen. Obviously, this does not mean that histamine plays a key role in the pathogenesis of peptic ulcer disease. In fact, its natural role in the regulation of acid secretion by the stomach has not been determined.[50,51] It is known, however, that enzymes for histamine synthesis reside in the mucosa of the stomach, and that repeated injections of histamine produce duodenal ulceration of the stomachs of guinea pigs[52] and rats.[53]

A number of other hormones and naturally occurring substances have been implicated either directly in peptic ulcer disease, or indirectly in the regulation of the secretory functions of the stomach. These include male and female sex hormones, thyroid hormone, parat-hormone, vasopressin, insulin, serotonin, the prostaglandins, and various gastroduodenal hormones.[20] Unfortunately, no definitive statement can yet be made as to just what part they play in the pathogenesis of peptic ulcer. Despite the fact that changes in levels of individual hormones have been noticed, no one has studied the patterning of hormonal changes over a period of time after the onset of the disease.

(b) *Essential hypertensions*

Recent research has shown that most of the physiological variables which have been seriously implicated in essential hypertension are autoregulated, and, in addition, are regulated by the C.N.S.

More specifically, as depicted schematically in Fig. 1, these variables are interrelated by a series of negative feedback loops: A fall in renal artery perfusion pressure causes the release of renin which, in the presence of angiotensinogen, produces angiotensin I and II. Angiotensin II causes the release of aldosterone, which may play a role at some stage in the course of essential hypertension. Angiotensin is the main, but not the only regulator of aldosterone production.[54-56] It is also regulated by a high intake of potassium which increases aldosterone production, and decreases renin secretion;[57,58] by pressure changes in thyrocarotid receptors; and, possibly, by the release of ACTH. By virtue of its effect on serum sodium, aldosterone may raise plasma volume, thereby diminishing renin release; and by increasing blood osmolality, aldosterone may cause the release of ADH, thereby increasing the renal reabsorption of water and lowering serum sodium—and osmolality. The possible interrelationship between the glucocorticoids and aldosterone, and salt and electrolyte metabolism are also noted in Fig. 1.

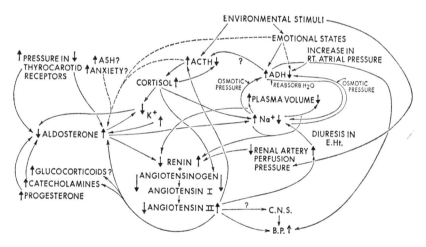

Fɪɢ. 1.   Diagrammatic representation of the factors which are believed to play a role in the pathogenesis of essential hypertension.

Psychophysiological studies of some or all of the variables mentioned above and shifts in their regulation may enable us to answer three obvious questions: (1) Can renal blood flow be increased in one renal artery and decreased in the other? In that event, the content in each renal vein of renin and/or angiotensin II could be measured. (2) Can the distribution

w

of blood flow within each kidney (measured by intra-arterial injections of Krypton-85 and intravenous injections of iodoantipyrine-I-131 be affected differently by operant methods? (3) If renal blood flow can be diminished by operant conditioning procedures, does hypertension ensue?

As mentioned above, apart from the fact that they regulate each other, the mechanisms which have been implicated in essential hypertension are regulated by environmental stimuli via the central nervous system. For example, in addition to changes in osmolality of the blood, the rate of ADH secretion is markedly increased by painful stimuli,[59] avoidance conditioning, and, possibly, by vagal afferent discharge. The infusion of an isotonic solution induces diuresis by the assumed medium of 'volume' receptors in the hypothalamus. In view of the hypothesis that, in essential hypertension, the circulation acts 'as if' there were volume expansion, and the finding that salt (and water) are lost in response to angiotensin and salt infusion, one might speculate that there is an aberrant response in ADH secretion, or of the kidney to ADH in essential hypertension. If this is so, it would link ADH to environmental and psychological stimuli by a chain of events mediated by the nervous system.

'Stressful' stimuli release both ACTH and ADH. Based on this fact, it has been suggested that vasopressin may also act as the corticotrophin releasing factor, which adds another link in the chain of psychological events whereby environmental stimuli may be translated into bodily changes in hypertension. All of the stimuli which cause changes in the release of ADH are mediated through the C.N.S. But two antidiuretic effects of environmental stimuli must be differentiated: a rapid, autonomically mediated, antidiuretic response, and one which is mediated by the hypothalamus and the neurohypophysis.[60] It is this latter mechanism which is regulated by changes in blood osmolality.[61]

No attempt has been made here to mention all the variables which may play a role in the pathogenesis of essential hypertension; nor have we attempted to discuss the variables which are specified in any detail. Rather, the purpose of this discussion was to provide some possible guide-lines for future research. In the past, clinical physiologists have failed to recognize that many of these important physiological variables are also regulated by psychosocial stimuli, acting through the C.N.S. Hopefully, this review has demonstrated the potential value of a combined behavioral–physiological approach.

(c) Graves' disease

In the course of the development of methods for the bio-assay of thyrotropin, a substance was discovered, now referred to as a long acting thyroid stimulator (LATS) which caused an increase in protein bound ^{131}I, its thyroid uptake, and in the release of thyroxine, even in hypohysectomized animals.[62,63] This increase in thyroid activity has been shown to occur in a number of animals, and LATS has been identified in the blood of 6–89 per cent of hyperthyroid patients with or without exophthalmos,[64,65] but not in patients with toxic adenoma, or malignant thyroid carcinomata.

Therefore, the most recent evidence suggests that LATS, which has been identified as an immunoglobulin, is pathogenetic of Graves' disease. The point is, of course, that if psychosocial stimuli do indeed antedate the onset of Graves' disease, and if LATS is the natural pathogenetic mechanism, how are these stimuli and LATS linked?

VI. ANIMAL STUDIES

Despite the weaknesses of clinical psychosomatic and psychophysiological research, many of the hypotheses derived therefrom have been verified in the laboratory. Animal research has clearly demonstrated that environmental stimuli modify or interact with experimental variables to produce physiological or structural changes analogous or homologous to clinical psychosomatic disease. Furthermore, such work has strongly supported, if not substantiated, the hypothesis that social stimuli may alter bodily functions by acting via the nervous system.

Animal studies in this area have, of course, two distinct advantages over human studies: Pure genetic strains of animals can be bred—strains which have a particular sensitivity, e.g. to restraint, which produces gastric ulceration. Moreover, in animals, early experiences can be manipulated to diminish or enhance susceptibility to later experimental manipulations.

(a) *Peptic ulcer*

Gastric ulcers can be produced in rats and monkeys by a wide variety of experimental manipulations, used singly or in combination. In rats, gastric ulcers have been produced by sensory stimulation, the administration of drugs, brain stimulation, diet, restraint or immobilization, and conditioning techniques.[66,67] When restraint is used, important parameters of the experiment are the species and age of the animal, the length of time it is immobilized, and the availability of food and water.[68]

In addition, rats may differ in their susceptibility to the same manipulation. As is true of man,[5] a high level of serum pepsinogen may be assumed to indicate an increased susceptibility to erosion in the glandular portion of the rat's stomach.[69,70] Rats bred by ADER[71] for susceptibility to gastric lesions upon restraint were found to have higher levels of serum pepsinogen prior to restraint than rats of other strains. In addition, these lesion-susceptible rats were more emotionally reactive,[72] and appeared to be more dominant in 'competitive' tasks.[73] On the other hand, susceptible animals who are handled early in life are less prone to develop gastric lesions upon restraint than those who are not. Life experiences in infancy, such as early weaning, may also be a critical variable in predisposing to gastric ulceration when male rats are later exposed to conflict situations[74] or immobilization.[75]

Despite the fact that the relationship between gastric ulceration in the rat and duodenal ulceration in man is enigmatic, the implications of these data cannot be disputed: Research on the production of ulcers in animals dispels many of the doubts that clinical psychosomatic research on human subjects leaves in the mind of the critical reviewer. A number of laboratory experiences and behavioral characteristics (such as activity cycles), in combination with physical stimuli and genetically determined physiological factors, do seem to interact to produce gastric ulcer.

Yet, one important question remains unanswered: On the one hand, different experimental manipulations have been shown to produce gastric secretion in different parts of the stomach: Immobilization restraint invariably produces lesions in the glandular portion of the rat's stomach, but conflict situations produce ruminal lesions in some rats,[76] and glandular lesions in others.[77] On the other hand, one may also conclude from the literature that a number of different experimental conditions produce the same anatomical lesion. This apparent contradiction clearly requires clarification. If the evidence indicates that different manipulations produce lesions only in the glandular portion of the stomach, this would facilitate our search for a common mediating mechanism. The study conducted by LEVINE and SENAY[78] is relevant in this regard: The authors found that when rats were restrained in a cold climate, intragastric pH fell and ulcers were produced, and that an antacid prevented ulcer production under these conditions. Presumably, then, these ulcers were caused by an increase in gastric acidity, which is believed to be mediated by histamine.[79] Interestingly, these authors also found that restraint and cold increase the activity of histidine decarboxylase, which increase is positively correlated with the incidence and severity of stress ulcers.[78] The mechanism of enzyme induction under these conditions is unknown.

The answer to the question of the mechanisms whereby restraint produces gastric ulceration might also be sought by available neurophysiological techniques, e.g. chronic unit recording of the nervous system. In fact, a restrained rat might be a particularly good experimental animal to use for this purpose.

(b) *Essential hypertension*

The most convincing and systematic study of the role of complex stimuli in producing prolonged systolic hypertension in mice was reported by HENRY et al.[80] The effects of mixing males from different boxes, of aggregating them in small boxes, of exposing mice to a cat for many months, and of producing territorial conflict in mixed males and females resulted in sustained elevations of systolic blood pressure which were higher in male than in female mice. Previous and early experiences of living together attentuated the effects on blood pressure when aggregation and territorial conflict were experimentally induced. Conversely, isolation from weaning to maturity exacerbated the effects of crowding on blood pressure.

In another area of research, salt has been shown to play a role in the pathogenesis of hypertension, a role which is hotly contested, however. The chronic ingestion of excess salt produces hypertension in rats of a particular strain, but it does not do so in all animals of that strain, and it takes time to do so.[81, 82]

The question of whether psychosocial stimuli elicit circulatory responses has been answered, in part, by the use of classical conditioning procedures.[83] When monkeys were placed on a continuous avoidance schedule, the change in blood pressure depended on the length or complexity of the schedule. In monkeys on the more complex schedules, blood pressure remained as high in the intervals between lever pressing sessions, as it had been during the experimental sessions.[84, 85]

Until recently, studies on conditioning of autonomic responses, and more specifically cardiovascular responses, were inconclusive. It was argued that the autonomic components of a response might be only a part of a more generalized pattern in which muscular action predominates.[86] This criticism lingered on until MILLER et al.[87] disposed of it by obtaining exquisite differential autonomic conditioning of vasomotor responses and systolic blood pressure in rats paralyzed with curare. They also showed that glomerular flow, renal flow, and urine formation could be brought under experimental control. In so doing, they have opened up a new area of investigation directly relevant to the study of hypertension.

Once again, the evidence derived from animal studies is much more convincing than that derived from human studies. Blood pressure, vasomotor tone, and many of the physiological variables which have been implicated in the pathogenesis of hypertension in man can be related to naturally occurring events and to behavior manipulated in the laboratory. The recent evidence brought forth by MILLER[87] and coworkers and by MASON,[45] raises exciting possibilities that we may be on the verge of a real breakthrough in understanding the pathogenesis and pathophysiology of hypertension.

VII. THE ROLE OF THE CENTRAL NERVOUS SYSTEM

Animal studies, and evidence of the role of the C.N.S. in the regulation of important hormonal variables in psychosomatic diseases, add credence to the belief that the nervous system is involved in these diseases. Unfortunately, however, too little is known about the neural circuits and the neuronal and neurochemical mechanisms which mediate the psychosocial stimuli which instigate autonomic and encocrine changes, and are, in turn, modified by feedback from the body.

(a) *Peptic ulcer*

Evidence derived from animal studies suggests that intracerebral stimulation and lesions may stimulate or inhibit the secretion of acid and pepsin, or change the production and quality of gastric mucus.[88,89] But it is hard to know what these findings mean. Obviously, animal species differ in their responses to brain stimulation.

Presumably, the excitatory effects of brain stimulation are mediated by the vagus nerve. An increase in neural activity in the vagus nerve causes an increase in gastric motility and secretion. But the vagus is not purely excitatory; it is also inhibitory.[90] And we still do not know just how these two opposing influences affect the stomach: For example, we do not know how increased vagal discharge can cause a dissociation of acid from pepsin secretion.[91] Nor are there any really good data available on differences in vagal activity which might account for the regulation of the various phases of acid secretion. One might ask whether there is a vagal, or some other mode of neural regulation of the phases of acid secretion, i.e., cephalic, interprandial, and postprandial. If so, which specific mechanisms perform this regulatory function? And do such mechanisms interact with the hormonal regulation of secretion?

(b) *Essential hypertension*

Answers to the questions of how environmental change is mediated, and how some of the pathogenetic mechanisms postulated in essential hypertension are affected by the nervous system must await further research. But we already know that the central nervous system is implicated in the regulation of autonomic nervous activity and of every possible etiological and pathogenetic mechanism in essential hypertension. Whether changes in these systems are primary or secondary in the disease are irrelevant at the moment. Once the initial pathogenetic process is set off, the nervous system may sustain that process by complex means.

The C.N.S. has even been implicated in experimental *renal* hypertension. In acute experimental renal hypertension, there is a decreased hypotensive response to sympathetic ganglion blocking agents and to attempts to reduce sympathetic vasoconstriction.[92,93] A number of workers have suggested that a dual mechanism is involved in experimental renal hypertension which is produced by interfering with the renal circulation:[94] At first, a pressor substance is released by the kidney; later, an additional, perhaps neural, mechanism is involved to sustain elevated B.P. levels.

This dual mechanism could be reduced to a single mechanism if it could be shown that a humoral substance, such as angiotensin, usually exerts its effects in part through the medium of the nervous system. Indeed this hypothesis seems now to be fairly well proven.[95,96] Further, McCubbin's[97] recent observations provide an example of the interaction of these mechanisms. After several days of infusing very small doses of angiotensin (which had no effect on B.P.) into dogs, their arterial pressure became elevated and labile. (Before the infusion the mean arterial pressure had been steady.) When surrounded by normal laboratory activity, their blood pressures, though labile, were high. If the laboratory was quiet, minor distractions caused marked increases in pressure due to increases in peripheral resistance. At the same time, a sensitization to an infusion of tyramine (which releases endogenous stores of noreprinephrine) caused further elevations of B.P. after angiotensin had been infused. Infusions of norepinephrine did not produce such an effect. These rather scattered observations suggest that a systematic study could be carried out of the role of psychosocial stimulation in animals made hypertensive by constricting the renal artery.

Folkow and Rubenstein[43] have been able to produce sustained hypertension by mild, intermittent stimulation, provided daily for several months in the area of the hypothalamus known to elicit the 'defense' reaction. In so doing, they demonstrated, for the first time, that brain stimulation alone will produce hypertension in animals. Of particular interest in this connection is the fact that acute stimulation of this hypothalamic locus produces a complex pattern of cardiovascular and behavioral responses, consisting of sympathetic vasodilation in muscle, increased heart rate, vasoconstriction in vascular beds (other than muscle), and increased secretion of catecholamines.[98] Analogous vascular changes occur in humans during states of fear and anticipation, and while they are performing mental arithmetic.

When the 'defense' reaction is elicited, cats growl, hiss, and run; their pupils dilate; and piloerection occurs. The 'defense' reaction occurs not only when the hypothalamus near the entrance of the fornix is stimulated, but also with stimulation of the dorsomedial amygdala and striae terminalis.[99,100] It is also known that the cerebral cortex attentuates the violence of the 'defense' reaction. Thus, the 'defense' reaction epitomizes a selective, yet correlated, vasomotor and behavioral response, produced by stimulation of a particular brain site.

Other neural mechanisms which have been implicated in hypertension are probably involved in adjustments to the elevated blood pressure. The evidence suggests that the carotid sinus reflex remains active and functioning in essential hypertension, but that the mechanoreceptors adapt to higher levels of B.P., and, therefore, no longer act maximally to reduce pressure levels. The nature of this adaptation is not yet clear. It is probably due to the direct effect of a high systematic arterial pressure, rather than a chemical substance.[93] WEINER[101] has pointed out that such an adaptation to an elevated mean B.P. would act to sustain it, and may, therefore, play a part in the 'neurogenic' stage of the illness.

There is still considerable controversy about the detailed anatomy of supramedullary and suprasegmental outflow from the brain responsible for vasomotor control. Another system involved in cardiovascular regulation which is better known has been described by a group of Swedish physiologists[102,103] as the sympathetic 'vasodilator' mechanism. Vasodilator nerves to skeletal muscles of mammals may be regulated by pathways from the motor cortex, via the hypothalamus, tectum of the midbrain, and the ventrolateral medulla oblongata, from where they travel to the spinal cord, When stimulated, vasodilation in skeletal muscle is accompanied by constriction in the splanchnic bed and skin. This system, which is activated by psychological factors and exercise, may mediate the effects of stimulation of the hypothalamus to produce the 'defense' reaction.

Obviously, the data described above do not tell us what ushers in essential hypertension. Neurogenic mechanisms are generally not thought to do so. But most workers in the field limit their remarks about 'neurogenic mechanisms' to those contained in the circuit from the mechanoreceptors to the medullary basomotor center and hence to the spinal centers. The interaction of this system and the sympathetic vasodilator system to alter peripheral resistance, or to affect the renal circulation, have never been studied. In fact, most workers still try to account for the increase in peripheral resistance in hypertension in the face of normal cardiac output by physiological means other than neural ones.

(c) *Graves' disease*

If it is true that LATS is the pathogenetic agent in Graves' disease, and if it is an immunoglobulin, one might ask how the nervous system could contribute to its regulation. In addition to the exposure to an antigen, do other factors control antibody formation, or do they contribute to the action of antibodies: At this point, one can only speculate that genetic factors may influence antibody formation in thyroid disease; LATS may act on cyclic AMP, as the corticosteroids and catecholamines do, to promote the entrance of iodine into thyroid cells.[104] There is also evidence that adrenalectomy[105] and the administration of thyroid hormone[106] enhance antibody formation. And some initial evidence has been accumulated which suggests that some immunological responses may be under the modulating influence of the central nervous system.[107] Whether LATS is among them remains to be seen.

VIII. CONCLUSION

One must conclude from an assessment of the current status of psychosomatic and psychophysiological research that there is little verified data at the clinical level. An attempt was made in this paper to delineate some of the factors which account for our lack of progress in this area. They include the major methodological weaknesses of past research, the study of single and often irrelevant variables, and the failure of investigators to acquaint themselves with new developments in related fields. It is only in the area of animal research that substantial progress has been made. The evidence that psychosocial stimuli elicit a wide range of physiological and biochemical responses and produce anatomical changes is fairly conclusive. In addition, animal studies have uncovered important etiological factors in these diseases.

It is, of course, well known that genetic factors play a role in the etiology of essential hypertension, Graves' disease, and probably in peptic ulcer. What we do not know is how much the etiological variance is also accounted for by experiential (e.g. social, familial, and economic) factors. In the area of psychosomatic disease, methodologies developed in other fields, such as the use of monozygotic twins separated at birth in the study of schizophrenia, might be employed in the area of psychosomatic disease to enhance our understanding of the interaction of the genotype with experience. Nor do we know enough about the specific genetic and experiential factors which make vulnerable the particular molecular and cellular configurations which terminate in a disease in one target organ and not another.

In the meantime, the work on animals permits the tentative conclusion that these diseases probably are neither caused nor sustained by any single pathogenetic factor. Psychosocial stimuli acting through the nervous system activate a wide range of inter-related responses. One can extrapolate from Ader's and Mason's work that no single factor alone can account for the pathogenetic or pathophysiological variance or the course of the disease. In essence, the presence of multiple factors and changes, and their interrelationships (as schematized in Fig. 1, for example), lead one to conclude that psychosomatic diseases are primarily diseases of physiological regulation. It is only because, in the past, analytic experiments were done and single dependent variables were studied by physiologists, who then conceptualized their results in linear causal terms, that this obvious point was missed, though not by Mason.

Admittedly, it is difficult to conceptualize such regulatory patterns. It is not enough just to state that psychosomatic diseases are diseases of regulation, in which the nervous system participates. The nature of the disturbance in regulation must be specified: It is possible that different disturbances are present in different diseases. But conceptual models do exist. Molecular biology may be one possible source of such models. In that field, several different kinds of regulatory devices for enzyme and protein synthesis and enzyme activity are known.

REFERENCES

1. ALEXANDER, F. *Psychosomatic Medicine*. Norton, New York, 1950.
2. KIRSNER, J. B. Peptic ulcer. A review of the current literature on various clinical aspects. *Gastroenterology* **54**, 610, 1958.
3. PICKERING, G. W. *The Nature of Essential Hypertension*. Grune & Stratton, New York, 1961.
4. MIRSKY, I. A., FUTTERMAN, P. and KAPLAN, S. Blood plasma pepsinogen—II: The activity of the plasma from 'normal' subjects, patients with duodenal ulcer and patients with pernicious anemia. *J. Lab. clin. Med.* **40**, 188, 1952.
5. WEINER, H., THALER, M., REISER, M. F. and MIRSKY, I. A. Etiology of duodenal ulcer—I: Relation of specific psychological characteristics to rate of gastric secretion (serum pepsinogen). *Psychosom. Med.* **19**, 1, 1957.
6. CROOG, S. H. Relation of plasma pepsinogen to ethnic origins. *U.S. arm. Forces med. J.* **8**, 795 1957.

7. DAMON, A. and BELL, B. Ethnic group and serum pepsinogen. *J. chron. Dis.* **20**, 803, 1967.
8. COHEN, S. I., SILVERMAN, A. J., WADDELL, W. and ZUIDEMA, G. D. Urinary catecholamine levels, gastric secretion and specific psychological factors in ulcer and non-ulcer patients. *J. psychosom. Res.* **5**, 90, 1961.
9. WEINER, H., THALER, M. T., REISER, M. F. and MIRSKY, I. A. (Unpublished observations).
10. STATE, D. Physiological factors: Chap. 3. *Adv. psychosom. Med.* **6** (in press), 1970.
11. SAMLOFF, I. M. Multiple molecular forms of pepsinogen and their distribution in gastric and duodenal mucosa. *Clin. Res.* **17**, 310, 1969.
12. SAMLOFF, I. M. and TOWNES, P. L. Heterogeneity and genetic polymorphism of human pepsinogen. *Gastroenterology* **56**, 1194, 1969.
13. SAMLOFF, I. M. and TOWNES, P. L. Pepsinogens: genetic polymorphism in man. *Science* **168**, 144, 1970.
14. TAYLOR, W. H. Pepsins of patients with peptic ulcer. *Nature, Lond.* **227**, 76, 1970.
15. MIRSKY, I. A. Physiologic, psychologic and social determinants in etiology of duodenal ulcer. *Am. J. dig. Dis.* **3**, 285, 1958.
16. DONGIER, M., WITTKOWER, E. D., STEPHENS-NEWSHAM, L. and HOFFMAN, M. M. Psychophysiological studies in thyroid function. *Psychosom. Med.* **18**, 310, 1956.
17. WALLERSTEIN, R. S., HOLZMAN, P. S., VOTH, H. M. and UHR, N. Thyroid 'hot spots': A psychophysiological study. *Psychosom. Med.* **27**, 508, 1965.
18. PERLMUTTER, M. and SLATER, S. Use of thyroid hormone to differentiate between hyperthyroidism and euthyroidism. *J. Am. med. Ass.* **158**, 718, 1955.
19. FLAGG, G. W., CLEMENS, T. L., MICHAEL, E. A., ALEXANDER, F. and WARK, J. A psychophysiological investigation of hyperthyroidism. *Psychosom. Med.* **27**, 497, 1965.
20. YAGER, J. and WEINER, H. Observations in man. *Adv. psychosom. med.* **6**, 40, 1970.
21. LACEY, J. I. and LACEY, B. E. The relationship of resting autonomic activity to motor impulsivity. *Res. Publs Ass. Res. nerv. ment. Dis.* **36**, 144, 1958.
22. LACEY, J. I. Psychophysiological approaches to evaluation of psychotherapeutic process and outcome. In: *Research in Psychotherapy*, RUBENSTEIN, E. A., *et al.* (Eds.), American Psychological Association, Washington, D.C., 1959.
23. LACEY, J. I. and LACEY, B. E. Verification and extension of the principle of autonomic response sterotypy. *Am. J. Psychol.* **71**, 50, 1958.
24. LACEY, J. I. and VAN LEHN, R. Differential emphasis in somatic response to stress. An experimental study. *Psychosom. Med.* **14**, 71, 1952.
25. LACEY, J. I., BATEMAN, D. E. and VAN LEHN, R. Autonomic response specificity. An experimental study. *Psychosom. Med.* **15**, 8, 1953.
26. COHEN, S. I., SILVERMAN, A. J. and BURCH, N. R. A technique for the assessment of affect change. *J. nerv. ment. Dis.* **124**, 352, 1956.
27. REISER, M. F. Reflections on interpretation of psychophysiological experiments. *Psychosom. Med.* **23**, 430, 1961.
28. WEINER, H., SINGER, M. T. and REISER, M. F. Cardiovascular responses and their psychological correlates. I: A study of healthy young adults and patients with peptic ulcer and hypertension. *Psychosom. Med.* **24**, 477, 1962.
29. WOLFF, C. T., FRIEDMAN, S. B., HOFER, M. A. and MASON, J. W. Relationship between psychological defenses and mean urinary 17-OHCS excretion rates. I: A predictive study of parents of fatally ill children. *Psychosom. Med.* **26**, 576, 1964.
30. WOLFF, C. T., HOFER, M. A. and MASON, J. W. Relationship between psychological defenses and mean urinary 17-OHCS excretion rates. II: Methodological and theoretical considerations. *Psychosom. Med.* **26**, 592, 1964.
31. SACHAR, E. J., MASON, J. W., KILMER, H. S., JR. and ARTISS, K. L. Psychoendocrine aspects of acute schizophrenic reactions. *Psychosom. Med.* **25**, 510, 1963.
32. BOURNE, P. G., ROSE, R. M. and MASON, J. W. 17-OHCS levels in combat. *Archs gen. Psychiat.* (*Chicago*) **19**, 135, 1968.
33. KATZ, J. L., ACKMAN, P., ROTHWAX, Y., SACHAR, E. J., WEINER, H., HELLMAN, L. and GALLAGHER, T. F. Psychoendocrine aspects of cancer of the breast. *Psychosom. Med.* **32**, 1, 1970.
34. KATZ, J. L., WEINER, H., GALLAGHER, T. F. and HELLMAN, L. Stress, distress, and ego defenses: The psychoendocrine response to impending breast tumor biopsy. *Archs gen. Psychiat.* **23**, 131, 1970.
35. HARLOW, H. F. Social deprivation in monkeys. *Scient. Am.* **207**, 137, 1962.

36. KAUFMAN, I. C. and ROSENBLUM, L. A. The reaction of separation in infant monkeys: Anaclitic depression and conservation-withdrawal. *Psychosom. Med.* **29**, 648, 1967.

37. MASON, W. A., DAVENPORT, R. K., JR. and MENZEL, E. W., JR. Early experiences and the social development of rhesus monkeys and chimpanzees. IN: *Early Experience and Behavior*, NEWTON, and LEVINE, S. (Eds.) C. C. Thomas, Springfield, Illinois, 1968.

38. HOFER, M. A. Physiological responses of infant rats to separation from their mothers. *Science* **168**, 872, 1970.

39. HOFER, M. and WEINER, H. Physiological responses to early maternal deprivation in the rat. Paper read at *Am. Psychosom. Med.*, Washington, D.C., 1970.

40. BROD, J. Essential hypertension—hemodynamic observations with bearing on its pathogenesis. *Lancet* **2**, 773, 1960.

41. BROD, J., FENCL, V., HEJL, Z. and JIRKA, J. Circulatory changes underlying blood pressure elevation during acute emotional stress (mental arithmetic) in normotensive and hypertensive subjects. *Clin. Sci.* **18**, 269, 1959.

42. BROD, J., FENCL, V., HEJL, Z., JIRKA, J. and ULRYCH, M. General and regional hemodynamic pattern underlying essential hypertension. *Clin. Sci.* **23**, 339, 1962.

43. FOLKOW, B. and RUBINSTEIN, E. N. Cardiovascular effects of acute and chronic stimulation of the hypothalamic defense area in the rat. *Acta physiol. scand.* **68**, 48, 1966.

44. LÖFVING, B. Cardiovascular adjustments induced from the rostral cingulate gyrus with special reference to sympatho-inhibitory mechanisms. *Acta. physiol. scand.* **53** (Suppl. **184**), 1, 1961.

45. MASON, J. W. Organization of psychoendocrine mechanisms. *Psychosom. Med.* **30**, 565, 1968.

46. MCGUIGAN, J. E. and TRUDEAU, W. L. Immunochemical measurement of elevated levels of gastrin in the serum of patients with pancreatic tumors of the Zollinger–Ellison variety. *New Engl. J. Med.* **278**, 1308, 1968.

47. MCGUIGAN, J. E. and TRUDEAU, W. L. Little gastrin in normal serum. *New Engl. J. Med.* **280**. 509, 1969.

48. ODELL, W. D., CHARTERS, A. C., DAVIDSON, W. D. and THOMPSON, J. C. Radioimmunoassay for human gastrin using unconjugated gastrin as antigen. *J. clin. Endocr. Metab.* **28**, 1840, 1968.

49. WILLIAMS, R. H. The pancreas. In: *Textbook of Endocrinology*, WILLIAMS, R. H. (Ed.), p. 613. Saunders, Philadelphia, 1968.

50. GLASS, G. B. J. *Introduction to Gastrointestinal Physiology*. Prentice-Hall, New Jersey, 1968.

51. HIRSCHOWITZ, B. I. The control of pepsinogen secretion. *Ann. N.Y. Acad. Sci.* **140**, 709, 1967.

52. GOBBEL, W. G., JR. and ADKINS, R. B. Production of duodenal ulcers by exogenous gastrin. An experimental model. *Am. J. Surg.* **113**, 183, 1967.

53. ROBERT, A. and STOUT, T. R. Production of duodenal ulcers in rats. *Fedn Proc. Fedn Am. Socs exp. Biol.* **28**, 323, 1969.

54. CONN, J. W., ROVNER, D. R. and COHEN, E. L. Normal and altered function of the renin–angiotensin–aldosterone system in man. *Ann. intern. Med.* **63**, 266, 1965.

55. DAVIS, J. O., HARTOFT, P. M., TITUS, E. O. and CARPENTER, C. C. J. The role of the renin–angiotensin system in the control of aldosterone secretion. *J. clin. Invest.* **41**, 378, 1962.

56. MULROW, P. J., GANONG, W. F., CERA, G. and KULJIAN, A. The nature of the aldosterone-stimulating factor in dog kidneys. *J. clin. Invest.* **41**, 505, 1962.

57. CANNON, P. J., AMES, R. P. and LARAGH, J. H. Relation between potassium balance and aldosterone secretion in normal subjects and in patients with hypertensive or renal tubular disease. *J. clin. Invest.* **45**, 865, 1966.

58. LEDINGHAM, J. G. G., BULL, M. B. and LARAGH, J. H. The meaning of aldosteronism in hypertensive disease. *Circulation Res.* **21** (Suppl. II), 177, 1967.

59. MIRSKY, I. A., STEIN, M. and PAULISCH, G. The secretion of an antidiuretic substance into the circulation of rats exposed to noxious stimuli. *Endocrinology* **54**, 491, 1954.

60. O'CONNOR, W. J. and VERNEY, E. B. The effect of increased activity of the sympathetic system in the inhibition of water diuresis by emotional stress. *Q. Jl. exp. Physiol.* **33**, 77, 1945.

61. VERNEY, E. B. Croonian lecture: The antidiuretic hormone and the factors which determine its release. *Proc. R. Soc.* **135**, 25, 1947.

62. ADAMS, D. D., PURVES, H. D. and SIRETT, N. E. The response of hypophysectomized mice to injections of human serum containing long-acting thyroid stimulator. *Endocrinology* **68**, 154, 1961.

63. MUNRO, D. S. Observations on the discharge of radioiodine from the thyroid glands of mice injected with human sera. *J. Endocr.* **19**, 64, 1959.

64. LIDDLE, G. W., HEYSSEL, R. M. and McKENZIE, J. M. Graves' Disease without hyperthyroidism. *Am. J. Med.* **39**, 845, 1965.
65. McKENZIE, J. M. Studies on the thyroid activator of hyperthyroidism. *J. clin. Endocr. Metab.* **21**, 635, 1961.
66. ADER, R. Experimentally induced gastric lesions. *Adv. psychosom. Med.* **6**, 1, 1970.
67. BRODIE, D. A. Experimental peptic ulcer. *Prog. Gastroenterology* **55**, 1968.
68. BRODIE, D. A. and HANSON, H. M. A study of the factors involved in the production of gastric ulcers by the restraint technique. *Gastroenterology* **38**, 353, 1960.
69. ADER, R. Plasma pepsinogen level in rat and man. *Psychosom. Med.* **25**, 218, 1963.
70. ADER, R. Plasma pepsinogen level as a predictor of susceptibility to gastric erosions in the rat. *Psychosom. Med.* **25**, 221, 1963.
71. ADER, R. (Personal communication).
72. SINES, J. O. Strain differences in activity, emotionality, body weight and susceptibility to stress induced stomach lesions. *J. genet. Psychol.* **101**, 209, 1962.
73. SINES, J. O. and EAGLETON, G. Dominant behavior and weight loss following water deprivation in normal rats and rats susceptible to stomach lesions. *Psychol. Rep.* **9**, 3, 1961.
74. SAWREY, W. L. and WEISZ, J. D. An experimental method of producing gastric ulcers. *J. comp. physiol. Psychol.* **49**, 269, 1956.
75. ERDÖSOVA, R., FLANDERA, V., KRECEK, J. and WIENER, P. The effect of premature weaning on the sensitivity of rats to experimental erosions of the gastric mucosa. *Physiologia bohemoslov.* **16**, 400, 1967.
76. SAWREY, W. L., CONGER, J. J. and TURRELL, E. S. An experimental investigation of the role of the psychological factors in the production of gastric ulcers in rats. *J. comp. physiol. Psychol.* **49**, 457, 1956.
77. LOWER, J. S. Approach-avoidance conflict as a determinant of peptic ulceration in the rat. Medical Dissertation, Western Reserve University, 1967.
78. LEVINE, R. J. and SENAY, E. C. Studies on the role of acid in the pathogenesis of experimental stress ulcers. *Psychosom. Med.* **32**, 61, 1970.
79. KAHLSON, G. and ROSENGREN, E. New approaches to the physiology of histamine. *Physiol. Rev.* **48**, 155, 1968.
80. HENRY, J. P., MEEHAN, J. P. and STEPHENS, P. M. The use of psychosocial stimuli to induce prolonged systolic hypertension in mice. *Psychosom. Med.* **29**, 408, 1967.
81. MENEELY, G. R., TUCKER, R. G., DARBY, W. J., BALL, C. O. T., KORY, R. C. and AUERBACH, S. H. Electrocardiographic changes, disturbed lipid metabolism and decreased survival rates observed in rats chronically eating increased sodium chloride. *Am. J. Med.* **16**, 599, 1954.
82. JAFFE, D., DAHL, L. K., SUTHERLAND, L. and BARKER, D. Effects of chronic excess salt ingestion: Morphological findings in kidneys of rats with differing genetic susceptibility to hypertension. *Fedn Proc. Fedn Am. Socs exp. Biol.* **28**, 422, 1969.
83. FIGAR, S. Conditional circulatory responses in men and animals. *Handbook of Physiology*, Vol. III, Sect. 2, p. 1991. American Physiological Society, Washington, D.C., 1965.
84. FORSYTH, R. P. Blood pressure and avoidance conditioning. *Psychosom. Med.* **30**, 125, 1968.
85. FORSYTH, R. P. Blood pressure responses to long-term avoidance schedules in the restrained rhesus monkey. *Psychosom. Med.* **31**, 300, 1969.
86. SMITH, K. Conditioning as an artifact. *Psychol. Rev.* **61**, 217, 1954.
87. MILLER, N. E. Learning of visceral and glandular responses. *Science* **163**, 434, 1969.
88. BROOKS, F. P. Central neural control of acid secreton. *Handbook of Physiology*, Vol. II, Sect. 6, p. 805. American Physiological Society, Washington, D.C., 1967.
89. FRENCH, J. D., PORTER, R. W., CAVANAUGH, A. B. and LONGMIRE, R. L. Experimental gastroduodenal lesions induced by stimulation of the brain. *Psychosom. Med.* **19**, 209, 1957.
90. CHRISTENSEN, J. The adrenergic nerves and gastrointestinal smooth muscle function. *Gastroenterology* **55**, 135, 1968.
91. LAMBERT, R., MARTIN, F. and VAGNE, M. Relationship between hydrogen ion and pepsin concentration in human gastric secretion. *Digestion* **1**, 65, 1968.
92. PAGE, I. H. and McCUBBIN, J. W. The pattern of vascular reactivity in experimental hypertension of varied origin. *Circulation* **4**, 70, 1951.
93. KEZDI, P. Mechanism of the carotid sinus in experimental hypertension. *Circulation Res.* **11**, 1962.
94. GOMEZ, A., HOOBLER, S. W. and BLAQUIER, P. Effect of addition and removal of a kidney transplant in renal and adrenocortical hypertensive rats. *Circulation Res.* **8**, 464, 1960.

95. SCROOP, G. C. and LOWE, R. D. Central pressor effect of angiotensin mediated by the parasympathetic nervous system. *Nature, Lond.* **220,** 1331, 1968.

96. FERRARIO, C. M., DICKINSON, C. J., GILDENBERG, P. L. and McCUBBIN, J. W. Central vasomotor stimulation by angiotensin. *Fedn Proc. Fedn Am. Socs exp. Biol.* **28,** 394, 1969.

97. McCUBBIN, J. W. Interrelationship between the sympathetic nervous system and the renin–angiotensin system. *Baroreceptors and Hypertension,* KEZDI, P. (Ed.) Pergamon, New York, 1967.

98. ABRAHAMS, V. C., HILTON, S. M. and ZEROZYNA, A. Effects of thyroxine on the synthesis of cholesterol and fatty acids by cell-free reactions of rat liver. *J. Physiol., Lond.* **154,** 491, 1960.

99. FERNANDEZ DE MOLINA, A. and HUNSPERGER, R. W. Central representation of affective reactions in forebrain and brain stem: Electrical stimulation of amygdala, stria terminalis and adjacent structures. *J. Physiol., Lond.* **145,** 251, 1959.

100. FERNANDEZ DE MOLINA, A. and HUNSPERGER, R. W. Organization of the sub-cortical system governing defence and flight reactions in the cat. *J. Physiol., Lond.* **160,** 200, 1962.

101. WEINER, H. Psychosomatic research in essential hypertension: Retrospect and prospect. *Biblthca Psychiat.* **144,** 581, 1970.

102. LINDGREN, P. and UVNÄS, B. Photo-electric recording of the venous and arterial blood flow. *Acta physiol. scand.* **32,** 259, 1954.

103. FOLKOW, B. and UVNÄS, B. The chemical transmission of vasoconstrictor impulses to the hind limbs and the splanchnic region of the cat. *Acta physiol. scand.* **15,** 365, 1948.

104. McKENZIE, J. M. Humoral factors in the pathogenesis of Graves' disease. *Physiol. Rev.* **48,** 252, 1968.

105. CHAR, D. F. B. and KELLEY, V. C. Serum antibody and protein studies following adrenalectomy in rabbits. *Proc. Soc. exp. Biol. Med.* **109,** 599, 1962.

106. LONG, D. A. and SHEWELL, J. The influence of the thyroid gland on the production of antitoxin in the guinea pig. *Br. J. exp. Path.* **36,** 351, 1955.

107. LUPARELLO, T. J., STEIN, M. and PARK, C. D. Effect of hypothalamic lesions on rat anaphylaxis. *Am. J. Physiol.* **207,** 911, 1964.

J. psychiat. Res., 1971, Vol. 8, pp. 499-512. Pergamon Press. Printed in Great Britain.

MILITARY PSYCHIATRY AND CHANGING SYSTEMS OF MENTAL HEALTH CARE

ALBERT J. GLASS

Department of Mental Health, State of Illinois, Chicago, Illinois

INTRODUCTION

HISTORICALLY, changes in systems of mental health care can be regarded as a complex resultant of the following four major influences:

(1) expanding concepts of the causation of mental disorders,

(2) widening of the sphere of mental disorders,

(3) the impact of social changes,

(4) new and improved techniques in intervention and treatment.

Less than 200 years ago, mental illness was limited to a relatively small incidence of severe, overt syndromes, commonly termed insanity or lunacy. These disorders were attributed to various occult influences, 'hereditary taint', or disease and injury. Prevailing attitudes permitted these obviously deviant persons to be driven from the community or isolated at home in cellars or attics, or incarcerated with other social and behavioral problems of the times. The system of mental health care was one of banishment from society with little concern for the comfort, needs, or the treatment of individuals so involved.

With recognition of human dignity and individual rights as exemplified by the American and French Revolutions, there arose growing concern for the welfare of the mentally afflicted. During this humanitarian era which began at the end of the eighteenth century, severe mental disorders were placed into asylums and retreats in which an environment of moral treatment was established that included kindness and consideration, usually without physical or mechanical restraint. However, the system remained one of banishment from the community, but with the considerable lessening of the previous degrading living conditions.

Moral treatment continued until the latter half of the nineteenth century. During this period, there was little essential change in the concepts of causation. Perhaps some widening of the scope of mental disorder occurred in that 'moral insanity' was included which added problems of abnormal behavior. Beginning in the early years of the nineteenth century, a medical care system for mental illness came into being which gradually replaced moral treatment by the establishment of public and private mental hospitals. With the rapid advances of scientific medicine, particularly in the latter half of the nineteenth century, mental disorders became diseases to be studied, classified, and investigated for causation and pathology, like that of physical illness. The medical model placed emphasis upon history, physical and laboratory examinations, diagnosis and prognosis, which were based upon uncovering organic causation. As a result, a widening of the sphere of mental disorders occurred which included severe mental disorders with demonstrable brain pathology; persistent deviant behavior often termed constitutional psychopathic states; senile, arteriosclerotic, and other disorders associated with aging; depressions, problems of alcohol, and drug addiction; and gross distortions of reality without apparent causation which became the functional psychoses. Also, less severe mental disorders or the neuroses gradually became recognized.

With the expanding dimensions of mental disorder, the industrial revolution, and the growth of urban populations, public mental institutions became more and more crowded and moral treatment steadily declined. The system remained one of banishment from the community now on the basis of incapacitating disease that produced deviant or unpredictable behavior for which little remedial treatment was as yet available. The banishment system was of a relatively closed type with almost all patients treated alike and few discharged. These conditions made the addition of physical facilities necessary at periodic intervals and large public mental institutions became commonplace. Situational or social-ecological causation played little or no influence in either the understanding or treatment of mental disorder.

MILITARY MEDICINE

Military medicine was born of a necessity to conserve personnel, particularly in combat operations. Experiences of warfare had repeatedly demonstrated a marked attrition of manpower from infectious disease, climatic extremes, and other non-battle injury and disease which was of even far greater magnitude than purely battle losses. However, it was not until the latter half of the last century that advances in medicine made available an increasing technical capability of safeguarding military personnel from externally induced disease and injury. Thus, military medicine was fated to pioneer in the development of prevention and treatment techniques for disease and injury of environmental origin. It was therefore a logical consequence that military psychiatry, a branch of military medicine was created in response to a need to curtail manpower losses from mental disorders when it became apparent that such conditions were of situational origin.

MILITARY PSYCHIATRY

Prior to World War I, mental diseases in military personnel, as in civil life, were narrowly defined to include mainly severe and bizarre abnormalities of psychotic proportions. Indeed it was not until 1912 that mental disorders in the U.S. Army were broadened from a single entity of the 'insanities' to the enlarged category of 'mental alienation' which included organic and functional psychoses, defective mental development, constitutional psycho-pathic states, hypochondriasis and nostalgia. Promptly thereafter the incidence of mental illness rose from 1–2 per 1000 troops per annum to 3–4 per 100 troops per annum.[1]

Because the low incidence of mental illness in military personnel as then defined was ascribed to pathology within the individual rather than environmental causes, there was little interest or concern for these problems by the expanding activities of military medicine. Such cases in the Army and Navy were either discharged from the service or transferred to the government hospital for the insane in Washington, D.C. (now St. Elizabeth's Hospital).[1]

Curiously, situational causation of mental illness in military personnel was clearly demonstrated during the Civil War by the prevalent syndrome 'nostalgia' which was characterized as a 'mild type of insanity caused by disappointment and a continuous longing for home.'[2] However, psychiatric sophistication at this time was insufficient to grasp the significance of situationally induced mental disorder. Instead emphasis was placed upon the innate vulnerability of youthful personnel as the cause for nostalgia. Also in the Japanese–Russian War (1904–06) where mental disorders of combat troops were first treated by psychiatric specialists, the somewhat increased frequency of these conditions were attributed to exposure to high explosives.[1] However, these observations excited little comment.

WORLD WAR I

From reports of the earliest fighting on the Western Front in 1914, there appeared accounts of a new psychiatric disorder termed 'shell shock' which was of such prevalence as to constitute a major military problem. These circumstances made mandatory the establishment of military psychiatry particularly since such mental disorders seemed clearly to be of environmental origin. Warfare had reached new heights of destruction and terror. In its early phases, optimum conditions existed in World War I for the emergence of psychiatric casualties. Troops new to battle were locked in intense prolonged combat associated with heavy concentrations of artillery and a high incidence of battle losses. Also advances in psychiatric knowledge, particularly in the understanding of neuroses by Freud and others in the decades prior to 1914, facilitated recognition of situationally induced mental illness. However, it was necessary that failure in battle be manifested by symptoms or behavior which were accepted by the combat reference group as constituting an inability, rather than an unwillingness to function in battle. Similar but less frequent failure of adaptation in previous wars were usually regarded as evidence of individual weakness and characterized as cowardice or other expressions of moral condemnation. For this reason, manifestations of psychiatric casualties beginning in World War I and usually their terminology have generally indicated a major causal relationship with traumatic conditions of the battle environment. Thus initially, psychiatric casualties of World War I seemed to be a direct result of enemy shelling. They appeared dazed and tremulous with or without dissociative behavior or major conversion reactions which were apparently the immediate consequence of nearby shell explosion—hence the terminology, 'shell shock'. By 1915–16, the Allied medical services clearly recognized that 'shell shock' was entirely a psychological disorder and terminology of the 'war neuroses' came into common usage. By this time, however, 'shell shock' had achieved legitimacy as a disease and thus an inability to function in battle.

LOCATION OF TREATMENT

In 1914, 'shell shock' cases from British combat troops were evacuated to England where they quickly overtaxed existing civil and military medical facilities. Consequently, military mental hospitals were created by taking over large civil mental hospitals.[3] Later, special neuropsychiatric hospitals and wards in general hospitals for 'shell shock' and functional nervous disorder were established. But under all of these circumstances, 'shell shock' cases were 'lost' or their symptoms became fixed and refractory due to secondary gain.[3]

Similar unsatisfactory results with 'shell shock' evacuees to rear facilities was experienced by the French medical services. After some months, advanced neuropsychiatric hospitals for the war neuroses were established in the zone of active military operations. Significant improvement was obtained by treatment in these forward locations.

When German submarines began sinking hospital ships, much work of the British medical services was shifted to France, including special facilities for functional nervous disorders. Here too, it was demonstrated that 'shell shock' was more effectively treated in advanced locations. These better results prompted a further extension of treatment to locations nearer the front in British casualty clearing stations and similar advanced posts of the French medical service. In 1916, Allied psychiatrists and neurologists reported that from 66 per cent (British) to 91 per cent (French) of the war neuroses were returned to combat duty by forward treatment. With further experiences, the British and French medical services showed conclusively that the war neuroses improved more rapidly when treated in permanent hospitals near the front than at the base, better in casualty clearing stations than even at advanced base hospitals, and better still, when encouragement, rest, persuasion and suggestion could be given in a combat organization itself.[3]

NETWORK OF SERVICES

Upon entry of the U.S. in World War I, the medical service of the AEF was fully aware of the war neuroses and the effective programs of the Allied medical services in coping with these problems. Upon the basis of the British and French experiences, Major Thomas Salmon, the chief psychiatrist of the AEF and his associates gradually implemented an integrated network of psychiatric services for the war neuroses. The three-echeloned system which became fully operational during the last several months of the war included: (1) divisional psychiatric facilities which held shell shock and similar mental disorders for 2–5 days of rest, encouragement and psychotherapy under the supervision of the division psychiatrist; (2) neurological hospitals which received refractory cases from the nearby divisional facilities and had a treatment capability of two to three weeks; and (3) a special psychiatric base hospital located in the advanced section of the communication zone which provided prolonged treatment for the most resistant of the war neuroses in order to prevent chronicity and evacuation to the United States.[3]

An important aspect of treatment at all echelons was described as "an intangible and mysterious therapeutic influence termed 'atmosphere'." By this was meant the feelings and attitudes of all medical personnel who came in contact with the war neuroses which sought to provide an urge or incentive for return to duty.[3]

CONTRIBUTIONS OF WORLD WAR I PSYCHIATRY

In retrospect, the accomplishments of military psychiatry in World War I provided much of the conceptional framework upon which has been based the current community mental health system. Major contributions in this regard include:

1. Repeated demonstrations that environmental stress and strain produced mental disease in so-called normal personnel as well as in those of neurotic predisposition. Previously, mental illness had been considered as originating almost exclusively from physical and/or psychological abnormalities within the individual.

2. Treatment of mental illness near or at its site of origin, although developed by trial and error, was a logical consequence of recognition that the war neuroses were caused by situational circumstances. It made practical sense to aid soldiers with emotional breakdown to cope with the demands of combat rather than withdrawal to remote hospitalization with its implication of failure, the development of fixed phobic avoidance symptoms, and subsequent chronic disability. In time, the crucial importance of location in the treatment of mental disorders has become the cornerstone of community mental health center operations as the principle of the maximum utilization of locally based mental health services.

3. A network of mutually supportive treatment facilities for the war neuroses from front to rear was established by the AEF medical services. Only recently has the value of such a comprehensive continuity of services for mild to severe mental disorders become appreciated by leaders of community mental health programs and is in various stages of implementation.

4. Probably for the first time, Salmon and his associates of the AEF noted and then utilized attitudes and behavior of treatment personnel as a therapeutic instrument. Later, this technique has formed the basis for various types of milieu therapy in civil psychiatry and in military psychiatry has become the principle of providing the atmosphere of 'expectancy' for return to duty.

BETWEEN WORLD WAR I AND WORLD WAR II

With the end of hostilities, the contributions of military psychiatry in World War I were largely disregarded. Psychiatry was not conceptually prepared to grasp either the significance of the situational causation of mental disorder or the importance of location and therapeutic 'atmosphere' in its treatment. Perhaps due to the relatively brief experiences of psychiatry in the AEF, the war neuroses became encapsulated as a special type of mental illness which occurred only under the extraordinary circumstances of combat and had little relevance for mental disorders of civil life. Moreover, extensive clinical experience with the common and persistent residual syndromes of the war neuroses in the postwar years created a widespread belief that these problems originated mainly from persons who were vulnerable to situational stress by reason of neurotic predisposition. The limited ability to cope with combat was deemed the result of faulty personality development and thus conformed to the prevailing psychoanalytic model of psychoneuroses and were so generally diagnosed.

Despite the foregoing events, World War I had a significant impact upon civil psychiatry. Many psychiatrists moved from almost exclusive function in mental institutions to outpatient clinics and office practice in the community. With increasing awareness of Freudian concepts, situational causation for mental disease became more acceptable, particularly for childhood neurotic and behavioral problems which influenced expansion of child guidance services. The utilization of interpersonal relationships along with the behavior of personnel in the treatment of schizophrenia by Sullivan, reintroduced the importance of a therapeutic milieu. However, for adult mental disorders, Freudian theory mainly confirmed previous concepts of an internal pathology or an intrapsychic etiology of mental disorders. The medical care system for mental illness became even more dominant than previously during this period, stimulated by the introduction of the somatic therapies such as fever therapy for general paresis, insulin coma, and electro-convulsive treatment. Somatic therapy increased discharges from mental hospitals, but made little change in the banishment system, as the patient population of public mental hospitals continued to rise.

Military psychiatry after World War I became a permanent component of military medicine. Psychiatric units consisting of open and closed wards, and outpatient services were provided as sections under the medical services at all U.S. Army general hospitals. The practice of military psychiatry at these large Army hospitals was similar to that of comparable civil mental facilities. But neither locally based treatment nor other concepts of social psychiatry as elaborated by the AEF survived after World War I.

Curiously, during this period, it was generally stated and believed that the major lesson learned by psychiatry in the World War I was the importance of psychiatric screening at induction to remove vulnerable individuals and thus prevent the emotional breakdown of troops in peace or war. Yet none of the experiences of World War I indicated that studies were conducted or observations made upon the validity of psychiatric screening. Indeed psychiatric screening was not performed in any extensive or uniform manner in World War I.[3]

WORLD WAR II

For the above-stated and other reasons of need and expediency before and during the early phases of World War II, the contributions of military psychiatry in World War I were completely ignored. Instead, reliance was placed upon psychiatric screening. Leading civil and military psychiatrists and other prominent medical authorities held that the war neuroses and other psychiatric disorders could be largely prevented by exclusion through screening examinations at induction of overt and potential mental disorders. The subsequent failure of the psychiatric screening program has been well documented.[1]

Emphasis upon psychiatric screening served to deny the magnitude of wartime mental disorders, for there was little preparation for the management of psychiatric illness, combat or otherwise. For example, the organization of psychiatric services in combat divisions which had been instituted in World War I was discarded immediately prior to World War II. The inevitable occurred. With expanding mobilization and the onset of war, a high incidence of mental disorders soon overwhelmed existing medical facilities and their meager psychiatric resources. The major available diagnostic category for these mainly situationally induced mental disorders was 'psychoneurosis' with its implication of unresolved internal conflict from which symptoms were unconsciously derived. The newly built cantonment hospitals of World War II were soon filled with patients, half or more with refractory psychiatric syndromes to which gain in illness had been added. The only solution to this mounting problem was medical discharge from the Army. Thus, mental illness became the major cause of manpower loss in the U.S. Army.

In the early combat experiences of the U.S. Forces after Pearl Harbor, during the Tunisia and Guadalcanal campaigns, mental disorders also occurred in large numbers. As initially in World War I, these casualties were evacuated hundreds of miles to distant medical facilities where their symptoms became fixed and few could be returned to combat duty. Again terminology for these cases was 'psychoneurosis'. With such labelling and its connotation of personality weakness, it was difficult for psychiatric disorders to be accepted by the combat group as being the result of battle conditions. Rather they were considered the consequence of failure in induction screening.

Because of the above stated events, efforts were made initially by individual psychiatrists and later in coordinated programs to move out of hospitals and establish locally based treatment services. However, two years elapsed in World War II before psychiatric services achieved sufficient organizational and operational capability to deal adequately with the large incidence of wartime mental disorders. These changes occurred during 1942, 1943 and 1944, initially in training bases in the U.S. and later in overseas combat theatres.

In the U.S., locally based psychiatric units, termed 'consultation services', were established at each of the training bases.[1] Here, psychiatric personnel worked with trainers in aiding newly inducted soldiers adjust to separation from family, lack of privacy, regimentation, unaccustomed physical activity and other deprivations and changes incident to the transition from civil to military life. Consultation services provided outpatient treatment for referred symptom disorders, participated in the orientation of trainees and worked with trainer personnel in upgrading their understanding of the problems of adjustment. More and more psychiatric personnel served the function of 'consultation' as later considered to be an essential element of comprehensive community mental health centers, With these prevention and intervention programs, the rate of hospitalization from troops in the U.S. was reduced considerably in the latter phases of the war and the value of locally based psychiatric services clearly demonstrated.

During the latter phase of the Tunisia campaign, in March, 1943, successful attempts were made to re-establish World War I forward type treatment for psychiatric casualties. As in World War I, it was found that 2–5 days of treatment program in a field facility near the fighting which included rest, sleep, food and opportunities to bathe, shave and discuss battle experiences, could return a majority of psychiatric casualties to combat duty.

Soon after this demonstration, a new terminology for psychiatric casualties was officially adopted. By directive, all psychiatric disorders in the combat zone were ordered to be designated as 'exhaustion' regardless of manifestations. Other and more definitive diagnosis were permitted in rear medical facilities.[4]

'Exhaustion' was readily accepted by the combat reference group. Almost all participants of battle could appreciate that anyone could be temporarily unable to cope with the stress and strain of continued battle. Again, as in World War I, psychiatric casualties became legitimized as a rational consequence of combat circumstances. Soon there appeared the simplistic generalization that 'every man has his breaking point'.

With the acceptance of 'exhaustion', manifestations of combat psychiatric breakdown became less dramatic. Psychiatric casualties did not need to portray 'psycho' to communicate inability to function in combat.

As the war proceeded, psychiatric services were expanded to include combat units. In March and April, 1944, an echeloned network of psychiatric services similar to that of World War I was established. Further experiences produced new insights as follows:

1. *Causation*

While the continued threat of danger was the essential element in the causation of combat psychiatric breakdown, the frequency of such casualties was related to social and environmental circumstances which either reduced or enhanced the capacity of individuals to cope with battle conditions. In this respect, most important was the sustaining influence of the small combat group or particular members thereof, termed group identification, group cohesiveness, the buddy system and leadership. Reapeated observations confirmed that the inadequacy of such sustaining relationships or their disruption during combat was mainly responsible for psychiatric breakdown in battle. These groups or relationship phenomena made it possible to explain marked differences in the psychiatry casualty rates of various combat units who were exposed to similar intensities of battle stress. Other circumstances of lesser but pertinent significance in combat adjustment included impairment of physiological capacity by reasons of fatigue, intercurrent illness, or inadequate physical conditioning and insufficient training in battle field tactics and the use of weapons.

2. *Treatment*

It was apparent in World War I and World War II that forward and early treatment had the advantage of providing prompt relief for fatigue, loss of sleep. and other temporary physical deficits. However, it was not until recognition of the sustaining influences of group and other interpersonal relationships that the significance of treatment near the site of origin was fully appreciated. Proximity of treatment to the combat unit maintained relationships and emotional investment in the core group. As a consequence, there existed in psychiatric casualties, under conditions of forward treatment, varying degrees of motivation to rejoin the combat group which was heightened by improvement in physical well-being by reasons of recuperative measures of sleep, food and the like. Also, treatment in the combat zone was of major importance in providing an atmosphere of expectancy for improvement and return to combat duty. Forward location and brief simplified treatment clearly communicated to both patients and treatment personnel that psychiatric casualties constituted only a temporary inability to function. Conversely, removal of psychiatric casualties to distant medical facilities weakened emotional ties with the combat group with implications of weakness or failure for which continuation of the sick role was the only honorable explanation.

3. *Diagnosis*

In World War I, Salmon and his associates were well aware of the deleterious effects of a definitive diagnosis for the early and fluid manifestations of psychiatric casualties. While 'shell shock' indicated situational origin, it also conveyed the impression of brain damage with potential residual defects. The diagnosis of 'neurosis' had a similar adverse effect of influencing psychiatric casualties to cling tenaciously to incapacitating symptomatology which required treatment in a rear hospital. For these reasons, field medical personnel were instructed to use only the term, 'N.Y.D.' (nervous)* for combat psychiatric disorders.[3] However, 'shell shock' was too firmly established to be changed.

Similarly, during the initial combat experiences of World War II, the diagnosis of 'psychoneuroses' for psychiatric casualties produced such deleterious effects that the designation of 'exhaustion' was created. 'Exhaustion', although a non-specific and non-psychological term was an apt description of a temporary fluid condition resulting from physical and emotional strain of combat, regardless of manifestations or predisposition. 'Exhaustion', later 'combat exhaustion' during the Korean War, and finally, 'combat fatigue' has become the established designation for the early stages of combat psychiatric disorders.

In World War II, 'psychoneurosis' was also utilized for situational emotional disorders of non-combat origin which had a similar adverse influence of facilitating fixation of symptoms with subsequent chronic disability. For this reason, late in World War II, a new Army psychiatric nomenclature was created which established new categories for situational disorders. One of these categories, the 'immaturity reactions', largely replaced the ubiquitous 'psychoneurosis' which had become the single major cause of medical discharge. As a result, during the Korean War, 'psychoneurosis' was infrequently utilized.[1]

CONTRIBUTIONS OF WORLD WAR II PSYCHIATRY

The prolonged and diversified experiences of psychiatry in World War II not only fully confirmed the validity of the concepts and practices of psychiatry in World War I, but further refined and elaborated upon these accomplishments. In this respect, the most significant contribution of World War II psychiatry was recognition of mutually supportive influences by participants in combat or other stress situations. World War II clearly showed that interpersonal relationships and other external circumstances were at least as important as personality configuration or the assets and liabilities of the individual in the effectiveness of coping behavior. For example, the frequency of psychiatric casualties seemed to be more related to the characteristics of the group than the character traits of the individual.

---

* N.Y.D. = Not Yet Diagnosed.

From this insight has come increasing awareness of the social determinants of adaption which has played a major role in changing systems of mental health care as will be later described.

Another important but as yet only a potential contribution of military psychiatry concerns the far reaching influence of diagnosis. World War I and World War II demonstrated that a definitive diagnosis in the early and fluid phase of a mental disorder can adversely affect the individuals so involved as well as exert a negative influence upon the attitudes and expectancy of treatment personnel toward improvement or recovery. Most psychiatric diagnoses indicate the existence of intrapsychic pathology such as personality disorder, psychoneurosis, and psychosis. As yet, there is no psychiatric designation for failure of adaptation which would include both external and internal determinants of causation. For this reason, it is suggested that civil psychiatry would be as equally benefitted as has been military psychiatry in avoiding the early use of a definitive diagnosis which place emphasis mainly upon liabilities of individuals and ignore the setting in which failure of adjustment occurred. In the initial states of patient contact, it would seem reasonable to utilize a general descriptive label and permit later events to determine the need for a more definitive diagnosis.

POST WORLD WAR II MILITARY PSYCHIATRY

Following cessation of hostilities, military psychiatry maintained the co-equal status with medicine and surgery which had been achieved in World War II. With other branches of military medicine, speciality training was instituted. In the course of several years, a cadre of career military psychiatrists was created which made possible a continuation of the gains made in World War II.

Following the abrupt onset of the Korean War in June, 1950, military psychiatry moved promptly to re-establish the World War II system of mental health care both at home and overseas. An echeloned network of services for psychiatric casualties was in operation within several months after the onset of the Korean fighting. The psychiatric screening of World War II was abandoned. A rotation policy of 9–12 months in the combat zone which had been successfully urged in World War II was implemented after the first year of the Korean War. In the United States, mental hygiene consultation services were established at all major Army bases with expanded and flexible usage of psychiatrists, social workers, psychologists and enlisted technicians to furnish both direct service for referred problems and indirect consultation services to supervisory personnel.

As a result of the rapid implementation of the psychiatric lessons learned in World War II, even during the initial year of severe combat in the Korean War, rates of psychiatric disorders were less than one-half of the high incidence in World War II. Thereafter, a steady decline of the psychiatric rate occurred which in the last year of the Korean War reached almost to previous peace time levels.

Following the Korean War, military psychiatry both in the U.S. and at overseas stations continued to further elaborate techniques of locally based mental health services. A collaborative effort with the office of the Provost Marshal General resulted in a stockade screening program of intervention for disciplinary offenders at all major posts which were conducted by personnel of the mental hygiene consultation services. This program markedly reduced the population of Army prisons.

A field approach by the various mental hygiene consultation services utilized enlisted technicians to deal directly with referred emotional disorders in the company area outside the clinic or hospital, which has served as a model for the current utilization of mental health workers in community mental health services.[5] The sustained emphasis of post World War II military psychiatry upon the concepts and practices of social psychiatry has been largely stimulated and influenced by the training and research activities of the Division of Neuropsychiatry, Walter Reed Institute of Research, headed by David McK.Rioch, which was established in 1951.

VIET NAM

According to recent reports[6,7] military psychiatry in the Viet Nam conflict has achieved its most impressive record. Psychiatric casualties are treated at forward areas often on an outpatient basis by enlisted specialists supported by general medical officers under the supervision as required by the division psychiatrist and the division social worker. As a result, so few mental disorders are evacuated to rear medical facilities as to create the impression that psychiatric casualties are rarely or infrequently produced by the unique nature of combat in Viet Nam. A full account of military psychiatry in Viet Nam has yet to be written.

REVERSAL OF THE BANISHMENT SYSTEM

In World War II, many thousands of medical and other personnel were exposed at first hand to the situational and social determinants of maladjustment and the success of brief treatment techniques for emotional disorders. Soon after World War II, there occurred a marked upsurge of interest and involvement in behavioral problems and mental disorders. Large numbers of demobilized physicians entered specialty training in psychiatry which produced a considerable expansion of such training programs. Similarly, there occurred a marked increase of applicants for graduate training in psychology, social work, and the other social sciences. Prior to World War II, psychiatry and the social sciences pursued parallel lines of endeavor, each having its own vocabulary and conceptual orientation. The demonstration in World War II of group process and the social determinants of behavior made impossible the isolation of psychiatry from the social sciences.

Under these changing circumstances, the post World War II old and new psychiatrists, social workers, psychologists, sociologists and nursing personnel were more and more dissatisfied with the traditional banishment–custodial system of mental health care with its emphasis upon psychopathology or other internal causation. The deleterious effect of prolonged care, often provided in locked wards, became increasingly recognized. In addition, this era also saw a widening of the scope of mental disorders to include defeatist patterns of behavior, character neuroses, alcoholism and drug abuse problems, delinquency, and even underachievement. But more important were the social changes of the post World

War II decades. These changes which are continuing, place emphasis upon self actualization, the rights of minority groups, including the mentally ill, and the insistence that patients be helped to achieve coping ability up to the limits of their potential. More and more the goal of prevention, intervention, and treatment has become adjustment within the community rather than the eradication of psychopathology or even organic pathology.

For the above reasons, in the early years after World War II, even without a clearly defined frame of reference, many members of the mental health disciplines moved toward the establishment of locally based services. Graduates of psychiatric training programs entered private practice and began a reversal of the banishment system for the more affluent mentally ill by treatment within the community, utilizing outpatient techniques and general hospitals or private psychiatric hospitals as needed.

But, the poor and the medically indigent continued to receive banishment–custodial type care in public mental hospitals. However, here, too, there was an increasing trend toward active treatment and discharge to the community so as to avoid institutional dependency. Soon there appeared various types of milieu therapy, including patient government and other techniques which endeavored to provide a positive treatment environment aimed at return of the short- and long-term hospitalized patient to the community. Then psychotropic drugs became available, which tranquilized patients, treatment personnel and the community, which facilitated discharge from the mental hospitals.

The above changes produced a continuing trend of decreasing public mental hospital inpatient populations with a corresponding increasing number of discharged mental patients in the community. Soon there arose a need for so-called aftercare services to provide sustaining type programs in the community for such discharged patients, in order to safeguard the gains made during hospitalization. Failure to furnish such sustaining support caused prompt readmission to the hospitals for the majority of discharged patients which has been critically termed the 'revolving door' policy. With further experiences, it became evident that many unnecessary admissions to public mental hospitals occurred only because the community provided little or no alternative to such hospitalization. Thus, it became more and more mandatory that community mental health services be established.

The slow rate of progress in changing the traditional delivery of mental health services led to a Commission established by Congress to study the problem and make appropriate recommendations. After five years of intensive work, their report, 'Action for Mental Health', was submitted.[8] As a direct consequence, in 1963, Congress enacted major legislation* providing for the construction and later the staffing of a nationwide system of comprehensive community mental health centers, which program is in various stages of implementation.

However, this effort to accelerate reversal of the banishment system is proceeding at a slow pace. Many difficulties are being encountered in ensuring sufficient finances and manpower for community services as well as overcoming resistance to such a major change. Even more important has been the need to develop techniques and organizational procedures which are relevant to the unique problems of the many diversified types of communities

---

* Public Law 88-164.

to be served. As was experienced in military psychiatry, the establishment of locally based services does not merely involve movement to the community of physical facilities and professional manpower. Upon leaving the structural hospital environment, mental health services are in a new arena, where many systems and sub-systems related to living and working conditions are in operation. Mental health services must become a part of this network of open systems and work with various community agencies and its power structure in order to effectively make its contribution. It is only through such experiences that psychiatric personnel can develop awareness and knowledge so as to develop practical techniques and programs of prevention, intervention, and treatment for the ever widening scope of mental disorders. Further, as in divisional and other local military services, mental health personnel must become an integral component of the community, and identify with the unique needs and problems of the community rather than providing only sterile intramural hospital or clinic services with a large waiting list. Also, as was demonstrated in World War I, a network of supporting services to community facilities must be established for the more difficult or special problems which cannot be reasonably managed by locally based services. Such community and support services must be organized into an integrated system so as to insure a continuity of care from forward to rear. Many difficulties have been and are being encountered in bringing together the many separate existing mental health facilities in attempting to establish such a mutually supportive network of services.

Despite the aforestated difficulties, reversal of the banishment system is proceeding even though progress is uneven. In this transition period, the contributions of military psychiatry, perhaps the first organized system of social psychiatry, are gradually being incorporated in civil programs of mental health services.

SUMMARY

The unique opportunities of military psychiatry in dealing with situationally-induced emotional disorders have provided operational concepts and procedures which have strongly influenced the development of social and community psychiatry. From the experiences of military psychiatry have come (1) recognition of social and environmental determinants in the causation of mental illness, (2) repeated demonstration that locally based facilities furnish optimum conditions for the prevention, intervention and treatment of mental disorders and, (3) awareness and utilization of therapeutic benefits that can be derived from personnel attitudes, administrative structure, and other aspects of the treatment environment. These contributions of military psychiatry have become incorporated in present day changes in the delivery of mental health services from prolonged care in remote institutions to treatment within the community by locally based facilities.

REFERENCES

1. GLASS, A. J. and BERNUCCI, R. J. *Neuropsychiatry in World War II*. Vol. 1. Office of the Surgeon General, Dept. of the Army, Washington, D.C., 1968.
2. *Medical and Surgical History of the War of the Rebellion. Medical Volume*, Part I, Vol. 1. Government Printing Office, Washington, D.C., 1870.

3. BAILEY, P., WILLIAMS, F. E., JOMORA, P. O., SALMON, T. W. and FENTON, N. *The Medical Department of the United States Army in the World War*, Vol. X. *Neuropsychiatry*. U.S. Government Printing Office, Washington, D.C., 1929.
4. MEDICAL DEPARTMENT, U.S. ARMY. *Neuropsychiatry in WWII*. Vol. 11, Part 1, Chap. 1. (in preparation).
5. GLASS, A. J., ARTISS, K., GIBBS, J. J. and SWEENEY, V. C. The current status of Army psychiatry. *Am. J. Psychiat.* **117**, 673, 1962.
6. TIFFANY, W. J., JR. Mental health of Army troops in Vietnam. *Am. J. Psychiat.* **123**, 1585, 1967.
7. OFFICE OF THE SURGEON GENERAL, DEPT. OF THE ARMY. The mental health of U.S. troops in Vietnam remains outstanding. Washington, D.C., 12 March, 1968.
8. Joint Commission on Mental Illness and Health. *Action for Mental Health*. Basic Books, 1961.

J. psychiat. Res., 1971, Vol. 8, pp. 513–520. Pergamon Press. Printed in Great Britain.

APPLICATIONS OF THE MILITARY MEDICAL MODEL TO CIVILIAN PSYCHIATRY

WILLIAM HAUSMAN

Department of Psychiatry, University of Minnesota Medical School, Minneapolis, Minnesota

AMONG the many contributions made by David Rioch during his twenty years at WRAIR, not the least of these has been his very significant role in mapping out for American psychiatry a new field which, in the very significant seminar held here at WRAIR in 1957, he labelled 'Preventive and Social Psychiatry'.[1] In the design of the program for that meeting, and in other publications by him prior to and since the date of that symposium, Rioch defined the scope of this new field and the importance of the relationship between psychiatry and the basic behavioral and social sciences. His interest in the development of this area has appeared to stem from his fascination with the implications of the unique observations and formulations of military psychiatrists from Thomas Salmon, in World War I, through those workers who have made contributions in all of the later wars and intervening periods up to and including the current struggle in Vietnam.

In 1967 I was privileged to write a paper with Dr. Rioch on Military Psychiatry in which the lessons of Thomas Salmon and of later military psychiatrists, particularly Albert J. Glass, were re-explored and restated.[2] We dealt with implications of the concepts of *immediacy*, *proximity* and *expectancy* which were first described, although in other terms, by Salmon and later, in these particular terms, by ARTISS;[3] and we drew attention to BUCHARD'S important statements on *commitment* and *concurrence*.[4] The three levels of prevention (primary, secondary and tertiary), the terminology of which probably originated in the Army motor pool, but which have become guidelines to the development of thinking about the various levels of intervention, were also elaborated in this paper. None of these issues was completely new. In addition to others,[3,5] Rioch had discussed some aspects of them in several papers during the previous years.[6,7] Subsequent to that paper several other authors have also commented on the significance of the lessons of military psychiatry for contemporary civilian practice.[8,9] I would like to take the opportunity here to further expand the implications of these contributions, particularly as they apply to education. My thoughts are drawn both from my service career and, more particularly, from my experiences since retiring from the Army in 1966.

To briefly repeat our restatement of the fundamental principles of *immediacy*, *proximity* and *expectancy*, as developed in the earlier paper, we viewed the civilian equivalent of *immediacy* essentially in terms of the temporal aspect of crisis intervention. *Proximity*, which on the battlefield related to the practice of treating the individual as close as possible to his unit of reference, usually his squad, and to working with him within the divisional boundaries and over short periods of time, relates, in civilian practice, to treating him close to home and job and in relatively short hospitalizations. While these two concepts lend themselves to relatively direct translation in civil psychiatry, *expectancy* is a somewhat more complex issue. In our view it basically relates to clarity of message. I believe that this is the most important of these concepts and one that is most easily lost in the setting of the contemporary psychiatric hospital, outpatient clinic or community mental health center even where other facets of social psychiatry are readily recognized and practiced.

My experiences and observations during the past four years are particularly related to these particular principles and to their employment in the context of developing a student mental health treatment and educational program in one medical school and in developing and restructuring a clinical, research, and educational program at another university. The latter task, though briefer in duration, will be the prime focus of my comments simply because I now find myself most preoccupied with it and also because my present position permits a greater degree of control and therefore a more effective test of the model. I will also touch on the relevance of the principles derived from military psychiatry to the community mental health center.

When I joined the faculty at Johns Hopkins University after retirement from service, I was asked to develop a program in student mental health, with a large part of my activity to be carried out at the Homewood undergraduate and graduate school campus. Although control over the screening of students and over some other important elements of the program was limited, there was the opportunity to develop a training program for residents in psychiatry in that setting. Each of the first-year residents was assigned for 3 hr of each week to working with students who had been previously screened by the psychologist-director of the service at Homewood, and the additional hour was devoted to supervision of the residents by a faculty member with experience in this area.[10]

This turned out to be an excellent opportunity to expose new residents to these basic principles of social psychiatry before they were encumbered with techniques and value systems based upon a more traditional view of the field. The residents were taught to recognize the value of early intervention with students who usually could be seen within a day or two of referral. After initial evaluation the student who was felt to need therapy was directed, with little delay, to a resident who saw him at a time when the student would not be in class. This in itself was important because we encouraged the residents to continue to view the students as 'students' rather than as 'patients'. Regardless of the intent of the psychiatrist, if the student had to make the choice of meeting therapy hour requirements at the expense of his student responsibilities, it was difficult for him not to see himself as a patient. Therapy, in almost all cases, was accomplished on a time-limited basis, usually in 10 hr or less. The student was encouraged to deal with here-and-now issues that focussed upon his view of himself, his school performance, his value system, and his *current* relationships with parents, peers and significant faculty members. The results were impressive not only in terms of fewer hospital admission and in reduction of the frequency of referral into long-term treatment but also in the dramatic recognition by the psychiatry resident of the importance of these concepts and in building into his therapeutic repertoire, at a critical point in his training, a recognition of these particular fundamentals of social psychiatry. A number of the residents who had been through this program sought further experiences in the community and on the campus and, in the process of doing so, demonstrated what I considered to be a genuine grasp of these principles and their implications for psychiatry in a variety of settings.

To return to our basic concepts, *immediacy* was satisfied by the ready availability of both the evaluatory psychologist and the resident-therapist. *Proximity* was built into the practice of seeing all students at Homewood, where the major environmental cues were those of the college campus, dormitory and other students. *Expectancy*, in this setting, involved the avoidance of labelling as 'patient', the focus on the here-and-now situation of the student and on the relevance of symptoms to current relationships and school programs. The time-limited therapy arrangement signaled our assumption that the student's therapy was not to go on indefinitely and that he was expected to continue in his full class schedule without interruption by therapy sessions or his being sent off campus by virtue of his difficulties.

After 3 years in Baltimore I was invited last year to head a Department of Psychiatry. This presented an opportunity to put these same principles into operation in a comprehensive educational and clinical program. I would like, in the remainder of this paper, to discuss my thinking and initial planning efforts, not only to amplify the relevance of these principles to civilian education and practice, but also to illustrate some of these translations with my own recent experiences.

Without going into great detail, my department, when I was appointed, consisted of a small (68 bed) three-ward adult psychiatric hospital, a smaller (16 bed) child psychiatry unit and an outpatient unit, all in the University Hospitals Building, and off-campus affiliate relationships with two County Hospitals and one VA Hospital. The department was traditionally oriented, with little investment in either classical psychoanalysis, community psychiatry (except for assignments to the County Hospital units) or in consultation or liaison relationships with other medical fields. Its faculty members, in a long-standing geographical full-time tradition, were permitted to earn part of their income with private patients. Medical students, for the most part, were not attracted to the field.

It appeared to me that certain changes were in order if we were to establish a modern and socially relevant psychiatry education program. The principles around which the new approach was to be developed were clear. The work has been in transformation of these principles into a viable system relevant to education and to patient care which can be accepted and carried out by a professional and subprofessional staff whose prior experiences and education have often differed from my own philosophy and orientation.

Our initial focus was on the adult clinical unit at the University Hospitals. By shifting the psychiatrists' basis for salary to a group practice-centered strict full-time arrangement, we have largely eliminated the entrepreneurial aspect of the system that made programmatic changes on our wards difficult, if not impossible. Parenthetically, I believe that this economic issue probably also relates to the difficulties elsewhere in the country in programming appropriate changes in psychiatric practice and education. What changes we have made have been designed in large measure to satisfy the basic philosophy behind the concepts of *immediacy*, *proximity* and *expectancy*.

In this new educational environment, with a self-imposed requirement to establish a socially appropriate program, it became important to rethink the non-military equivalents of our terms.

As noted before, *immediacy* on the battlefield relates to how quickly the soldier can be brought into the forward psychiatric treatment program after he becomes incapacitated for duty. At the student health service it means how soon the student can be seen after contacting the service. On the traditional teaching hospital service one saw such impediments to *immediacy* as clinic waiting lists, apparent non-availability of beds, particularly when students or residents were not on tap as 'primary therapists' in a system that emphasized prolonged one-to-one therapy, and delay, after admission, before definitive therapeutic efforts were begun. It became clear that in this setting the invoking of *immediacy* involved not only fewer impediments to intial acceptance of the patient for treatment but also the reduction of ambiguity in the staff's commitment to his treatment. It required institution of a system of more rapid evaluation and the early commitment of the staff to a consistent set of therapeutic procedures. The relevance of this approach, particularly for the hospitalized patient, is supported by the work of BRANDON and GRUENBERG in Duchess County, where the length of time of intial hospitalization was correlated with the subsequent degree of chronicity and where, when these factors were considered in modifying a state hospital program the incidence of what they called 'chronic severe social breakdown syndrome' was reduced.[11] Resolution of the requirement for *immediacy* obviously insists upon a recognition of its importance by all team members, including the admissions clerk, resident and staff psychiatrist, psychologist, nurse, social worker and others.

The issue of *proximity* in combat basically relates to keeping the soldier as close as possible to his unit of reference. It considers distance, environment (where he remains in the divisional sector, with its familiar terrain, insignia and language cues), and time, in that the stay in the medical unit is sufficiently brief that the man's identification with his unit will not be reduced and so that the unit will not have the opportunity to 'close ranks' behind him. On the college campus the issue relates to the maintenance of the student role, and the scheduling of visits to the therapist on campus and in times other than that scheduled for classes.

When I came to the University Hospitals, the pattern of hospital admissions on all services had required referral by a physician prior to admission. This, in effect, meant that a large proportion of patients were admitted from distant parts of the state, anywhere from 100–250 miles off, inasmuch as many of the local psychiatrists hospitalized their own patients in local private hospitals and we had developed no adequate emergency room facilities. A recent administration-approved relaxation of referral requirements for admission should help to increase the proportion of our patients from the local area, as should the development of an enlarged Emergency Room Service, now on the drawing boards. For all patients, greater awareness by the staff of the importance of reducing hospital time is likely to alter in a favorable manner the disruption of family and job (or school) relationships.

With those patients who still come from outlying parts of the state and are not discharged quickly, concern over *proximity* is not so readily resolved. A part of the answer to this issue may be worked out by establishing stronger ties between our staff and the personnel of the many community mental health centers located throughout the state. Through better liaison with local treatment facilities, we hope it will be possible not only to shorten hospitalization but also to maintain better contact of both patients and staff with family units. The doctor, through his relationship with the center near the patient's home, can more effectively relate to the realities of the home situation and can feel more assured of a consistent treatment program after discharge.

As we have previously indicated, *expectancy*, the principal ingredient of battlefield management of the psychiatric casualty, relates, in the non-military setting, to the clarity of message to the patient. The translation of this concept to the college campus is discussed above. In our plans for redeveloping our clinical services, and in our first attempts to communicate the fundamentals of social psychiatry to students at all levels, *expectancy* again represents our most significant cornerstone.

One of the dilemmas of education in modern psychiatry is in the variety of different treatment approaches available. This results in the presentation of a confusing myriad of models to the student and also creates the likelihood that the patient will be presented by the staff with a variety of messages, often with significant apparent discrepancy between them. The teaching hospital must offer to the student a comprehensive view of available therapeutic modalities while it is also our obligation to provide the best possible treatment for our patients. This is essential not only for the well-being of the patients but also because we have a responsibility to demonstrate the best examples of therapy to our students. In attempting to resolve this apparent dilemma we are invoking a 'firm' or team system which provides for one child and three adult firms, each with assigned staff and students. This will create small clinical and teaching units, each of whose staffs are being asked to organize around a common philosophy of treatment encompassing both in- and out-patient areas. Our hope is that the firm, with a relatively small staff that meets together frequently, can reduce ambiguity of message to the patient as the staff strives to find an agreed-upon and consistent approach to the various therapeutic activities with each patient on that unit. I have made use of the authority of my role in the department to repeatedly emphasize to psychiatric staff and residents, to psychologists, students and staff nurses, and to others working on our service, the special importance to the patient of clarity of message.

The effect of this emphasis has been interesting. The student nurses, for instance, have in the past focussed almost exclusively on one-to-one relationships with patients on our wards, while their instructors and all of their educational programs have been separate from and unrelated to the Department of Psychiatry. With the interested agreement of their instructors, I have arranged to talk with each group of students assigned to psychiatry. In meeting each group to date, I have conveyed to them my belief that the single most important principle of any therapeutic endeavor in psychiatry, and probably also on other medical services, is the clarity of message. As a result, the students and their instructors recently have been requesting participation in the planning of the new firm programs as they recognize the likelihood that what they been doing on the ward may have been unrelated to other events involving their assigned patients and therefore possibly might be deleterious to the best interests of those patients. They were also concerned at the apparent discrepancy between the content of their program and what was happening in the field as exemplified by our newer program.

In one of our recent semi-monthly informal forums for the clinical staff, the issue of admission procedures led to the interesting and cogent observation by one of the residents that the decision about admission of a patient to the hospital was particularly critical because 'once they are admitted, they are in the hospital for at least three to six weeks.' In terms of *expectancy* he was saying that the staff's assumptions about illness are significantly modified by the *fact* of admission, whether or not the basis for admission was valid. This permitted us to look collectively at the role of *expectancy* in terms of our own practices and led to our establishing an important guideline that all new admissions were for evaluation, that the patient, at the time of admission, was to be told of this, and that appropriateness for hospitalization must be re-assessed soon after admission by the ward staff. Further, we agreed that, when possible, all emergency admission should be made to one particular firm, which considers its primary task to be that of crisis intervention and which, therefore, has a set that better permits such *patient-oriented* decisions to be made. Hopefully, the model of this firm will be contagious, to further augment the other firms' approaches to patients on other wards.

Other issues in the hospital setting that involve *expectancy* include several facets of an effective milieu therapy program. The issue of patient responsibility for events on the ward, the clothing patients and staff wear, the tendency of all staff members in a variety of situations to focus on adaptive rather than sick behavior and the willingness of the staff to expose their own doubts, difficulties and personal characteristics to the patients are all related to this important principle.

We have seen a shift, in our recently-instituted community meetings on each ward, from their initial focus that often emphasized simple reassurance of individual patients in the group to an approach that demonstrates the staff's willingness to demand of the patient behavior that permits more meaningful social interaction both with other patients and with staff. An example of this occurred a short while ago at a community meeting which I attended. Early in the session the patient group, which was discussing patient job assignments, appeared to 'ignore' the behavior of a relatively new patient who sat on the floor, coughed loudly, groaned, threw water around her and left the room several times over the objections of the group. The only comments about her, usually in negative and despairing terms, occurred when she was out of the room. The group generally agreed that no one on the ward could communicate with her. I finally observed to the group that she seemed to be communicating very actively with them, even to the extent that she blocked them from attending to other business. On the other hand, they did not seem to be able to deal with her except in her absence. Their response to my intervention was to send some patients out for her and then, on her return, to insist that she sit on a chair and talk with them. After a few weak attempts to maintain her prior behavior, she complied and then began to talk with the group, admitting her difficulty in relating with them despite her fear of loneliness. After talking with the group about herself for 10–15 min, she indicated that she was now ready for the group to return to their previous agenda. When she later interrupted the discussion of ward assignments to ask what job she was to be given, she again gained their attention, but this time in a way that was more consistent with the group's objectives.

Although *expectancy* seems to be a clearly defined and obvious concept, in the terms noted previously, I am impressed with the difficulty that the more conventionally trained worker, whether psychiatrist, nurse, or of other discipline, has in accepting and making use of it even when it is accepted intellectually as a criterion of effective therapeutic intervention. Rather, as one analyzes more traditional psychotherapeutic procedures, there is ample evidence that the message to the patient is anything but clear. Also, there is a great deal to suggest that the implicit expectancy in most conventional psychotherapy tends toward rein-forcement of pathology, of incapacity, and of dependency on the therapist and the milieu.

I have emphasized, in this part of my paper, the relationship of these important concepts to the restatement and redevelopment of psychiatric education and practice in the more conventionally oriented university hospital. Before concluding, I would like to make a few remarks on their application to community psychiatry. These will be based more on observations than on personal experiences, and for this reason, and also because there is a great deal of overlap between what I have described in the hospital and what I see in the community mental health center, I will limit my comments in this area.

We have recognized that *immediacy* is almost directly translated from the military to certain outpatient settings. It is obvious that when the so-called community mental health center arranges appointments at the convenience of the therapists' schedule and when 50-min hr and long-term psychotherapy take precedence over crisis-oriented intake and management, we must have serious doubts about the social and preventive orientation of that center. If the center is located in the community it serves; if its setting emphasizes contact with that neighborhood and its values; if the treatment team emphasizes awareness of the current environment and of the adaptive potential of the client; and if the entire staff places particular priorities in understanding the identified patient in his family, work and other social contexts, then we can assume that *proximity* becomes a meaningful basis for that center's operations.

If *expectancy* is as important in the community mental health center as it is in the teaching hospital, the student mental health service, or the military situation, we must expect to see the staff organized and oriented in a way that emphasizes clarity and consistency of message to the patient. While this sounds relatively straightforward, it is obvious that the busy service-oriented center often finds its workers begrudging the time necessary for the all-staff meetings that are essential if the treatment philosophy of a given center is to be established and reinforced in a consistent manner. While strong leadership in such a center is essential, the apparent agreement of a staff that is manifested by passive response to unilateral guidance, whether by memo or in more direct personal contact, is not equivalent to the staff's honest appraisal of their individual and collective responsibilities, attitudes, biases and agreements. More commonly than not the staff may unconsciously collude to permit various team members to present significantly different messages to the same patients. This is often more pronounced when the issue is tied to disciplinary differences so that a challenge of one's views and behavior evokes the time-honoured protection of the professional sentient group. Leadership of such a task group must recognize these tendencies and group characteristics and must attempt to make the many subtle barriers to exploration of these factors explicit and subject to study. In my view it is only when these steps are taken that the community mental health center becomes what it ideally should attempt to be—a place where a socially-relevant type of practice is conducted in a way that respects the important basic principles of social and preventive psychiatry.

Y

At this point I would like to say that in my view the directions of change in American psychiatry since the passage of legislation to support Community Mental Health Centers, has been disappointingly slow and ineffective. I believe that this is, in part, a failure of leadership in the training programs in our field to make use of basic principles such as I have discussed here in establishing more relevant and innovative designs for training mental health personnel and in establishing model programs that are in consonance with these philosophies. Perhaps the newer concepts of health care maintenance and delivery recently proposed by the Department of Health, Education and Welfare[12] will serve to expedite such change. But this alone will not achieve these objectives without more forceful leadership within our own field.

While change to a new orientation in psychiatric education and practice is difficult, I believe we are demonstrating that it is not impossible to achieve. Despite the expected discomfort on the part of most of our own professional workers, their enthusiasm for learning these 'new' concepts and for effective implementation of new programs is clear. I believe that, in a university setting, learning is more important than is the rapid achievement of a final product. There is evidence that a great deal of learning is taking place in our staff as they struggle with a changing model of patient care, and that this process of change is focussing around these basic principles—*immediacy, proximity* and *expectancy*. For this, and for all I have learned in the process, I am grateful for the opportunity I have had for working in and thinking about military psychiatry, to the pioneer insights of Thomas Salmon and, most of all, to David Rioch who made their translation so possible and so important.

REFERENCES

1. *Symposium on Preventive and Social Psychiatry*, 15–17 April, 1957, Walter Reed Army Institute of Research, Walter Reed Army Medical Center, Government Printing Office, 1958.
2. HAUSMAN, W. and RIOCH, D. McK. Military psychiatry, a prototype of social and preventive psychiatry in the United States. *Archs gen. Psychiat.* 16, 727, 1967.
3. ARTISS, K. L. Human behavior under stress—from combat to social psychiatry. *Milit. Med.* 128, 1011, 1963.
4. BUCHARD, B. L. The U.S. Army's mental hygiene consultation service. In: *Symposium on Preventive and Social Psychiatry*, Government Printing Office, 431, 1958.
5. GLASS, A. J. Principles of combat psychiatry. *Milit. Med.* 117, 27, 1955.
6. RIOCH, D. McK. Problems of preventive psychiatry in war. *Psychopathology of Children*, p. 146. Grune & Stratton, New York, 1955.
7. RIOCH, D. McK. Recent contributions of neuropsychiatric research to the theory and practice of psychotherapy. *Am. J. Psychoanal.* 20, 115, 1955.
8. GLASS, A. J. The role of psychiatry in the development of comprehensive community health services. *Milit. Med.* 135, 345, 1970.
9. TALBOTT, J. A. Community psychiatry in the Army. *J. Am. med. Ass.* 210, 1233, 1969.
10. HAUSMAN, W. The uncommitted student: A social approach to therapy in the college and graduate school setting. Proc. XI Interamerican Congress of Psychology, Mexico City, 1967.
11. BRANDON, S. and GRUENBERG, E. M. Measurement of the incidence of chronic severe social breakdown syndrome. In: *Evaluating the Effectiveness of Community Mental Health Services*, E. M. GRUENBERG (ed.) Mental Health Materials Center, New York, 1966.
12. FINCH, R. H. Medicare and medicaid reforms, public statement, Washington, D.C., 1970.

J. psychiat. Res., 1971, Vol. 8, pp. 521–530. Pergamon Press. Printed in Great Britain.

OCCUPATIONAL SOCIALIZATION IN THE PROFESSIONS: THE CASE OF ROLE INNOVATION*

EDGAR H. SCHEIN

Sloan School of Management, Massachusetts Institute of Technology, Cambridge, Massachusetts

INTRODUCTION

THE TOPIC of occupational socialization in the professions is particularly pertinent in the present world because of the increasing rate of change in our institutions and total society. Rapidly advancing technology and increasing social complexity have created a situation where even the most conservative professions like teaching and law are under great strain. The traditional models of professional practice have come under challenge from students and young practitioners within the professions, and have been found to be increasingly inadequate to deal with the complex problems with which society has confronted the professional.

If the professional of today finds himself unprepared to deal with the demands which society is placing upon him, it is not for lack of technical training in the profession. Scientific knowledge and technology have more than adequately kept pace in most professions. If there is a problem, it is more in the conservative attitude and role rigidity of the professional, those traits which we associate more with the *socialization process* than with education or training. Hence I would like to focus this analysis on occupational *socialization*, on those events in the development of the professional which provide him with his motives, values, ethical standards, and norms of where, how, and on whom to practice.

TYPES OF PROFESSIONAL CAREERS

In any profession the individual can pursue three broadly different types of careers:

(1) *Custodianship*

This type of career is characterized by the total acceptance on the part of the practitioner of the currently existing norms of that profession, and by the practitioner's basic acceptance of the current levels of knowledge and skill in that profession. He is content to use his

---

* This paper is based on research being conducted under the sponsorship of The Carnegie Commission on Higher Education.

technical training in the performance of a traditionally defined role; he works hard at maintaining present professional norms; he accepts whatever licensing procedures may exist; and he favors the development of strong professional associations ruled essentially by elected colleagues.

(2) *Content innovation*

This type of career is characterized by the acceptance of the traditional norms of the profession pertaining to practice, but by a *dissatisfaction* with the existing levels of knowledge and skill which underlie the profession. Thus, the content innovator will concentrate on science, technology, or scholarship to improve the knowledge base and technology which underlie the profession. Often he will be a professor in a professional school or in a department related to a profession (e.g. microbiology relative to medicine). The content innovator will be oriented more to academic standards and associations of scholars or scientists; he will be relatively indifferent to professional associations unless their norms make it difficult to upgrade standards or practice by utilizing the knowledge which the innovator produces, in which case he will be hostile to such norms; he will view licensing procedures as conservative forces which make it difficult for the practitioner trained in the most modern manner to become easily licensed; he will assume that the profession will be best served by giving to the practitioner the most current knowledge and skill training, and will be indifferent to how such knowledge and training is used by the practitioner or what values the practitioner learns.

(3) *Role innovation*

This type of career is hardest to describe because of its relative rarity and the ease of confusing it with *content* innovation. The essence of role innovation is a basic rejection of the norms which govern the *practice* of the profession combined with a concern for the role of the professional in society. The role innovator redefines: (a) who is a legitimate client; (b) who can or should initiate the contact between client and practitioner; (c) what is an appropriate setting for conducting professional practice; and (d) what are the legitimate boundaries of the professional's areas of expertise. Underlying each of these is a concern with making the profession more relevant to the pressing problems of society.

Let me illustrate from the professions of psychiatry, law, and architecture. In psychiatry, role innovation occurred dramatically when a number of military psychiatrists, many of whom participated in the symposium to which this paper contributed, decided to move the locus of their practice to the front lines and to involve entire patrols in group discussions rather than talking just to an individual who exhibited specific symptoms. Furthermore, they did this on their own initiative rather than waiting for a referral from some other source, and they involved themselves as much in the sociology of life in the combat zone as in the mental health of individual soldiers.[1]

In the case of law, perhaps the best example is Ralph Nader, with his concern that the law should become an instrument of constructive social change, that the consumer should be defined as a client though he may never have thought of going to a lawyer over an automobile safety issue, that legal aid should be available to the poor powerless individual as well as to the rich powerful corporation, and that legal training should put much more emphasis on value issues than it has traditionally done.[2]

In the case of architecture, many young architects coming out of school today face the dilemma of whether they should design for the *client* who hired them (e.g. the real estate developer), or the ultimate *user* of the buildings (e.g. the low income black family). Does the poor black family wish to live like a middle class white family? If economic resources are scarce, is the marginal utility of an extra 5 per cent of safety in building construction equal to the marginal utility of more buildings for the poor? Is functionality an aesthetic variable?[3] Recent architecture graduates are even beginning to question the relevance of an apprenticeship period preceding licensing examinations, and are looking for States in which they can practice without a license.

We can find in every major profession, practitioners who wish to conduct their practice in a drastically different manner. Such individuals are usually *not* content innovators, though the new areas of practice which they define may then stimulate the development of new knowledge and techniques such as medical sociology; environmental, consumer, and poverty law; and environmental psychology or 'socio–physical design'.

OCCUPATIONAL SOCIALIZATION FOR THE ROLE INNOVATOR

The remainder of this paper will deal with several questions pertaining to *role* innovation: (1) What is the relationship of role innovation to content innovation? (2) How does role innovation come about in a profession? (3) What kind of educational and socialization process will increase role innovation in a profession? The third of these questions is especially important to answer, because in our rapidly changing society, professions will have to become more adaptive to the changing needs of that society, and the key to such adaptation will be the availability of an increasing number of role innovators in the professions.

(1) *How do content and role innovation interact?*

The present analysis will not pretend to make a thorough epistemological investigation of this complex question, but several points should be brought out. First of all, the inter-action of content and role innovation seems to be different depending upon whether the field underlying the profession is basically convergent or divergent. For example, in engineering with its essentially convergent underlying base, content innovation has usually preceded role innovation. As new knowledge became converted to new technology, new roles for engineers were developed such as computer specialists, systems theorists, and the like.

In the more divergent behavioral and social sciences almost the reverse trend has taken place. Psychiatrists, sociologists, social workers, and psychologists have consistently found themselves facing social problems for which the existing levels of knowledge and technology were inadequate. In trying to cope with such problems they developed new roles and new concepts of legitimate practice, and these new roles in turn stimulated new areas of research and scholarship. Two striking examples in psychology are (1) the development of humanistic psychology as an outgrowth of the role innovations of the applied behavioral scientists doing various kinds of group training, and (2) the development of organizational psychology as an outgrowth of Lewin's concept of "action research" and the development by organization consultants of new data-gathering methods as a part of their effort to change the organization.[4,5,6,7]

In architecture and law we see a more complex interaction because these fields are based in part upon convergent fields (engineering and the law of precedent) and in part upon divergent fields (design and the law as an instrument of social change). As architects and lawyers find themselves increasingly facing social problems which cannot be solved by the simple application of existing technology or precedents from earlier decisions, the balance within both the practice of the profession and the underlying content base as taught in the professional school is shifting toward the divergent fields. Both architecture and law schools are beginning to hire applied behavioral scientists onto their faculties, and both are beginning to stimulate value discussions among their students. As these discussions proceed and as more disciplines interact within the professional school, new areas of content will be identified and new research methods will be invented.

In the case of Walter Reed's Neuropsychiatry Division, its high rate of content and role innovation is partly attributable to the forces of (1) proximity to pressing medical and social problems deriving from continuing military operations, (2) the encouragement of an interdisciplinary approach to problems, and (3) the presence of both convergent and divergent fields within a single laboratory.

In summary, one can find various different patterns of interaction between role and content innovation, and these differences are attributable to the degree of severity of new problems to be solved, the nature of the underlying disciplines, and the degree to which the field is exposed to inter-disciplinary forces.

(2) *How does role innovation come about in a profession?*

We can identify three basically different sources of role innovation. They are not mutually esclusive or independent of each other, but are logically distinct.

First, changes in the environment or society may create new problems which must be solved—new diseases are discovered or unsolved social problems come to be identified and pinpointed. For example, large urban centers breed ghetto dwellers who require a different form of law, architecture, social service, and health care; educationally disadvantaged groups such as blacks are identified and pinpointed as targets for new forms of education, training, counseling, and management. Role innovation occurs in these cases through 'role suction', in the sense that custodially-oriented practitioners may find themselves being pulled in new directions by the gravity of the problems with which society confronts them. The doctor who works in the ghetto community health center finds himself becoming part social worker, part community sociologist, and part politician, in addition to his traditional medical role.

Second, certain classes of individuals have cognitive styles and value systems which are in varying degrees out of line with the role demands of their job. Such individuals will begin to redefine the job to suit their personal style and in that process create some new ways of doing that job.

In the cognitive area, we are exploring the dimension of convergence–divergence both as it applies to a field of study or profession and as it applies to an individual's cognitive approach to problems.[8,9] A number of investigators have linked creativity to divergence, i.e. the ability to recall, re-combine, and create new cognitive elements.[10] Both content and role innovators should therefore have divergent styles. What may distinguish these two types of innovators is (1) level of talent and (2) the degree to which professional practice permits the expression of *content* creativity within traditional concepts of practice. Those creative individuals who either have insufficient talent for content innovation or are professionally blocked from content innovation by conservative professional norms may begin to re-define professional practice and through role innovation find greater congruence between their cognitive style and their occupation.

In the value area, we find the role innovator to be the person who accepts the *pivotal* or *central* norms of the professional organization in which he works, but who rejects the peripheral norms.[11] For example, there is the psychiatrist who believes that no one should practice without an M.D. (pivotal norm), but who rejects the notion that the patient must always take the initiative in coming to the psychiatrist (peripheral norm), or the norm that psychiatrists should not reveal their own personal feelings in the context of a therapeutic relationship. If such a person rejected the pivotal norms of the profession as well, he would no longer be part of that profession. The important theme in role innovation is that the innovator retains his membership in the profession, but stretches the concept of what is legitimate professional practice.

Third, role innovation results from professional school training which is deliberately aimed at changing the profession. In a previous paper, I have pointed out that professional schools can be classified in terms of whether they are custodially or innovatively oriented.[11] Some schools attempt to teach their students the present concepts of how the profession should be practiced; other schools attempt to predict what the profession of the future will have to know and be able to do, and deliberately train in terms of that future concept. To the extent that such latter schools are successful, they are producing graduates who will, from the outset, reject many of the traditional peripheral norms and attempt to invent new ones.

The socialization which occurs in the early part of the professional's career can either enhance or undo the norms which he learned in an innovative professional school. We have clear evidence in the case of managers who graduate from innovative management schools, that if they work for large traditionally oriented business enterprises, they tend to unlearn some of the norms learned in school. If the graduates are sensitive to this kind of organizational socialization, they often resolve the conflict by leaving the traditional organization and going into a smaller innovative organization or setting up their own company or consulting practice. This process is comparable to the architecture graduates refusing to take three-year drafting jobs in preparation for licensing examinations, and the law graduates refusing to work for traditional law firms as very junior 'partners'.

For the young professional to be able to sustain values which are in opposition to some of the norms of his profession requires a strong socialization process in school supported by early career routes which support the deviant values. Thus young law graduates must have opportunities such as joining 'Nader's Raiders', and young psychiatrists must have opportunities to work in creative settings such as the Neuropsychiatry Division of the Walter Reed Army Institute of Research.

(3) *What kind of socialization process will increase role innovation in a profession?*

Let me now pull together some of the above points by focusing on some of the conditions which must obtain during the education and early career of the professional, if he is to become a role innovator. The conditions are to be viewed as a set of hypotheses about how professional education and training should be organized if we are to increase the number of role innovators in our society.

Underlying the specific hypotheses which I will present is a model of the socialization process which must be made explicit. I am assuming that in most professions there are powerful socialization forces which work toward a custodial orientation in the profession. This is especially true in professions like teaching, management, and engineering which are pursued in large bureaucratically organized settings rather than through private practice or small professional offices. In order to counteract these forces, it is necessary for the professional school to stimulate in its students the development of a strong value system which will be capable of withstanding conservative socialization forces. In addition, it is necessary for the profession itself to stimulate or at least tolerate early career paths which may deviate in varying degrees from the traditional ones. The profession itself and the professional schools will jointly have to create *half-way houses* in which the young practitioner can become exposed to some of the major social problems facing the profession without being so overwhelmed by them that he falls back on the tried and true models and, in sheer panic, develops a safe custodial orientation. In other words, professional socialization occurs both during school and the early career. If norms supportive of role innovation are to be developed, one must look *both* to the school and the early part of the career.[12]

Condition 1: The professional school faculty must be anchored in *underlying disciplines* and must be oriented toward content innovation (research/scholarship), rather than being anchored in professional practice *per se*. In other words, the professional schools should avoid hiring the successful practitioner and concentrate instead on hiring scholars and researchers. If too many teachers are successful practitioners, they will simply perpetuate the existing norms which govern the practice of that profession. Having successful businessmen or lawyers teach management or law enhances conservative custodial orientations, especially since the successful practitioner will be the more seductive teacher. In medical schools this phenomenon has been well documented by BECKER[13]—if students have a choice between listening to the research microbiologist and the successful internist, they will always pay attention to the latter, even though this may curtail their professional education in important ways.

Condition 2: The professional school faculty must be *inter-disciplinary*, even if professional practice rests on only one or two fields. In particular, the faculty should include the behavioral sciences and the humanities in order to stimulate intensive analysis of value issues, of humanistic questions, and of the role of the profession in society. The inter-disciplinary emphasis should be retained, even if it is difficult for students to integrate the various points of view during their time in school. It is my assumption that a premature integration can be genuinely harmful in a rapidly changing society. Basically, the student does not know during his period of professional training what demands will be put upon him 5–10 yr hence when he is a practitioner. The broader the base of knowledge from which he is operating, the better equipped he will be to cope with changing environmental demands. The greater his understanding of value issues and the human consequences of professional practice, the better he will be able to deal with new and as yet unanticipated social problems. For example, one hopes that doctors being trained today will know how to handle the social problems of experimental genetics when our technology makes it possible to breed whatever kind of human being we choose to breed.

Condition 3: The professional school curriculum must be organized in such a manner that the student obtains frequent opportunities to enage in *projects which force him to make intellectual and personal commitments, and in which he obtains immediate and relevant feedback on the consequences of these commitments.* I believe strongly that self-knowledge and self-confidence are key ingredients to successful role innovation, and that the only way to build such knowledge and confidence is to provide opportunities for personal involvement combined with accurate and timely feedback. Another way to put this point is to say that the role innovator must take a 'pro-active' role toward his career, and that his professional education must stimulate and encourage pro-activity rather than passive learning.[14] Even though most of school has overtrained the average student to be reactive, it is my hypothesis that this trend can be reversed at any time by creating a learning environment which stimulates active involvement of the learner and gives him effective feedback on the consequences of his own behavior.

Condition 4: The professional school curriculum must train the student in the *ability to diagnose complex social systems.* In all professions it is becoming clear that both the client and the practitioner are parts of larger social systems, and that these systems interact within society. The potential role innovator must be able to see clearly the connections between various social systems of the community and the society, and he must begin to think in terms of 'client systems' such as organizations, groups, populations of people with a common interest, and the like. He must know about the probable effects of different kinds of interventions which he may make, and he must take into account the entire social nexus which surrounds his client.

Condition 5: The professional school curriculum must train the student in the *skills of intervening in social systems and initiating constructive change processes through the utilization of behavioral science knowledge about change.* For example, it is becoming clear that the delivery of health care, legal aid, and housing in the urban ghetto is as much a problem of initiating change in the *social system* of the city as it is a problem of medicine, law, or architecture. The practitioner who wants to work on such problems must have applied behavioral science skills along with his other professional skills if he is to reach his client in any effective manner. If he is to develop such skills, he must have both theoretical training in change theory and opportunities to engage in complex change projects. The Case-Western Reserve Medical School concept of having every medical school student work with an entire family during his school years is an example of such a project focus.

Condition 6: The professional school curriculum must create opportunities to *learn to work with other people in team or other group settings.* As society becomes more complex, one can see an increasing need for social problems to be attacked by teams of professionals who come from different disciplines—the architect or doctor working with the social worker and sociologist on urban problems, or the juvenile court judge working with the psychiatrist and social worker on problems of delinquency. Most present-day professional training puts far too much emphasis on individual project and thesis work. Students do not learn any social psychology, and they do not learn the attitudes and skills which go with team effort. When they later find themselves having to collaborate on practical problems with practitioners from other professions they have neither the inclination nor the skills for such collaboration, thus cutting off one very important avenue toward role innovation.

Condition 7: The professional school must help to *manage the early career of its graduates to insure that the values and skills which are nurtured during school continue to be nurtured in the early formative years of the career.* I have already mentioned professional half-way houses, settings where real clients and real problems can be faced, but under the tutelage of members of the professional school. Internship and residence in a University Teaching Hospital is probably one good model for such half-way houses. Community health centers or legal aid centers partly staffed by professors from the nearby medical or law school would be another example. If it is not possible to develop special settings, the professional school should develop a program on *continuing education* which permits the graduate to return to school at annual or bi-annual intervals to discuss and review his work experiences, to be brought up-to-date on new developments, and to re-solidify the norms and values taught in school. If it is too difficult to bring graduates back to the school setting, it would still be possible to organize *alumni activities* regionally in such a way that revitalization and re-affirmation of norms takes place through continued contact with fellow graduates and visitors from the school.

If the socialization which occurs during professional school is to have enduring effects, the psychological contract between student and school should not be terminated at graduation. The school should think of itself as having a longer-range responsibility to its graduates, this responsibility to be discharged in a variety of ways: (1) More active help from the faculty in locating jobs which will permit role innovative activities; (2) Periodic coaching and counseling help from the faculty as graduates need it and call for it during their early career; (3) More involvement of the faculty with professional associations and large organizations in which their graduates work, i.e. the schools will have to begin to influence the environment within which their graduates work as well as influencing the graduates themselves; (4) More concern about and review of licensing procedures which may exist in the profession to insure that graduates are not placed into a situation of having to unlearn some of the very things which they learned in professional school.

SUMMARY

I have argued that in our rapidly changing society we will increasingly generate social problems which the professions, as presently constituted, will be unable to handle. Therefore, we must stimulate and make possible an increasing rate of role innovation in all the professions. Role innovation involves certain attitudes, values, and skills which can be developed and nurtured during professional school and in the early career. Such nurturance will require special efforts on the part of professional schools. Schools will have to employ faculties which are committed to *basic research*; they will have to put more emphasis on *inter-disciplinary curricula* and on *project-centered education* which will permit the growth of self-insight, self-confidence, diagnostic skill, and a humanistic value orientation; they will have to increase the use of the *applied behavioral sciences* in order to train skills of working in and with complex social systems; they will have to maintain a relationship with graduates through better career counseling, continuing education activities, and consulting services to alumni; and, finally, they will have to monitor more closely the operation of the profession through its licensing procedures, professional association, and other related activities.

As a final note, I would like to mention that the kind of professional education for role innovation which I have tried to describe above will, of course, require professors who are themselves motivated to be role innovators vis-a-vis their own teaching role. To become involved with students in project-centered education, to work in an inter-disciplinary setting, to maintain relationships with graduates, and to become interested in social problems outside of the University will require a different set of attitudes on the part of professors. We must look, therefore, to the graduate training which we currently give to the individuals who will ultimately become the teachers, scholars, and researchers in our professional schools. If we cannot loosen up the concept of what is a professor, we will ultimately fail in loosening up the concept of what is a role-innovative professional. Most of us involved in the symposium to which this paper is a contribution are professors in professional schools. I would like to close this paper by challenging all of you to re-examine your own educational goals, values, and practices. Are you training custodians, content innovators, or role innovators? Does your own teaching style and the organization of your own professional school put sufficient emphasis on training role innovators? If not, our professions may be in trouble, because I do believe that we will need role innovators in ever larger numbers if our professions are to play a useful role in our increasingly complex society.

REFERENCES

1. HARRIS, F. G. and LITTLE, R. W. Military organizations and social psychiatry. *Symposium on Preventive and Social Psychiatry*. Walter Reed Army Institute of Research, Washington, D.C., 173, 1957.
2. NADER, R. Law schools and law firms. *The New Republic* **161**, 20, 1969.
3. O'HARE, M. Designer's dilemma. *Daedalus* **98**, 765, 1969.
4. BENNIS, G., BENNE, K. D. and CHIN, R. *The Planning of Change*. 2nd Ed. Holt, Rinehard & Winston, New York, 1969.
5. SCHEIN, E. H. and BENNIS, W. G. *Personal and Organizational Change Through Group Methods: The Laboratory Approach*. John Wiley, New York, 1965.
6. SCHEIN, E. H. *Organizational Psychology*. Prentice-Hall, 1965.
7. SCHEIN, E. H. *Process Consultation: Its Role in Organization Development*. Addison–Wesley, Reading, Mass., 1969.
8. GUILDFORD, J. P. *The Nature of Human Intelligence*. McGraw-Hill, New York, 1967.
9. HUDSON, L. *Contrary Imaginations*. Penguin, Middlesex, England, 1967.

10. GETZELS, J. W. and JACKSON, P. W. The highly intelligent and the highly creative adolescent: a summary of some research findings. In: *Scientific Creativity: Its Recognition and Development*, TAYLOR, C. W. and BARRON, F. (Eds.), p. 161. John Wiley, New York, 1963.
11. SCHEIN, E. H. Organizational socialization and the profession of Management. Third Douglas M. McGregor Memorial Lecture, Cambridge, Mass., 1967. *Ind. Mgmt Rev.* 9, No. 2, 1, 1968.
12. SCHEIN, E. H. The individual, the organization, and the career. *J. appl. behavioral Sci.* (in press).
13. BECKER, H. S., GEER, B., HUGHES, E. C. and STRAUSS, A. *Boys in White: Student Culture in Medical School*. University of Chicago Press, Chicago, 1961.
14. KOLB, D., WINTER, S. and BERLEW, D. Self-directed change: two studies. *J. appl. behavioral Sci.* 4, 453, 1968.

J. psychiat. Res., 1971, Vol. 8, pp. 531–537. Pergamon Press. Printed in Great Britain.

PSYCHOLOGICAL ISSUES IN TRAINING FOR RESEARCH IN PSYCHIATRY

MORTON F. REISER

Department of Psychiatry, Yale University School of Medicine, New Haven, Connecticut

THE PAST twenty years have been prosperous ones for academic psychiatry. As the pre-emptory pressures for training of clinicians (that followed World War II) began to ease, serious interest in research and research training emerged and commanded generous support from NIMH and from the private Foundations. A wide variety of training programs developed, symposia and institutes on the special problems of research training were held, and career research models were designed. A generation of research psychiatrists has come into being and has taken over leadership of many academic departments. Until recently, prospects have been good for the continuing development of an increasingly rational and scientific psychiatry that would progressively articulate more effectively and meaningfully with an ever widening spectrum of biological and social sciences.

Suddenly, we are faced with the deplorable prospect of serious and drastic curtailment of support both for research and for research training. This makes it more urgent than ever to re-examine some of the unresolved issues embedded in the process of selection of candidates for research training since severely limited resources will place increasingly higher premium on identifying those most likely to be truly creative. Likewise, it is important to focus renewed attention on development of training patterns that can be expected to maximize the potential for creative work and productive activity in those selected. Full consideration of these questions would require more extensive and comprehensive discussion of the nature of scientific creativity than I am qualified to undertake. Rather, what I wish to accomplish in this paper is to call attention to three issues that I regard as fundamental in selecting psychiatrists for research training and in arranging the context of training programs in ways that might insure optimal development of innate talent and creative potential. By so doing, I hope to stimulate interest in these as cogent and relevant subjects that warrant more serious attention and study than they have heretofore received. It is not likely that they will be automatically taken care of or solved simply by more effective design of the form structure and curriculum content of training programs—matters which have received more of our attention to date.

There are, of course, many basic attributes required of the researcher in psychiatry such as intelligence, energy, ingenuity, feeling for experimental design, dedication, integrity, stamina, selflessness, ability to communicate and publish, and capacity for continuing change and growth. These are basic requirements for research in any field, but they do not insure scientific creativity. True creativity in research requires, in addition, that a man be driven, even obsessed, by a compelling sense of curiosity (hopefully combined with ability to ask researchable questions). Curiosity as a trait is *so fundamental* a requirement that it surely warrants development of sensitive and sophisticated methods for its assessment, and special methods for its nurturance. A second trait which I consider fundamental for research in psychiatry, particularly clinical psychiatry, is psychological-mindedness—a trait closely allied to and more familiar in discussions of clinical skills. Finally a third issue that is fundamental to any discussion of scientific creativity is the highly complex mental process called "regression in the service of the ego" that was first described and discussed by ERNST KRIS as being involved in artistic creativity.[1]

For the purposes of this discussion, curiosity and psychological-mindedness can be regarded as enduring personality traits or, in HARTMANN's terms as clusters of autonomous ego functions operating optimally in the conflict-free sphere.[2] When well developed, they manifest themselves as highly individualized personal styles or postures that characterize the individual's way of addressing, perceiving, and evaluating the world in all of its dimensions and manifestations. In other words, they constitute innate automatized perspectives that the individual brings to all his experiences, but especially important in this context to those that are new and novel. They are part of the most intimate fiber of a man and they color to a degree all phases of his experience: approach, encounter, reflection, response and conclusion. Highly specific traits or styles such as these probably make their appearance very early in life. For example, W. W. Sawyer has described school boys who are born mathematicians as being mentally venturesome in a special way. "When one of them is told that no one has ever trisected an angle by means of a ruler and compass alone, he attempts to carry out this operation. When he has been shown how to solve a quadratic equation by completing the square, he tries to solve a cubic equation by completing the cube. He has the desire to explore that marks the creative mathematician. And he may, throughout his life, have an unconscious that concerns itself day after day and also night after night, with the field of mathematics."[3]

Perhaps the most important characteristics of curiosity in the context of this discussion are: (1) its compelling, urgent, driven quality, i.e. the constant hunger for new sensory experience, for new observations and new facts; (2) its outward directedness and (3) its essentially active nature. SZENT-GYÖRGI emphasizes that it is just not truth that the creative scientist seeks, but *new* truth,[4] and POPPER emphasizes the *quest*, "It is not his possession of knowledge of irrefutable truth that makes the man of science, but his persistent and recklessly critical *quest* for truth."[5] The search is accompanied by strong inner excitement, and the gratification and pleasure that goes with discovery is powerful internal reward for the scientist. This restless *quest* for *new* truth must in some way be prerequisite for the kind of readiness to perceive new perspectives in displays of data that facilitates the experience of serendipity. I wonder whether this capacity may not be detectable on psychological testing as a perceptual-cognitive fluidity in assessing figure ground relationships. (This is a question that could be put to empirical test.)

The most cogent characteristics of psychological-mindedness to emphasize here are: (1) sensitivity to symbolic meanings, to situational resemblances between life events in historical context, and to human qualities of experience; (2) intense interest, sensitivity and empathy for people and particularly for their affective experiences and, (3) interest and curiosity about behavior and the motives that underly it. In contrast to curiosity, psychological-mindedness has a much larger inwardly directed component and it is more passive in its emphasis, more receptive and reflective; and does not have the same driving, urging, compelling quality as does curiosity. To whatever degree it represents innate talent and interest, it probably exerts an important influence on the individual's selection of clinical psychiatry as a career choice. Since it may well be fundamentally important, if not absolutely prerequisite for creative research in clinical psychiatry, training programs should provide opportunity for fullest development of these talents. This is the reason I feel that provision of adequate time for continuing maturation and deepening experience as a clinician is so important in clinical research training programs.

If we ask how these two traits may interact in psychiatric research process, we encounter first more general questions about the nature of scientific discovery, and more specifically, questions about the state of mind that may be conducive to inspiration and discovery. Psychiatry is one of the biological sciences. The approach of the biologist to his research problems is strongly influenced by the fact that he is faced by very complex, multiple, and often unknown factors in his experimental field, and it is therefore quite different from that of the mathematician or theoretical physicist. The biologist is accustomed to having his ideas forced upon him by the nature of his observations and he must therefore be somewhat passive and receptive to the facts and realities of nature as they register and force their way into consciousness—a phenomenon very familiar to the mature, experienced, psychologically-minded clinician. The sudden emergence of new ideas into awareness from deep within the investigator is a phenomenon very well known in the history of scientific discovery. SZENT-GYÖRGI describes his behavior on the threshold of discovery, ". . . the first thing I notice is that I find myself running every morning at an early hour, very impatiently, to my laboratory. My work does not finish when I return from my workbench in the afternoon. I go on thinking about my problems all the time and my brain must be going on thinking about them even when I sleep, because I usually get the answer to my problems ready made at the moment when I wake up, and sometimes in the middle of the night. My brain must do as the laxative that was advertised by saying 'while you sleep, it does the work.' As far as I can remember, very rarely have I found the answer to any of my problems by conscious thinking. This conscious thinking only acted as a primer for my brain, which seemed to work much better without my muddling, when I was asleep. I think that without such concentration and devotion, nothing serious can be achieved, be it in art or in science."[4] LINUS PAULING feels that is is possible to train the unconscious to help in the discovery of new ideas. And this, of course, is particularly important in connection with our interest in training programs. He writes, "My own experience, which I may illustrate by some examples, has suggested to me that it is possible to train the unconscious to help in the discovery of new ideas. I reached the conclusion some years ago that I had been making use of my unconscious in a well-defined way. I had developed the habit of thinking about certain scientific problems as I lay in bed, waiting to go to sleep. Sometimes I would think about the same problem for several nights in succession, while I was reading or making calculations about the problem during the day. Then I would stop working on the problem, and stop thinking about it in the period before going to sleep. Some weeks or months might go by, and then, suddenly, an idea that represented a solution to the problem or the germ of a solution to the problem would burst into my consciousness."

"I think that after this training, the subconscious examined many ideas that entered my mind, and rejected those that had no interest in relation to the problem. Finally, after tens or hundreds of thousands of ideas had been examined in this way and rejected, another idea came along that was recognized by the unconscious as having some significant relation to the problem, and this idea and its relation to the problem were brought into consciousness."[3]

Both Pauling and Szent-Györgi are saying that the investigator must devote his conscious efforts fully to the solution of the problem and that without these efforts, the inspiration does not emerge. Poincaré, the famous French mathematician, said essentially the same thing, but added that inspiration, accompanied by a sense of absolute certainty and unsupported by any full demonstration, must in its turn also *be followed* by a period of conscious work when the mind must implement the inspiration, deduce and order its immediate consequences, arrange proof, and above all, verify the results. Thus, inspiration does not just happen simply. Rather, it implies previous intellectual effort, and it must in turn be followed by a period of checking the validity of the sudden insight, since strong solutions can also come clad in an aura of subjective certainty.

Taton, in his volume, *Reason and Chance in Scientific Discovery*, quotes the experience of Charles Nicole, who discovered in 1909 the secret of transmission of epidemic typhus, which illustrates the fact that the moment of illumination may accompany an actual perceptual experience, in this case, a proprioceptive one. Although the disease had reached epidemic proportions in the village, it was not being passed from patients to hospital personnel; within the hospital, it seemed not to be contagious. "One day, just like any other, immersed, no doubt, in the puzzle of the process of contagion in typhus, in any case not thinking of it consciously—of this I am quite sure—I entered the doors of the hospital when a body at the bottom of the passage arrested my attention. It was a customary spectacle to see poor natives suffering from typhus, delirious and febrile as they were, gain the landing and collapse on the last steps. As always, I strode over the prostrate body. *It was at this moment the light struck me.* When a moment later I had entered the hospital, I had solved the problem. I knew beyond all possible doubt this was it. This prostrate body and the door in front of which he had fallen had suddenly shown me the barrier by which typhus had been arrested . . . for it to have remained harmless once the patient had passed the reception office, the agent of infection must have been arrested at this point . . . The patient had already been stripped of his clothing, of his underwear, he had been shaved and washed. It was therefore something outside himself, something that he carried on himself in his underwear or on his skin which caused the infection. This could be nothing but a louse."[6] The precipitating sensory experience may be proprioceptive or visual or a combination of the two as in the apocryphal tale of Archimedes' discovery of the solution to the problem of specific gravity. It would seem that the solution when first achieved may be formed in the mind in a non-verbal mode, i.e. in a form characteristic of preconscious and unconscious modes of mentation, as in dreams, daydreams and hypnogogic images.[7] As Kris has pointed out, it is probably not due just to chance or the mere workings of probability that the new idea appears suddenly in consciousness. The scientist's previous work and preoccupation with the problem prepared the ground, and in fact, the new idea had been already worked out. The solution was, in fact, there but in non-verbal and therefore unrecognized form. The point I am underscoring is that the idea then gets pushed over into recognizable form by the incidental, unexpected proprioceptive or visual perception. Even a dream image may on occasion function in similar fashion as evidenced again by the legend of the discovery of the benzene ring. The main point I wish to make is that a *very important* part of scientific endeavor may very well be to seek actively (in the service of curiosity) a state of passive receptivity to inner preconscious experiences and to the results of preconscious and unconscious data processing. To put it another way, it is an active striving for self-regulated 'regression in the service of the ego.' But it must be achieved under appropriate circumstances, i.e. *after* previous conscious thought and activity has properly prepared the ground. This means that the scientist must develop the capacity to shuttle appropriately back and forth between the passive-receptive state and the 'hard-headed' activity of full consciousness, each at its proper time—as with astronauts, who must work very actively in preparation for the mission but at the time of lift-off, must become extremely passive only to again take over active control once flight has been achieved.

The traits of curiosity, psychological-mindedness, and a capacity to maneuver oneself into a properly receptive frame of mind should be present at least to some degree in all who undertake a research career in psychiatry. The major problems are first to detect those who possess them and then to nurture and develop them to their fullest capacity, remembering that they can probably be easily squelched.

It is easier to specify factors that tend to squelch these traits in the young investigator, than it is to delineate conditions that encourage their growth. The stunting potential of over-emphasis on method for its own sake ('methodolotry'), of grantsmanship, and of the scientific pecking order that favors the investigator with hard data are all obvious. On a site visit for the career investigator program, a number of years ago, I encountered a young man who had abandoned a magnificently imaginative and creative and important research problem because someone at a meeting had said that his data were soft. He had turned, instead to a relatively sterile project in order to get data that could be 'digitized'. Academic publication pressures often act in the same direction. There can be great pressure to do research in areas that will yield respectable publications and concomitantly discouragement for engaging in pursuit of questions that might be regarded as 'not researchable' in a narrow sense. Fads in research may operate in the same fashion. ABELSON has deplored the common tendency to go with the crowd and to rush into glamorous areas following an instrumental breakthrough.[8] IRVINE PAGE has pointed out that excessive dependence on instrumentation, especially through the medium of a technician, can also squelch the investigator's own capacities, "How can investigators keep the possibilities of fresh and creative approaches open for study? My suggestion is simple and, I am sure for many, simple-minded. When a young man starts his research, let him get his butterfly net out and put his thinking cap on. Sit down with the problem as it exists in nature—see and feel the problem—then decide how it can best be solved. With simple equipment and a clear plan, first he should try some preliminary orienting experiments with his own eyes and hands, not those of a technician. Then he should buy, or design, the necessary equipment and hire the technicians who may accelerate the work. Thus a problem might get solved, instead of just a paper being written."[9]

What, then, can the major recommendations be for the nurturence of creativity in the research scientist. Clearly, the first one is the avoidance of the counter influences, the discouraging factors noted above. That is the easy part of the answer. We must also ask what, if any, are the positive features in a training environment that may enhance the young scientist's ability to be creative. Pauling believes that it is likely that young men can be given some training in having ideas. Certainly, instruction in the art of having ideas would be just as valuable to the young experimental scientist as instruction in laboratory technique. But, unfortunately, we do not yet know enough to be able to prepare a formal course of instruction in the art of having ideas.

Most of those who have thought about this aspect of the problem, emphasize the importance of the training environment—the desirability of providing an environment in which originality can thrive. Such an environment implies training in asking questions and in the habits of reflection. The training environment should provide models of investigators with these very qualities and must provide reinforcement and reward for curiosity and receptivity. It should encourage the scientist to take some distance from an immediate problem and to ask, if you like, the silly questions—the questions that can result in a fresh, creative approach. It is also most desirable for training to take place in a multi-disciplinary setting where there is exposure to multiple approaches to the questions in the field. Seminars, conferences, and problem-solving workshops and retreats are of great importance, retreats being particularly helpful since they provide an atmosphere in which people have a chance to pursue problems in a continuing informal way, unrestrained by fixed agenda and rules of procedure. I have already indicated that I believe continuing immersion in clinical training to be of value in that it helps with the development of receptivity to inner thought processes; and the same, of course, applies to personal psychoanalysis as well as to psychotherapeutic work with patients.

These are the interesting, challenging, relatively intangible aspects of the problem. They relate to the human dimension—personalities, atmosphere, attitudes, individual values, capacities to support and be supported, capacities to nurture and be nurtured, etc. Despite the fact that we are forced to create formal structures such as programs and curricula in order to train in institutional settings, the central, or core essence of the research training experience still derives from the apprentice, preceptorship model. This means that the hard-to-define, but all-important qualities of the programs rest with the senior leadership—with the values and goals of the director. The degree to which the program director and his staff embody the essential and desirable traits of the creative research psychiatrist is bound to influence greatly the program's success in selecting candidates and in creating a training environment that will support the creative potential of its trainees.

Although the Neuropsychiatry Division of the Walter Reed Army Institute for Research has not been charged with the task of training psychiatrists for research careers, it has, in fact, trained a great many, as all of you here know. My prescription for desirable leadership qualities turns out to include many of the qualities that I observed in David Rioch during my tour of duty here. I hasten to add that this is an unofficial prescription-portrait. I certainly cannot and do not expect his full agreement or approval. This, by the way, illustrates the last quality of a great research teacher that I want to mention, namely, the capacity to question, to challenge constructively and to teach students to expect and be prepared for it.

REFERENCES

1. KRIS, E. *Psychoanalytic Explorations in Art.* Int. Univ. Press, New York, 1952.
2. HARTMANN, H. *Ego Psychology and the Problem of Adaptation.* Image, London, 1958.
3. PAULING, L. *The Genesis of Ideas.* Proceedings of the Third World Congress in Psychiatry, Vol. 1, pp. 44–47, 1961.
4. SZENT-GYORGI, A. *On Scientific Creativity.* Proceedings of the Third World Congress of Psychiatry, Vol. 1, pp. 47–50, 1961.
5. POPPER, K. *The Logic of Scientific Discovery.* Basic Books, New York, 1959.
6. TATON, R. *Reason and Chance in Scientific Discovery.* Science Editors, New York, 1962.
7. LEWIN, B. *Dreams and the Uses of Regression.* Int. Univ. Press, New York, 1958.
8. ABELSON, P. Government support of research. *Science* 139, No. 3553, 1963.
9. PAGE, I. Technicians, equipment and originality. *Science* 140, No. 3566, 251, 1963.

INDEX